Tamoxifen

FOR THE TREATMENT
AND PREVENTION
OF BREAST CANCER

Tamoxifen
FOR THE TREATMENT AND PREVENTION OF BREAST CANCER

Edited by V. Craig Jordan, PhD, DSc
Northwestern University Medical School

Note to the reader

The information in this volume has been carefully reviewed for correctness of dosage and indications. Before prescribing any drug, however, the clinician should consult the manufacturer's current package labeling for accepted indications, absolute dosage recommendations, and other information pertinent to the safe and effective use of the product described. This is especially important when drugs are given in combination or as an adjunct to other forms of therapy. Furthermore, some of the medications described, as well as some of the indications mentioned, may not have been approved by the US Food and Drug Administration at the time of publication. This possibility should be borne in mind before prescribing or recommending any drug or regimen.

Library of Congress 98-068150

ISBN 1-891483-00-5

For information on obtaining additional copies of this volume, contact the publishers, PRR, Inc., 48 South Service Road, Melville, NY 11747.

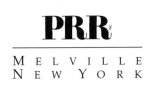

M E L V I L L E
N E W   Y O R K

Publishers of
ONCOLOGY
Oncology News International
Primary Care & Cancer
Managed Care & Cancer
In Touch: The Good Health Guide to Cancer
   Prevention and Treatment
Cancer Management:
   A Multidisciplinary Approach
Myths and Facts About Cancer

To Monica...

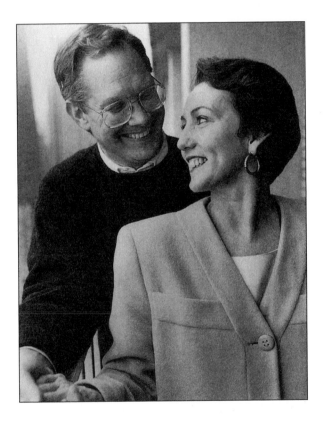

About the Author and Editor

Professor Jordan is one of the many who have contributed to the successful development of tamoxifen. However, his credentials for writing and editing this book are unique. For more than 30 years, he has been involved in the research and development of antiestrogens and has been a strong advocate for the clinical evaluation of tamoxifen—now the world's leading cancer medicine.

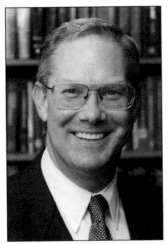

His work in the early 1970s promoted the development of ICI 46,474 from a laboratory curiosity to its position today as the most important drug for the treatment and prevention of breast cancer. Professor Jordan formulated the concepts of prevention, long-term adjuvant therapy, and selective estrogen-receptor modulation in his laboratory, and then proceeded to successfully translate these ideas to clinical trials and practice.

Professor Jordan has received numerous prestigious national and international awards. Most importantly, in 1993, Professor Jordan received the Cameron prize from the University of Edinburgh. Recipients of this award are a select group of medical researchers from any field who have changed the practice of therapeutics. The 100 awardees are considered to have made the most important medical contributions to the world during the past century.

Professor V. Craig Jordan

Professor Jordan is Director of the Lynn Sage Breast Cancer Research Program at the Robert H. Lurie Comprehensive Cancer Center at Northwestern University. He lives in Chicago with his wife, Dr. Monica Morrow.

Contents

	About the Author and Editor	9
	Contributors	15
	Acknowledgments	17
	Foreword *Nancy Brinker*	19
	Introduction—Foundations *V. Craig Jordan, PhD, DSc*	23
Chapter 1	Why Tamoxifen? *V. Craig Jordan, PhD, DSc*	31
Chapter 2	The Clinical Development of Tamoxifen *V. Craig Jordan, PhD, DSc*	41
Chapter 3	Current Approved Uses and Recommendations of Tamoxifen in the United States *V. Craig Jordan, PhD, DSc*	53
Chapter 4	Early Overviews of Adjuvant Tamoxifen Therapy *I. Craig Henderson, MD*	57
Chapter 5	Tamoxifen for Early Breast Cancer—1998 *V. Craig Jordan, PhD, DSc*	79
Chapter 6	Tamoxifen for Adjuvant Therapy and for the Treatment of Advanced Disease in Premenopausal Breast Cancer Patients *Peter M. Ravdin, MD, PhD*	87
Chapter 7	Additional Benefits of Tamoxifen for Postmenopausal Patients *Malcolm M. Bilimoria, MD* *Monica Morrow, MD* *V. Craig Jordan, PhD, DSc*	97
Chapter 8	Endometrial Cancer and Tamoxifen *Richard R. Barakat, MD*	109
Chapter 9	Tamoxifen and Endometrial Cancer: The Worldwide Clinical Database *Vasileios J. Assikis, MD* *V. Craig Jordan, PhD, DSc*	117

continued on the following page

Contents *continued*

Chapter 10   **Controversies on the Duration of Tamoxifen**   127
              Administration in an Adjuvant Setting
              Norman Wolmark, MD

Chapter 11   **The Duration of Tamoxifen**   141
              V. Craig Jordan, PhD, DSc

Chapter 12   **What To Do After Tamoxifen?**   145
              V. Craig Jordan, PhD, DSc

Chapter 13   **Talking With the Breast Cancer Patient**   153
              About Tamoxifen
              Amy S. Langer, MBA

Chapter 14   **Questions and Answers About Tamoxifen**   162
              V. Craig Jordan, PhD, DSc; Richard R. Barakat, MD;
              I. Craig Henderson, MD; Amy S. Langer, MBA;
              Monica Morrow, MD; C. Kent Osborne, MD;
              Joseph Ragaz, MD; Norman Wolmark, MD

Chapter 15   **Breast Cancer: Who and Why?**   187
              Monica Morrow, MD

Chapter 16   **Tamoxifen for Breast Cancer Prevention**   207
              V. Craig Jordan, PhD, DSc
              Monica Morrow, MD

Chapter 17   **The STAR Trial**   225
              V. Craig Jordan, PhD, DSc

Chapter 18   **Y-ME Hotline: The 20 Most Frequently**   235
              Asked Questions About Tamoxifen
              V. Craig Jordan, PhD, DSc
              Monica Morrow, MD

Appendix 1   **Translational Research: Applying**   247
              Laboratory Discoveries to Patient Care
              V. Craig Jordan, PhD, DSc

Appendix 2   **How Does Tamoxifen Work?**   257
              V. Craig Jordan, PhD, DSc

Appendix 3   **Breast Cancer Susceptibility Gene BRCA-1**   265
              V. Craig Jordan, PhD, DSc

Appendix 4   **How Are Drugs Developed?**   271
Ruth O'Regan, MD
V. Craig Jordan, PhD, DSc

Appendix 5   **The IARC Evaluates Carcinogenic Risk**   281
Associated With Tamoxifen

Appendix 6   **Recommended Further Reading**   283
and References for Physicians and Scientists

Acknowledgments in Five Photocollages   285

Index   305

Contributors

V. Craig Jordan, PhD, DSc
Director
Lynn Sage Breast Cancer
  Research Program
Robert H. Lurie Comprehensive
  Cancer Center
Northwestern University Medical School
Chicago, Illinois

Vasileios J. Assikis, MD
Resident in Medicine
Department of Medicine
Cook County Hospital
Chicago, Illinois

Richard R. Barakat, MD
Associate Attending Surgeon
Gynecology Service
Memorial Sloan-Kettering Cancer Center
New York, New York

Malcolm M. Bilimoria, MD
Fellow in Surgical Oncology
Division of Surgery
M. D. Anderson Cancer Center
The University of Texas
Houston, Texas

Nancy Brinker
Founding Chairwoman
Susan G. Komen Breast Cancer
  Foundation
Dallas, Texas

I. Craig Henderson, MD
Adjunct Professor of Medicine
The University of California
San Francisco, California

Amy S. Langer, MBA
Executive Director
National Alliance of Breast Cancer
  Organizations (NABCO)
New York, New York

Monica Morrow, MD
Director
Lynn Sage Comprehensive Breast Cancer
  Program
Department of Surgery
Northwestern University Medical School
Chicago, Illinois

Ruth O'Regan, MD
Fellow
Hematology/Oncology Division
Robert H. Lurie Comprehensive
  Cancer Center
Northwestern University Medical School
Chicago, Illinois

C. Kent Osborne, MD
AB Alexander Distinguished Chair/
  Chief of Medical Oncology
The University of Texas Health
  Science Center
San Antonio, Texas

Joseph Ragaz, MD, FRCPC
Senior Medical Oncologist/
  Associate Professor
Vancouver Cancer Centre
The University of British Columbia
Vancouver, British Columbia

Peter M. Ravdin, MD, PhD
Associate Professor of Medicine/Oncology
The University of Texas Health
  Science Center
San Antonio, Texas

Norman Wolmark, MD
Chairman
National Surgical Adjuvant Breast and
Bowel Project (NSABP)

Chairman/Professor
Department of Human Oncology
Allegheny University of the Health Sciences
Pittsburgh, Pennsylvania

Acknowledgments

This book began as the result of conversations with hundreds of women with breast cancer who wanted to learn more about tamoxifen. I owe a great debt of gratitude to each of these women for the help and insight they have provided. Most importantly, without the constant support and encouragement of my wife, Monica, the manuscript for this book could not have been written. Further, this book would not have been published without the tireless efforts of the editorial/art/production team at PRR: Jack Gentile, Jim McCarthy, Quinn Kaufman, Jeannine Coronna, Cara Glynn, Andy Nash, Michelle Chizmadia, Andrea Green, and Madeline McCarthy. I owe each person a great debt of gratitude for their dedication to this project. I especially thank Nancy Brinker for agreeing to contribute the Foreword for my book, as well as Sharon Green, Michelle Meline, and Judy Perotti of Y-ME in Chicago for all of their help in identifying patients' specific concerns about tamoxifen.

I must also thank the more than 70 staff, students, and fellows of the "tamoxifen teams," who, over the past 30 years, have translated ideas into results in my laboratories in England, Switzerland, and the United States. Special thanks must also go to my many colleagues at ICI Pharmaceuticals (now Zeneca), whose friendship and support have transformed laboratory concepts into clinical facts.

I must also thank my secretary, Gloria Duncan, for patiently typing the numerous versions of the manuscript; Alexander de los Reyes for completing some of the figures; Dr. Michael Dukes of Zeneca for locating the pictures of Dr. Dora Richardson and the Queens Award for Technological Achievement. Jim Ziv also deserves special thanks for the photograph of my laboratory.

Finally, rather than list all the names of those who have made possible the success of tamoxifen over the past 30 years, I have chosen to acknowledge their contributions in the five photographic collages shown at the back of this book. In those *Acknowledgments*, you will find photographs of the many investigators and clinicians, friends and colleagues who were important in the discovery and development of tamoxifen, and who have made important contributions in the field of antiestrogens and the fight against cancer.

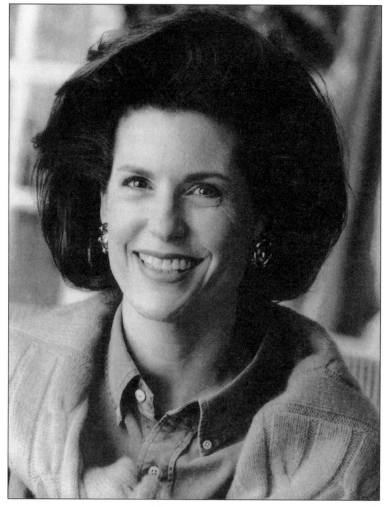

Nancy Brinker

Foreword

Nancy Brinker
Founding Chairwoman
Susan G. Komen Breast Cancer Foundation
Dallas, Texas

Tamoxifen has changed the treatment of breast cancer and brought hope to millions of women who develop the disease. In 1973, tamoxifen was approved in the United Kingdom for the treatment of advanced breast cancer, and in 1978, it was finally introduced to the United States. Though originally indicated for the treatment of advanced disease in postmenopausal women, the Food and Drug Administration (FDA) has since approved tamoxifen for the treatment of all stages of breast cancer. In 1998, the FDA also approved tamoxifen for reducing the incidence of breast cancer in well women at high risk for developing the disease.

Tamoxifen's success was the result of a close collaboration between Zeneca Pharmaceuticals—the agent's discoverer and manufacturer—and the academic and clinical communities. However, it was the investigators themselves who believed in tamoxifen's strength and took the time to probe it to its full potential. It was their steadfastness and will to fight the battle against cancer that gave reign to tamoxifen, and in turn, literally saved the lives of thousands of women.

We at the Komen Foundation are committed to finding a cure for breast cancer. To achieve this goal, we have made a pledge to raise financial resources to enable first-class laboratory and clinical research in our nation's finest universities and cancer centers. We are committed to providing fellowships to the best and brightest young doctors and scientists, giving them the opportunity to start their careers in centers of scientific excellence.

Achievements in research are the milestones by which we can measure our progress. We believe in recognizing great achievements, and in 1992, to mark the 10th anniversary of the Susan G. Komen Foundation, we established the Brinker International Breast Cancer Award for completed research. A blue-ribbon panel of scientists and doctors assembled to select a recipient for the Inaugural Brinker International Breast Cancer Award for Basic Research. The committee selected Dr. V. Craig Jordan for his dedication to breast cancer research and for guiding the successful clinical development of tamoxifen. The citation reads: "Dr. Jordan has been tireless in his sustained effort to provide underlying scientific strategies for the clinical value of tamoxifen which have resulted in improved survival for thousands of women with primary breast cancer." The Komen Foundation is pleased to have supported research on tamoxifen for Dr. Jordan's laboratories at the University of Wisconsin (Madison) and Northwestern University Medical School (Chicago); and in Dr. C. Kent Osborne's laboratory at the University of Texas in San Antonio. Both doctors are contributors to this book.

Tamoxifen is the strongest warrior yet in our continuing battle against breast cancer. Yet only through cooperation, research, and the propagation and advancement of knowledge can we look forward to the ultimate conquest of breast cancer and a brighter future.

Nancy Brinker
Founding Chairwoman
Susan G. Komen Breast Cancer Foundation

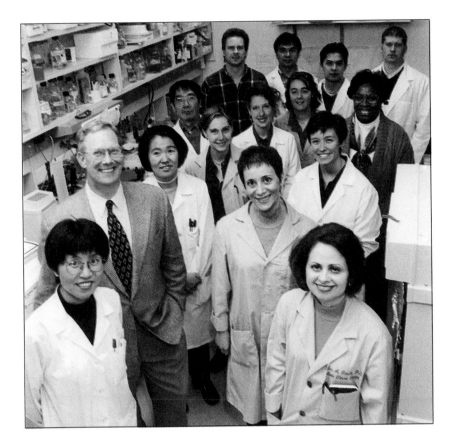

The 1999 Tamoxifen Team

*Clockwise: Hong Lui, V. Craig Jordan, Eun-Sook Lee,
Sarah Blink, Yasuo Hozumi, Jennifer MacGregor,
Greg Herbert, Jun Horiguchi, Ruth O'Regan,
Alex de los Reyes, Mike Chisamore, Gloria Duncan,
Kathy Yao, Anait Levenson, and Debra Tonetti.*

Introduction

Foundations

V. Craig Jordan, PhD, DSc
Director
Lynn Sage Breast Cancer Research Program
Robert H. Lurie Comprehensive Cancer Center
Northwestern University Medical School
Chicago, Illinois

In 1967, I met three scientists at ICI Pharmaceuticals Ltd. (now Zeneca) in Cheshire, England, who would alter the course of my life and start my involvement in the development of drugs for the treatment of breast cancer. At the time, I was working as a summer student with Dr. Steven Carter, who headed the anticancer screening program. My project was to study an exciting new natural product, called cytochalasin B, that causes nuclear extrusion from the cell.

The compound had no potential as an anticancer agent, but it subsequently found universal use in the laboratory as a tool in cell biology. Twenty years later, Dr. Wade Welshons, working in Dr. Jack Gorski's laboratory and later in my laboratory at the University of Wisconsin, would use the compound to demonstrate that the estrogen receptor was a nuclear protein.

Dr. Arthur Walpole (Figure 1) worked in the laboratory across the corridor from Steven Carter and was head of Reproduction Research. He had just published work on a new antiestrogen, ICI 46,474, that was a potent postcoital contraceptive in the rat. Although there was enormous potential for a new agent to regulate fertility, it was also recognized that antiestrogens could be used to treat breast cancer.

This was one of Dr. Walpole's interests.

In the laboratory next to Carter's was Dr. Michael Barrett, then in charge of developing new heart drugs as part of the cardiovascular program. He was responsible for the discovery of practolol and Tenormin. When he became chairman 5 years later, in 1972, Dr. Barrett offered me a faculty position in the Department of Pharmacology at the University of Leeds. He suggested Dr. Arthur Walpole as the external examiner for my PhD on antiestrogens, entitled "Structure Activity Relationships of Some Substituted Triphenylethylenes and Triphenylethanols."

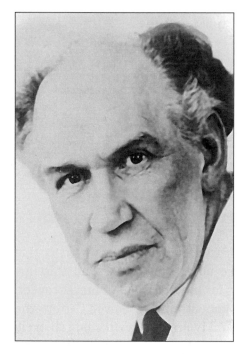

FIGURE 1   Dr. Arthur L. Walpole, who died suddenly on July 2, 1977   At the time of his death, he had retired as Head of the Fertility Control Program at ICI's Pharmaceuticals Division in Alderley Park, near Macclesfield, Cheshire; but he had continued to work as a consultant on the Joint Research Scheme between ICI and the Department of Pharmacology at the University of Leeds, England.

In 1969, supported by a research scholarship from the Medical Research Council, I decided to study the estrogen receptor with Dr. Edward Clark in the Department of Pharmacology at the University of Leeds. Dr. Jack Gorski had published an exciting series of reports showing that the estrogen receptor could easily be extracted from the rat uterus and isolated by sucrose density gradient analysis. My project was going to be simple: I was to establish the new technique of sucrose density gradient analysis, isolate the receptor, and crystallize the protein with an estrogen and an antiestrogen. Through x-ray crystallography in the Astbury Department of Biophysics at the University of Leeds, we would then establish the three-dimensional shape of the complexes to explain antiestrogenic action. The goal was to solve a fundamental question in pharmacology: What is the molecular mechanism of action for a drug?

Progress was slow in establishing the receptor purification technique of sucrose gradient analysis, and I switched my thesis topic to study the structure activity relationships of antiestrogens. As it turned out, this was a good, strategic decision, as it has taken the best efforts of the research community nearly 30 years to achieve success. The structure of the estrogen-receptor complex was solved by scientists at York University, England, in 1997.

In 1972, however, there was little academic interest in the pharmacology of antiestrogens. Enthusiasm in the pharmaceutical industry was chilled because these drugs had not fulfilled their promise as contraceptive "morning after" pills. It was clear that no one was recommending antiestrogen research as a sound career choice; it was perceived as a dead end. To make matters worse, the University of Leeds encountered difficulty in securing a qualified examiner for my thesis. (Sir Charles Dodds, the discoverer of the synthetic estrogen, diethylstilbestrol [DES], declined with regrets because he had not kept up with the literature during the 20 years since his retirement!) This led Professor Barrett to select Dr. Arthur Walpole from ICI, and thus, indirectly, the door was opened for the future development of ICI 46,474 into tamoxifen.

When I accepted my faculty position at the University of Leeds in 1972, I was first required to obtain additional research experience elsewhere. Professor Barrett solved this problem by arranging for me to work with Dr. Michael Harper at the Worcester Foundation for Experimental Biology in Massachusetts (Figure 2). Dr. Harper is a reproductive biologist, who, some years earlier, had worked with Dr. Arthur Walpole at ICI. He is also the co-patent holder for ICI 46,474. However, at that time, Dr. Harper was heading a team

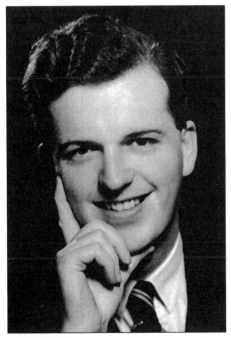 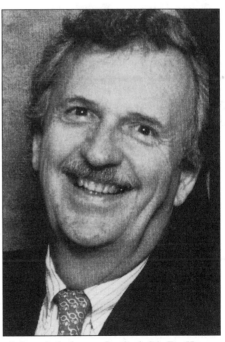

FIGURE 2   Dr. Michael J. K. Harper, co-patent holder for ICI 46,474 He discovered the opposing biological activities of the *cis* and *trans* isomers of substituted triphenylethylenes. On the left is Dr. Harper in the mid 1960s; and on the right, on the occasion of his 60th birthday.

at the Foundation working on the potential of prostaglandins to be used as a "once-a-month" contraceptive pill.

When I arrived at the Worcester Foundation in September, 1972—incidentally, not knowing anything about prostaglandins—I discovered that Dr. Harper had accepted a job with the World Health Organization in Geneva. My new boss, Dr. Ed Klaiber, said I could do anything I liked as long as some of my work included prostaglandins. I immediately found myself as an independent investigator and planned my work on prostaglandins. However, my new circumstances would also allow me to explore my passion—to develop a drug for breast cancer.

The Development of ICI 46,474 Into Tamoxifen

By 1971, ICI 46,474 had shown modest activity in a preliminary clinical study for the treatment of advanced breast cancer. It was still clear, however, that much remained to be done to develop antiestrogens as acceptable therapeutic agents. ICI did not have a breast cancer research program, but Dr. Walpole agreed to help with my request for assistance to conduct a systematic laboratory study of the antitumor properties of tamoxifen at the Worcester Foundation. I, on the other hand, had no experience with laboratory models of breast cancer. Fortunately, the Worcester Foundation was a marvelous place to learn, as well as find help in new areas of scientific endeavor.

Dr. Elwood Jensen, then director of the Ben May Laboratory for Cancer Research in Chicago, was a member of the scientific advisory board for the Foundation. Quite generously, he agreed to help me prepare for my study of tamoxifen. The short time I spent in his laboratory, with the help of Dr. Gene DeSombre, was exceptional and provided me with the skills to evaluate the antitumor actions of tamoxifen back in Massachusetts.

To facilitate our progress, Dr. Walpole suggested I contact Ms. Lois Trench, the clinical drug monitor for tamoxifen at one of ICI's companies in Wilmington, Delaware. She admitted, however, that no one knew much about the new drug in the United States clinical department, and insisted that I become a consultant to encourage clinical trials with tamoxifen.

Full of energy and drive, Lois arranged for me to study the interaction of tamoxifen with the estrogen receptor. In 1974, she also arranged for me to explain the antitumor effects of tamoxifen at meetings of the Eastern Cooperative Oncology Group (ECOG). Thereafter, she invited me to introduce tamoxifen to the National Surgical Adjuvant Breast and Bowel Project (NSABP) at an international symposium she organized in 1976 in Key Biscayne, Florida.

The work at the Worcester Foundation went exceptionally well. Lois supplied human breast tumors to resolve the controversy of whether tamoxifen inhibited the binding of estrogens to the human estrogen receptor. The first laboratory studies of tamoxifen as a breast cancer preventive were successfully completed in 1974, and Lois sponsored me to present the work at the International Congress of Steroidal Hormones meeting in Mexico City. There was still little interest in the concept at that point (it was 10 years too early!), but most importantly, a series of papers was commenced.

These papers fully described the antitumor effects of tamoxifen in animals. Some of that work was included in the handbook given to clinicians in America to support their clinical studies in 1974. The work was also used to support licensing of tamoxifen in Japan and Germany. But, I felt no urgency to publish the results since there was still no particular interest in antiestrogens.

Contributing to the clinical development of tamoxifen was my interest and goal. However, my strategic error was ultimately pointed out by Dr. Eliahu Caspi, a senior scientist at the Foundation. He taught me his simple adage: "Tell them what you have done so far." He explained that each paper should take no more than 2 weeks to complete.

Taking his advice, I have not stopped writing since that day in 1974.

A New Strategy: Long-Term Adjuvant Tamoxifen

Upon my return to England in September of 1974, my principal interest was to understand the pharmacology of tamoxifen and to devise a strategy for the best clinical application of an antiestrogen treatment. The drug had been available for the treatment of advanced breast cancer in Britain since 1973, but similar approval would not occur in the United States until 1978. Throughout this period, ICI Pharmaceuticals and the Yorkshire Cancer Research Campaign supported my laboratory at the University of Leeds in England. There, the "tamoxifen group" devised the strategy of long-term (greater than 1 year) adjuvant tamoxifen therapy that was taken into clinical trials on both sides of the Atlantic. My group also discovered that a metabolite of tamoxifen, 4-hydroxytamoxifen, had a high affinity for the estrogen receptor, but still retained antiestrogenic activity. This set the stage for the subsequent discovery of numerous new antiestrogens that are currently being tested in clinical trials around the world.

The scientific basis for prevention and long-term (greater than 1 year) adjuvant therapy had been established in the laboratory by 1977. In turn, ICI 46,474 became tamoxifen. This data would provide the rationale for the clinical development of antiestrogens for the next 25 years.

This book is intended for the physician whose primary discipline is not medical oncology, but whose practice includes women at risk for breast cancer and/or women who are either taking tamoxifen to treat breast cancer, or women who are taking raloxifene to prevent osteoporosis. This book is also recommended for nurses in breast care centers who are responsible for the day-to-day care of women. It was written to provide answers to numerous questions about breast cancer treatment and prevention.

Additionally, this book was designed to provide a foundation of the most current information for the surgeon or the physician-in-training, who, by the time they come to practice, will be called upon for advice from their patients about the risks and benefits of a diverse menu of selective estrogen-receptor modulators for a number of clinical applications.

This new knowledge will be derived from a comparison with the gold standard of tamoxifen.

Victory—

does not depend entirely upon numbers or courage; only skill and discipline will ensure it.

—Flavius Vegetius, AD 378

Chapter 1

Why Tamoxifen?

V. Craig Jordan, PhD, DSc
Director
Lynn Sage Breast Cancer Research Program
Robert H. Lurie Comprehensive Cancer Center
Northwestern University Medical School
Chicago, Illinois

One hundred years ago, Dr. George Beatson[1] made the astonishing decision to treat advanced breast cancer in a premenopausal woman by removing her ovaries. Beatson was aware that farmers in Scotland could affect lactation in their animals by removal of the ovaries, so after completing preliminary studies in rabbits, he reasoned that the "ovarian irritation" of the mammary glands—breast cancer—in a woman might be influenced by the removal of her ovaries. Beatson initially reported that one of his patients had a dramatic response to the procedure, and by 1900, Stanley Boyd[2] at Charing Cross Hospital in London had collected the records of 46 premenopausal women (excluding 8 Edinburgh cases) with advanced breast cancer to document their responses to oophorectomy.

He observed, however, that only 1 in 3 patients (actually 37%) responded to the procedure. The reason for this was to remain obscure for the next 60 years.

Estrogens: The Circulating Messengers of the Ovaries

What was remarkable about Beatson's original report in 1896 was that the endocrine role of the ovaries was completely unknown. In 1923, Drs. Allen and Doisy[3] in St. Louis described their finding of an "estrus stimulating principle" in the follicular fluid of pig ovaries. The ovaries were known to control reproductive functions, and it was also known that female animals came into heat and accepted males only at certain times in their reproductive cycles.

Allen and Doisy's studies illustrated the close relationship that was necessary between the laboratory and the clinic to unlock the mysteries of human physiology. They devised a test system for examining follicular fluid by first ovariectomizing mice and eliminating the reproductive cycle. They discovered that the vaginal epithelium underwent the same cellular changes (called cornification) in response to injections of ovarian follicular fluid as the vagina

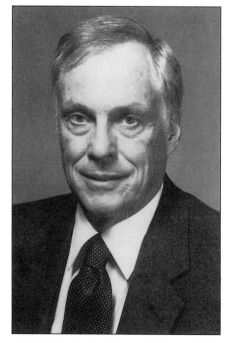

FIGURE 1 Professor Elwood V. Jensen He proposed the estrogen-receptor system to explain responses to estrogens at estrogen target tissues. Later, he devised the estrogen-receptor assay to predict the hormonal dependency of breast cancer.

did when the unovariectomized mouse went into heat or "estrus" (from the Latin word meaning *frenzy*). The chemicals produced by the ovaries—that were subsequently identified as circulating messengers—were named estrogens. It was thus discovered that these estrogens could selectively activate estrogen target tissues (uterus, vagina, breast) in a woman. The concept of endocrine control of one organ by a distant organ became an established fact.

Now, we should return to the original question regarding why some breast tumors responded to the removal of ovarian influence whereas others did not. In 1962, Drs. Elwood Jensen (Figure 1) and Herb Jacobson[4] synthesized radioactive estradiol—the most potent of the natural estrogens in a woman's body. With this breakthrough, these investigators were able to address the question of differing tissue responses to estrogen. Although natural estrogens circulate throughout the female body, only target tissues become activated. Jensen and Jacobson injected radioactive estradiol into immature female rats (ie, animals that have no estrogen because their ovaries are inactive) and killed the animals at different times over the next 24 hours to find out where the estrogen had gone. They found that the radioactivity was initially bound to all tissues, but was only retained in the estrogen target tissues (uterus and vagina). There must be a mechanism, they reasoned, a receptor, perhaps, that enabled the target tissues to retain estrogen.

The Estrogen-Receptor Hypothesis

The estrogen-receptor (ER) protein was subsequently isolated from the rat uterus in 1966 by parallel research ventures by Jensen's group at the University of Chicago, and by Dr. Jack Gorski's group at the University of Illinois. The work rapidly translated to the clinic and established the concept of a

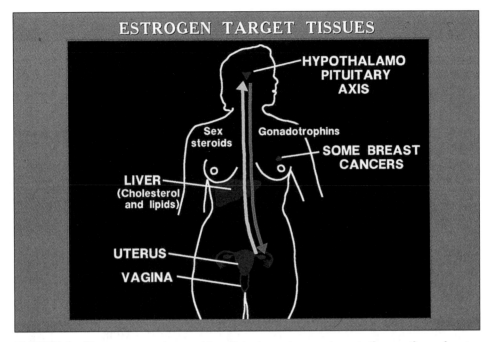

FIGURE 2 **Sites commonly considered to be estrogen target tissues throughout a woman's body** Each site contains estrogen receptors within the cell to control the function of the tissue. The menstrual cycle is controlled through the hypothalamo-pituitary axis via feedback mechanisms that regulate ovarian steroidogenesis and ovulation. Similarly, estrogen regulates uterine biochemistry to prepare the tissue for progesterone action following ovulation in anticipation of successful ovum fertilization and implantation. Without implantation, steroidogenesis fails and menstruation occurs. Estrogen also controls circulating cholesterol through the regulation of liver metabolism, and estrogen maintains bone density (not shown). Some breast cancers contain the estrogen receptor and are considered to be estrogen target tissues.

pattern of estrogen target tissues containing the estrogen receptor throughout a woman's body (Figure 2).

Jensen's work, however, did not stop there. He reasoned that since estrogen controls estrogen action via the estrogen receptor, then perhaps breast cancer growth was regulated by the same mechanism. In the laboratory, he established that some breast cancers did indeed contain the estrogen receptor. He forged forward, conducting the initial clinical studies that illustrated the principle that patients whose tumor contained the estrogen receptor would respond to an endocrine maneuver, but that those whose tumor was "estrogen receptor negative," would be unlikely to respond.[5] This principle was established in Bethesda, Maryland in 1974 at a National Cancer Institute-sponsored meeting. Investigators from around the world were invited to pool their clinical data on the usefulness of the estrogen-receptor assay to predict hormone-responsive breast cancer. This conference was enormously successful and the consensus revolutionized the treatment of breast cancer.[6] A patient with an estrogen receptor-positive tumor has a 60% chance of responding to endocrine ablation, but a patient with an estrogen receptor-negative tumor has only a 10% chance of a response. Surgeons now had a test that could help them select women most likely to respond to endocrine ablation, and therefore, reduce the cost and morbidity of treating everyone with ovarian or adrenal ablation.

The test would avoid disappointing results in two thirds of patients.

Dramatic progress was also being made in a parallel research venture that would make endocrine ablation obsolete. There was a better way to treat patients—by blocking estrogen action in the tumor itself. If estrogen was the key that unlocked the growth mechanism in breast cancer, perhaps a drug that blocked the lock could be found and ablative surgery to remove the source of hormones could be avoided.

The First Antiestrogens

In 1958, Dr. Leonard Lerner[7] and coworkers at the William S. Merrell Company in Cincinnati reported their laboratory results with the first nonsteroidal antiestrogen MER, 25 or ethamoxytriphetol. The pharmacological properties of the drug were unique. Ethamoxytriphetol was antiestrogenic in every species tested[7] and the researchers could not detect any other hormonal or antihormonal activity. Theoretically, an antiestrogen could have many uses in gynecology or for the treatment of breast cancer. But it was the discovery that an antiestrogen could prevent pregnancy in laboratory animals—after they had mated—that seized the imagination of the pharmaceutical industry. Oral contraceptives had already been established as effective agents to regulate fertility, but the tablets had to be taken daily throughout the cycle to suppress ovulation. Perhaps the antiestrogens would be effective "morning after pills" for occasional use?

Early clinical trials with ethamoxytriphetol demonstrated that the drug was active as an antiestrogen, but had low potency and persistent troublesome side effects. These factors prevented further clinical evaluation. However, a successor compound, clomiphene, an analogue of the estrogen triphenylethylene (Figure 3), was found to be more potent than ethamoxytriphetol, and clinical trials were initiated.[8] Rather than acting as an antifertility agent, however, clomiphene appeared to actually induce ovulation, thus guaranteeing the precise effect it was supposed to prevent! To this day, clomiphene is used to induce ovulation in subfertile women.

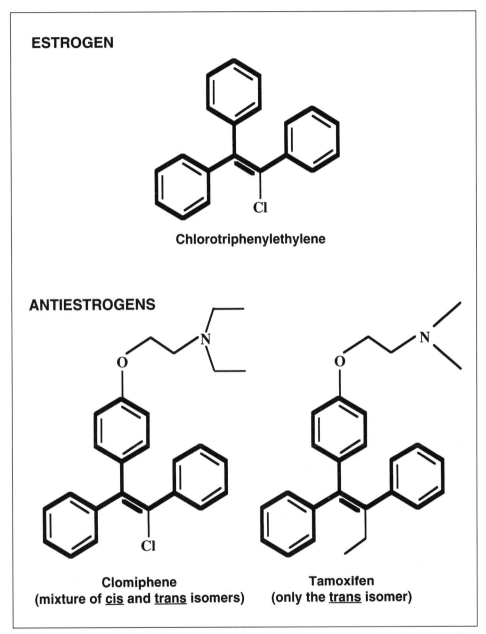

ESTROGEN

Chlorotriphenylethylene

ANTIESTROGENS

Clomiphene
(mixture of <u>cis</u> and <u>trans</u> isomers)

Tamoxifen
(only the <u>trans</u> isomer)

FIGURE 3 **Structural formula of triphenylethylene compounds (shown in bold) that have either estrogenic or antiestrogenic properties** The key to antiestrogen activity is a correctly positioned alkyaminoethoxy side chain, illustrated by the two drugs in the lower part of the figure. Clomiphene is a mixture of two isomers with opposing biological properties. The *trans* isomer is an antiestrogen, whereas the *cis* isomer is an estrogen. The diagram shows only the formula of the antiestrogenic *trans* isomer. The mixed isomers are used as an inducer of ovulation originally under the trade name, Clomid. For comparison, the formula of tamoxifen is shown on the bottom right. It is the pure *trans* isomer only and is sold under the trade name of Nolvadex for the treatment and prevention of breast cancer.

Antiestrogens and Breast Cancer

During the 1960s, many pharmaceutical companies around the world were involved in the study of the structure activity relationships of the antiestrogens. Each compound was an effective antifertility agent in the laboratory rat, but it was clear that the properties scientists were observing in animals did not translate into a clinically useful contraceptive. A number of preliminary clinical trials in breast cancer were conducted with several new antiestrogens because of the recognized link between estrogen and the growth of some breast cancers. It had also been found in the laboratory that antiestrogens could block the binding of radioactive estradiol in its target tissues, so the rationale for clinical studies in the 1970s was strong.

The Upjohn Company in Kalamazoo, Michigan conducted extensive tests on their new antiestrogen, nafoxidine; but in the 1970s, after numerous clinical studies around the world, development was abandoned because all patients suffered severe toxic side effects.[9] Similarly, clomiphene, an impure mixture of geometric isomers, was tested, but concerns about potential side effects or toxicities, particularly cataracts, prevented further clinical development for long-term treatment. Clinical studies were abandoned in the early 1970s.[8]

ICI 46,474 to Tamoxifen

Scientists in the fertility control program of the pharmaceuticals division of Imperial Chemical Industries (ICI) in England were particularly interested in the discovery of the new nonsteroidal antiestrogens. The most potent nonsteroidal estrogen, diethylstilbestrol, had been discovered by Sir Charles Dodds in the late 1930s. Structural analogues, the triphenylethylenes (Figure 3), were subsequently found to be potent, long-acting estrogenic drugs. ICI Pharmaceuticals (now Zeneca) had already provided the triphenylethylenes to Sir Alexander Haddow for his pioneer-

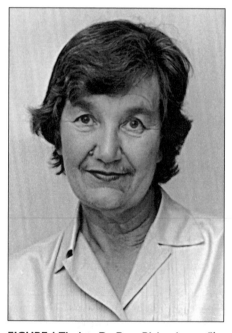

FIGURE 4 The late Dr. Dora Richardson She was the co-patent holder for ICI 46,474 and the organic chemist responsible for the synthesis of triphenylethylenes at ICI Pharmaceuticals, Macclesfield, England. This photograph was taken on the occasion of her retirement in 1979.

ing studies[10] on the value of high-dose estrogen therapy to treat advanced breast cancer in postmenopausal women and to treat prostate cancer in men. This breakthrough in 1944 established a somewhat paradoxical, but effective, therapeutic option that is still used today.

What interested the scientists at ICI was the fact that the new antiestrogens were derivatives of the estrogen, triphenylethylene (Figure 3); but it was clear that improvements in the toxicity profiles and potencies had to be made before any clinically useful agent could be developed for long-term therapy.

Dr. Dora Richardson (Figure 4) began the process by systematically synthesizing numerous analogues of triphenylethylene. The breakthrough came in the mid 1960s when Drs. Harper and Walpole discovered that the *trans* isomer of a triphenylethylene, ICI 46,474, was the antiestrogenic compound of choice, whereas its *cis* geometric isomer ICI 47,699 was an estrogen in all tests.[11] Although the option as a fertility regulator was kept open—in fact, tamoxifen, as it became known, was marketed during the 1970s in Great Britain and Ireland for the induction of ovulation—Walpole suggested using tamoxifen as a treatment for breast cancer. Earlier in his career, Walpole had established a solid reputation as a cancer researcher, and had conducted clinical studies with triphenylethylenes in the treatment of breast cancer in the 1940s.[12] ICI 46,474 had antiestrogenic activity in rats and primates, but would it work as an antitumor agent in women with breast cancer?

Table I

Comparison of Early Clinical Experience With Antiestrogens as a Treatment for Advanced Breast Cancer

Antiestrogen	Daily Dose	Year	Response Rate	Toxicity
Ethamoxytriphetol	500-4500 mg	1960	25%	acute psychotic episodes
Clomiphene	100-300 mg	1964-1974	34%	fear of cataracts
Nafoxidine	180-240 mg	1976	31%	cataracts, ichthyosis, photophobia
Tamoxifen	20-40 mg	1971-1973	31%	transient thrombocytopenia*

*"The particular advantage of this drug is the low incidence of troublesome side effects." Cole et al: *Br J Cancer* 25:270-275, 1971.

"Side effects were usually trivial." Ward: *Br Med J* I:13-14, 1973.

Dr. Mary Cole and coworkers at the Christie Hospital in Manchester, England, conducted the first preliminary evaluation of ICI 46,474 for the palliative treatment of breast cancer. Initially, 46 postmenopausal patients with late-stage disease were treated with the drug; 10 patients responded.[13] These results were subsequently confirmed in a small dose-response study by Dr. Harold Ward in Birmingham, England.[14]

Tamoxifen Goes Forward Alone

The late Dr. Arthur Walpole deserves the credit for pursuing the application of tamoxifen as a potential palliative treatment for advanced breast cancer in postmenopausal women.[12] Tamoxifen, however, was only one of numerous compounds being tested by pharmaceutical companies during the 1960s. Table 1 compares and contrasts the different compounds that underwent evaluation.

ICI Pharmaceuticals had the good fortune to discover a potent antiestrogen with a low profile of toxic side effects. At the onset, it was clear that tamoxifen had several advantages compared to the other contenders. Tamoxifen had higher antitumor potency (ie, a lower dose could be used) compared with other compounds being evaluated at the time. Moreover, while side effects represented a major problem with the other antiestrogens, tamoxifen had virtually no side effects. In fact, tamoxifen seemed to have none of the troublesome side effects observed with high-dose estrogen therapy or androgen therapy that were the standard treatments of the time. Based on experience with drugs, such as clomiphene, investigators were also concerned about the potential of long-term therapy leading to cataract development. Even during the 1960s, however, the Zeneca scientists believed that tamoxifen would not produce cataracts. This has proved to be true after 25 years of use.

Back in the 1960s and '70s, Zeneca was the only company that had chosen to develop an antiestrogenic drug for the treatment of advanced breast cancer. However, there was little enthusiasm from the clinical community about this innovation—All hopes seemed pinned instead on the discovery and application of new cytotoxic chemotherapeutic agents. Thirty years ago, clinical researchers reasoned that their only hope of curing breast cancer lay in the development of better and stronger cytotoxics. That perspective would eventually change when tamoxifen was successfully developed as a treatment for all stages of breast cancer and as the first drug to reduce the incidence of breast cancer in high-risk women. ■

References

1. Beatson GT: On the treatment of inoperable cases of carcinoma of the mamma: Suggestions for a new method of treatment with illustrative cases. *Lancet* 2:104-107, 1896.

2. Boyd S: On oophorectomy in cancer of the breast. *Br Med J* 2:1161-1167, 1900.

3. Allen E, Doisy EA: An ovarian hormone: Preliminary report on its localisation, extraction, and partial purification and action in test animals. *JAMA* 81:819-821, 1923.

4. Jensen EV, Jacobson HI: Basic guides to the mechanism of estrogen action. *Recent Prog Horm Res* 18:387-414, 1962.

5. Jensen EV, Block GE, Smith S, et al: Estrogen receptors and breast cancer response to adrenalectomy, in Hall TC (ed): Prediction of response in cancer therapy. *Monogr Natl Cancer Inst* 34:55-70, 1971.

6. McGuire WL, Carbone PP, Vollmer EP (eds): *Estrogen Receptors in Human Breast Cancer.* New York, Raven Press, 1975.

7. Lerner LJ, Holthaus FJ, Thompson CR: A nonsteroidal estrogen antagonist 1-p-2 diethylaminoethoxyphenyl -1- phenyl 2-p- methoxyphenyethanol. *Endocrinol* 63:215-318, 1958.

8. Lerner LJ, Jordan VC: Development of antiestrogens and their use in breast cancer: Eighth Cain Memorial Award Lecture. *Cancer Res* 50:4177-4189, 1990.

9. Jordan VC: Origins of antiestrogens, in: Lindsay R, Dempster DW, Jordan VC (eds): *Estrogens and Antiestrogens: Basic and Clinical Aspects,* pp 9-20. Philadelphia, Lippincott-Raven, 1997.

10. Haddow A, Wakinson JN, Patterson E, et al: Influence of synthetic oestrogens upon malignant disease. *Br Med J* 2:4368-4371, 1944.

11. Harper MJK, Walpole AL: A new derivative of triphenylethylene: Effect on implantation and mode of action in rats. *J Reprod Fertil* 13:101-117, 1967.

12. Jordan VC: The development of tamoxifen for breast cancer therapy: A tribute to the late Arthur Walpole. *Breast Cancer Res Treat* 11:197-209, 1988.

13. Cole MP, Jones CTA, Todd IDH: A new antiestrogenic agent in last breast cancer: A preliminary appraisal of ICI 46,474. *Br J Cancer* 25:270-275, 1971.

14. Ward HWC: Antiestrogen therapy for breast cancer—A trial of tamoxifen at two dose levels. *Br Med J* 1:13-14, 1973.

Chapter 2

The Clinical Development of Tamoxifen

V. Craig Jordan, PhD, DSc

In 1973, Nolvadex, the ICI Pharmaceuticals Division (now Zeneca) brand of tamoxifen (as its citrate salt), was approved by the Committee on the Safety of Medicines in the United Kingdom for the treatment of breast cancer. Similarly, approval was given in the United States for the treatment of advanced disease in postmenopausal women by the Food and Drug Administration on December 30, 1977. Nolvadex is now available in more than 110 countries as first-line endocrine therapy for the treatment of breast cancer. To mark this achievement, ICI Pharmaceuticals was presented with the Queen's Award for Technological Achievement by the Lord Lieutenant of Cheshire, Viscount Leverhulme, on July 6, 1978 (Figures 1 and 2). The remarkable success of tamoxifen encouraged a closer examination of its pharmacology with a view to further development and wider applications.

Tamoxifen's Metabolism

The metabolism of tamoxifen in animals and humans was first described by Fromson and coworkers at Zeneca. The major metabolic route to be described was hydroxylation to form 4-hydroxytamoxifen, which was subsequently shown to have high binding affinity for the estrogen receptor (ER) and be a potent antiestrogen in its own right, with antitumor properties in the dimethylbenzanthracene (DMBA) model. Indeed, it was an advantage for tamoxifen to be metabolically activated to 4-hydroxytamoxifen, but this was not a prerequisite for antiestrogen action. The metabolite was subsequently shown to localize in target tissues after the administration of radioactive tamoxifen to rats.

Originally, 4-hydroxytamoxifen was believed to be the major metabolite of tamoxifen in patients, but Hugh Adam at Zeneca demonstrated that N-desmethyltamoxifen was the principal metabolite found in patients (Figure 3). There was usually a blood-level ratio of 2:1 for N-desmethyltamoxifen to tamoxifen in patients maintained on tamoxifen therapy, since N-desmethyltamoxifen had twice the plasma half-life of tamoxifen (14 days vs 7 days).

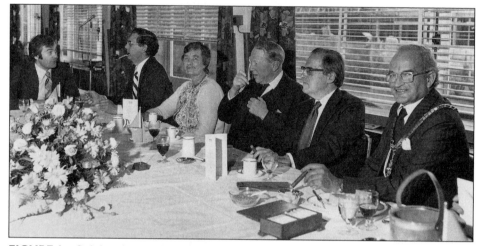

FIGURE 1   Celebrations at ICI Pharmaceuticals Division on the occasion of the 1978 presentation of the Queen's Award for Technological Achievement   At the head table are seated (left to right) Dr. Barry Furr, Deputy Chairman Alan Hayes, the late Dr. Dora Richardson, Viscount Leverhulm, Division Chairman Peter Cunliff, and the Mayor of Macclesfield.

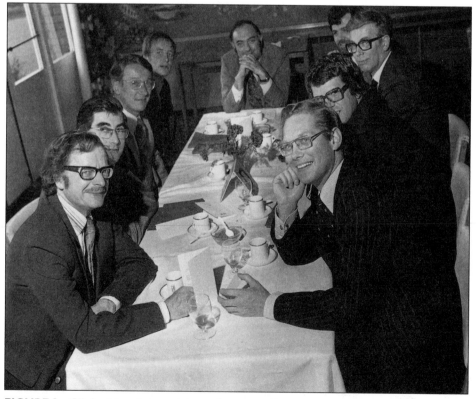

FIGURE 2   Clinical development team for tamoxifen present at the 1978 presentation of the Queen's Award for Technological Achievement   Front left, Dr. Roy Cotton, who was initially in charge of clinical development; front right, the author, and behind, Dr. Sandy Todd.

The ubiquitous use of tamoxifen in recent years has resulted in the publication of numerous methods to estimate tamoxifen and its metabolites in serum.[1] The metabolites that have been identified in patients are shown in Figure 4. The minor metabolites—metabolite-Y, metabolite-Z, and 4-hydroxy-N-desmethyltamoxifen—all contribute to the antitumor actions of tamoxifen because they are all antiestrogens that inhibit the binding of estradiol to the estrogen receptor.

Blocking Growth of Breast Cancer Cells

The next significant advance in the understanding of tamoxifen action in breast cancer came with the availability of hormone-dependent human breast cancer to study antitumor mechanisms in the laboratory. In 1975, Marc

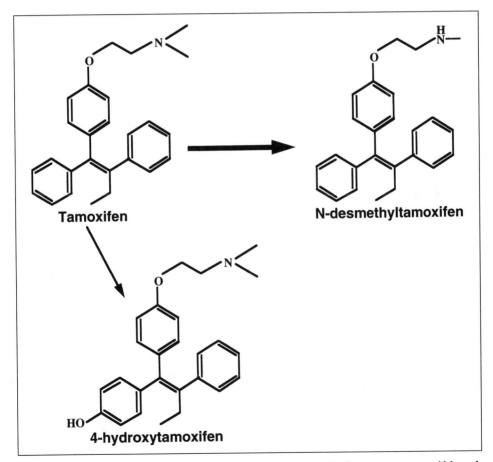

FIGURE 3 Original metabolites of tamoxifen found in human serum Although N-desmethyltamoxifen is the major metabolite and is present at about twice the concentration of tamoxifen in patient's serum, the minor metabolite 4-hydroxytamoxifen, has a high-binding affinity for the estrogen receptor and may contribute significantly to antitumor effects.

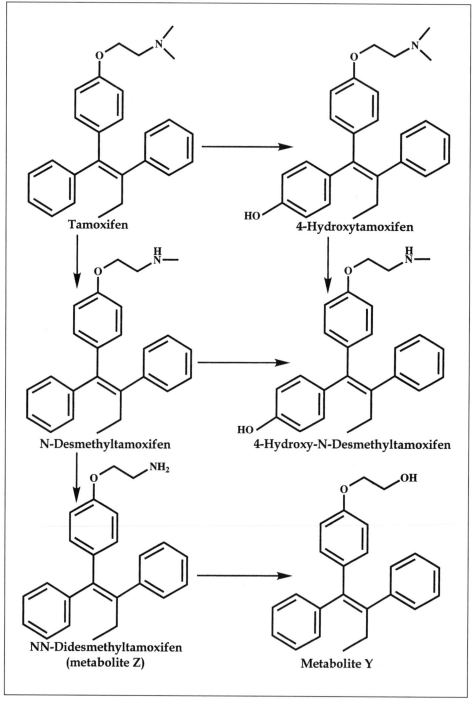

FIGURE 4   Metabolites of tamoxifen found in humans

Lippman[2] at the National Cancer Institute was the first to describe the ability of tamoxifen to inhibit the growth of MCF-7 estrogen receptor-positive breast cancer cells in culture. He was also the first to demonstrate that the addition of estrogen could reverse the action of tamoxifen. Nearly a decade later, C. Kent Osborne[3] in San Antonio and Rob Sutherland[4] in Australia independently described the blockade by tamoxifen of breast cancer cells at the G1 phase of the cell cycle.

Adjuvant Tamoxifen: Laboratory Studies to Clinical Trials

Throughout the 1970s and '80s, the development of tamoxifen became a conversation between the laboratory and the clinic (see Figure 5). The initial

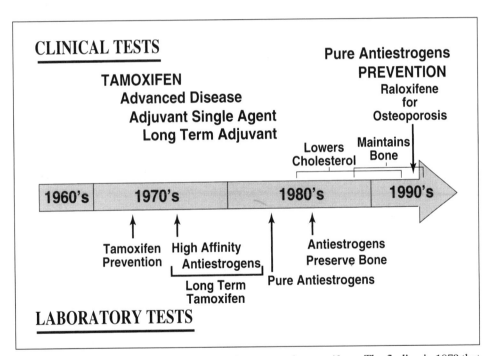

FIGURE 5   Laboratory and clinical development of tamoxifen   The finding in 1973 that tamoxifen could prevent mammary cancer in rats ultimately led to breast cancer prevention trials in the 1990s. The 1977 laboratory finding that long-term treatment was superior to short-term treatment led to longer-than-1-year tamoxifen arms in adjuvant clinical trials. The discovery in 1976 of compounds with a high affinity for the estrogen receptor led to the development of new compounds like raloxifene that are now being tested in clinical trials as a preventive for breast cancer and osteoporosis. Although it appears to be paradoxical that an "antiestrogen" could maintain rather than decrease bone density, the principle was first illustrated in our laboratory in 1987. It was tested with tamoxifen in clinical trials in postmenopausal women in the late 1980s, and subsequently used as justification for the development of raloxifene as a new targeted antiestrogen or selective estrogen-receptor modulator (SERM) to prevent osteoporosis.

success of adjuvant monotherapy with L-phenylalanine mustard or combination chemotherapy in the mid 1970s to delay the recurrence of node-positive breast cancer helped encourage the investigation of other, perhaps less toxic, therapies. Laboratory studies using the DMBA-induced rat mammary carcinoma model were first used to explore whether tamoxifen would be effective and whether the drug produced a tumoristatic or tumoricidal effect in vivo.

Previous in vitro studies by Marc Lippman had indicated that tamoxifen could be a tumoricidal drug; but the results from the in vivo DMBA studies (first reported at a breast cancer symposium at King's College, Cambridge, England in September 1977—Figure 6) demonstrated that a 1-month course of tamoxifen therapy given 1 month after the carcinogenic insult only delayed the appearance of mammary tumors; continuous therapy for 6 months, on the other hand, resulted in 90% of the animals remaining tumor free (Figure 7). Indeed, tumors appeared whenever tamoxifen therapy was stopped.[5] Thus, tamoxifen was shown to have a tumoristatic component to its mode of action, and the laboratory results indicated that long-term (up to 5 years) or indefinite therapy might be the best clinical strategy for adjuvant tamoxifen treatment.[6,7]

Subsequent laboratory studies using DMBA or N-nitrosomethylurea (NMU)-induced rat mammary tumors or human breast cancer cell lines inoculated into athymic mice have all supported that initial observation. However, attention now focused on the clinical evaluation of the laboratory concept.

Several trials of tamoxifen monotherapy as an adjuvant to mastectomy were initiated in the mid to late 1970s. The majority of clinical trials organizations selected a conservative course of 1 year of adjuvant tamoxifen therapy. This decision was based on a number of reasonable concerns. Patients with

FIGURE 6 (right)   Participants at a Breast Cancer Symposium in September 1977 at Kings College, Cambridge, England   The concept of extended adjuvant tamoxifen treatment was first proposed at this meeting. Clinical studies of 1-year adjuvant tamoxifen were in place; regrettably, a decade later, this approach was shown to produce little survival benefit for patients. In the insets (top), the author, who presented the new concept (bottom left); Professor Michael Baum, the session chairman, who was about to launch the Nolvadex Adjuvant Trial Organization (NATO) 2-year adjuvant tamoxifen trial; and (bottom right) Dr. Helen Stewart, who was a participant at the conference. She would initiate a pilot trial in 1978, and, led by Sir Patrick Forest, would later guide the full randomized Scottish Trial of 5 years' adjuvant tamoxifen treatment vs control in the 1980s. Both clinical trials were later proven to produce survival advantages for patients. The concept of longer tamoxifen treatment producing more survival benefits for patients was eventually established indirectly by the Oxford Overview Analysis in 1992[8] and directly by the Swedish group led by Dr. Lars Rutqvist.[9]

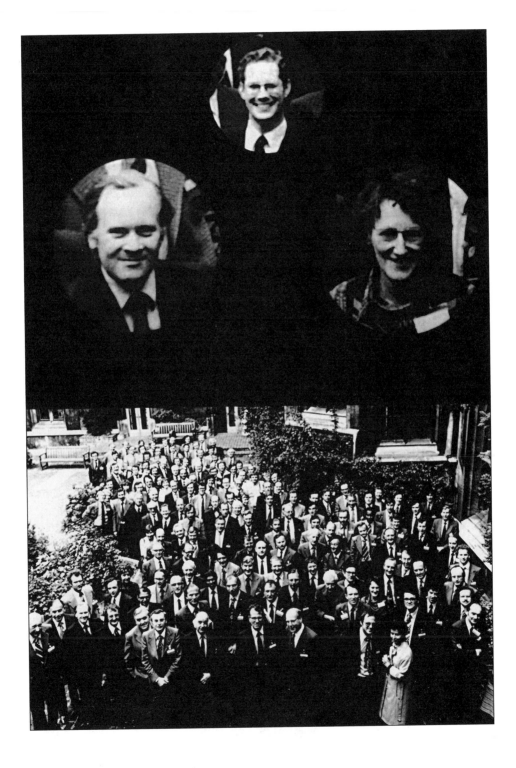

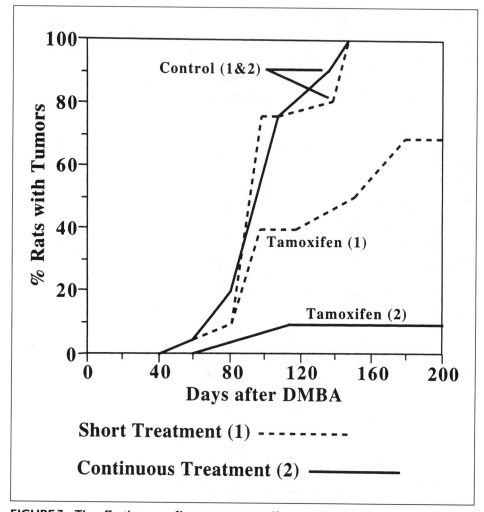

FIGURE 7   The effectiveness of long-term tamoxifen treatment in the dimethylbenzan-thracene (DMBA)-induced rat mammary carcinoma model   The administration of 20 mg DMBA by gavage to 50-day-old female Sprague Dawley rats results in all animals developing mammary tumors 160 days later. The short-term (30 days) administration of different daily doses (12.5-800 µg) of tamoxifen between days 30 and 60 after DMBA results in a delay of tumor formation. However, not all animals are protected from the carcinogen. In contrast, the daily administration of a clinically relevant dose (50 µg daily = 0.25 mg/kg in rats or 20 mg daily to a 70 kg woman) of tamoxifen continuously, starting 30 days after DMBA, results in 90% of animals remaining tumor free.

advanced disease usually respond to tamoxifen for 1 year, and it was expected that estrogen receptor-negative disease would be encouraged to grow prematurely during adjuvant therapy. If this growth occurred, then the physician would have already used a valuable palliative drug and would have only combination chemotherapy to slow the relentless growth of recurrent disease. A related argument involved the changing strategy for the application of adjuvant combination chemotherapy. Recurrent treatment cycles (2 years) were found to be of no long-term benefit for patients. In contrast, it seemed that aggressive, short-term courses of treatment (6 months) with the most active cytotoxic drugs had the best chance to kill tumor cells before the premature development of drug resistance. The same intuitive sense that "longer might not be better" contributed to a reluctance on the part of the researchers to start with long-term tamoxifen therapy.

The remarkable success of tamoxifen encouraged a closer examination of its pharmacology.

Finally, there were sincere concerns about the side effects of adjuvant therapy and the ethical issues of treating patients who might never have recurrent disease. Although this argument primarily focused on chemotherapy and node-negative patients, it is fair to say that few women in the mid 1970s had received extended therapy with tamoxifen—therefore, long-term side effects were largely unknown. Most tamoxifen-treated patients had only received about 2 years of treatment for advanced disease before drug resistance developed. Potential side effects, such as thrombosis and osteoporosis, were only of secondary importance.

The use of tamoxifen in the disease-free patient, however, would change that perspective.

In 1977, Dr. Douglas C. Tormey and I organized the first evaluation of long-term tamoxifen therapy in node-positive patients treated with combination chemotherapy plus tamoxifen.[10] This pilot study was initiated to determine whether patients could tolerate 5 years of adjuvant tamoxifen therapy and whether metabolic tolerance would occur during long-term treatment. No unusual side effects of tamoxifen therapy were noted, and blood levels of tamoxifen and its metabolites, N-desmethyltamoxifen and metabolite-Y, remained stable throughout the 5 years of treatment. Although this study was not a randomized trial, those patients who received long-term tamoxifen therapy continued to make excellent progress, and many patients were to take the drug for more than 14 years. We have reported that tamoxifen does not produce metabolic tolerance during 10 years of administration. Serum levels of tamoxifen and its metabolites are maintained.[11]

Randomized Trials

These data and the DMBA rat mammary carcinoma data were used to support randomized Eastern Cooperative Oncology Group (ECOG) trials EST 4181 and 5181. An early analysis of EST 4181, which compares short-term tamoxifen with long-term tamoxifen (both with combination chemotherapy), has demonstrated an increase in disease-free survival with long-term tamoxifen therapy.[12,13] In fact, the 5-year tamoxifen arm has now gone through a second randomization, either to stop the tamoxifen or to continue the antiestrogen indefinitely[14] (see Chapter 11).

Building on the success of these earlier trials that demonstrated the efficacy of tamoxifen in receptor-positive postmenopausal patients, the National Surgical Adjuvant Breast and Bowel Project (NSABP) has conducted a 2-year registration study of combination chemotherapy (L-PAM, 5FU) plus tamoxifen, with an additional year of tamoxifen alone. Overall, these investigators concluded that 3 years of tamoxifen confers a significant advantage over 2 years of tamoxifen.[15]

A 1994 report from Italy has demonstrated that the addition of combination chemotherapy (CMF for 6 cycles followed by 5 courses of epirubicin) to long-term tamoxifen (5 years) therapy does not seem to significantly improve the clearcut effectiveness of tamoxifen alone to prevent recurrence in estrogen receptor-negative and node-positive disease.[16]

While the 2-year adjuvant tamoxifen study conducted by the Nolvadex Adjuvant Trials Organization or NATO (an acronym chosen to encourage American investigators to read *Lancet* papers because they might believe the work had been done by the North Atlantic Treaty Organization!)[17] was the first to demonstrate a survival advantage, clinical trials are still evaluating a longer duration of tamoxifen therapy (see Chapter 11).

A small randomized clinical trial conducted in France has demonstrated a survival advantage for estrogen receptor-positive patients who received 3 years of tamoxifen vs no treatment. Similarly, a Scottish trial that evaluated 5 years of tamoxifen vs no treatment demonstrated a survival advantage for patients who take tamoxifen.[18] The Scottish trial is particularly interesting because it addresses the question of whether to administer tamoxifen early as an adjuvant or to save the drug until disease recurs. This comparison was possible because most patients in the control arm received tamoxifen at recurrence. Early concerns that long-term adjuvant tamoxifen would result in premature drug resistance were unjustified, since patients on the adjuvant tamoxifen arm had a survival advantage.

Conclusion

During the past 30 years, tamoxifen has moved from the laboratory to become the endocrine treatment of choice for all stages of breast cancer. The drug has a remarkable profile of interesting pharmacological effects: On one hand, tamoxifen can inhibit estrogen-stimulated breast cancer growth, while on the other hand, it can also mimic some of the physiological functions of estrogen to support bone and lower circulating cholesterol.

The following chapters in this volume are intended to provide an up-to-date appraisal of the effectiveness and side effects of long-term tamoxifen therapy and to discuss the success of tamoxifen as a preventive for breast cancer in high-risk women. The clinical trials that have tested the worth of tamoxifen as a preventive now provide the physician with a new therapeutic dimension. ■

References

1. Langen-Fahey SM, Jordan VC, Fritz NF, et al: Clinical pharmacology and endocrinology of long-term tamoxifen therapy, in Jordan VC (ed): *Long Term Tamoxifen Treatment for Breast Cancer,* pp 27-56. Madison, University of Wisconsin Press, 1994.

2. Lippman ME, Bolan G: Oestrogen responsive human breast cancer in long-term tissue culture. *Nature* 256:592-593, 1975.

3. Osborne CK, Boldt DH, Clark GH, et al: Effects of tamoxifen on human breast cancer cell cycle kinetics accumulation of cells in early G1 phase. *Cancer* 43:3583-3585, 1993.

4. Sutherland RL, Reddel RR, Green MD: Effects of oestrogens on cell proliferation and cell cycle kinetics: A hypothesis on the cell cycle effects of antiestrogens. *Eur J Cancer Clin Oncol* 19:307-318, 1983.

5. Jordan VC: Use of the DMBA-induced rat mammary carcinoma system for the evaluation of tamoxifen as a potential adjuvant therapy: *Reviews on Endoc Rel Cancer* (10 Suppl) 49-55, 1978.

6. Jordan VC, Dix CJ, Allen KE: The effectiveness of long-term treatment in laboratory model for adjuvant hormone therapy of breast cancer, in Salmon SE, Jones SE (ed): *Adjuvant Therapy of Cancer,* pp 19-24. New York, Grune and Stratton, 1979.

7. Jordan VC: Laboratory studies to develop general principles for the adjuvant treatment of breast cancer with antiestrogens: Problem and potential for future clinical applications. *Breast Cancer Res Treat* 3(Suppl):73-86, 1983.

8. Early Breast Cancer Trialists' Collaborative Group: Systemic treatment of early breast cancer by hormonal, cytotoxic, or immunotherapy. *Lancet* 339:1-15, 1992.

9. Swedish Breast Cancer Cooperative Group: Randomized trial of two versus five years of adjuvant tamoxifen for postmenopausal early stage breast cancer. *J Natl Cancer Inst* 88:1543-1549, 1996.

10. Tormey DC, Jordan VC: Long-term tamoxifen adjuvant therapy in node positive breast cancer: A metabolic and pilot clinical study. *Breast Cancer Res Treat* 4:297-302, 1984.

11. Langan-Fahey SM, Tormey DC, Jordan VC: Tamoxifen metabolites in patients on long-term therapy for breast cancer. *Eur J Cancer* 26:883-888, 1990.

12. Falkson HC, Gray R, Wolberg WH, et al: Adjuvant trial of 12 cycles of CMFPT followed by observation or continuous tamoxifen versus 4 cycles of CMFPT in postmenopausal women with breast cancer: An Eastern Cooperative Oncology Group phase III study. *J Clin Oncol* 8:599-607, 1990.

13. Tormey DC, Gray R, Abeloff MD, et al: Adjuvant therapy with a doxorubicin regimen and long-term tamoxifen in premenopausal breast cancer patients: An ECOG group trial. *J Clin Oncol* 10:1848-1856, 1992.

14. Tormey DC, Gray R, Falkson HC (for the Eastern Co-operative Oncology Group): Postchemotherapy adjuvant tamoxifen therapy beyond 5 years in patients with lymph-node positive breast cancer. *J Natl Cancer Inst* 88:1828-1833, 1996.

15. Fisher B and the National Surgical Adjuvant Breast and Bowl Project Investigators: Prolonging tamoxifen therapy for primary breast cancer. *Ann Int Med* 106:649-654, 1987.

16. Boccardo F, Amorosso D, Rubagotti A, et al: Prolonged tamoxifen treatment of early breast cancer: The experience of the Italian Co-operative group for chemohormonal therapy of early breast cancer, in Jordan VC (ed): *Long-Term Tamoxifen Treatment for Breast Cancer*, pp 159-179. Madison, University of Wisconsin Press, 1994.

17. Nolvadex Adjuvant Trial Organization: Controlled trial of tamoxifen as a single adjuvant agent in the management of early breast cancer: Interim analysis at four years. *Lancet* i:257-261, 1983.

18. Breast Cancer Trials' Committee, Scottish Cancer Trials Office (MRC): Adjuvant tamoxifen in the management of operable breast cancer: The Scottish Trial. *Lancet* ii:171-175, 1987.

Chapter 3

Current Approved Uses and Recommendations of Tamoxifen in the United States

V. Craig Jordan, PhD, DSc

Medicines are approved for use in the United States by the Food and Drug Administration (FDA). Approval for use in humans is only made after a vigorous evaluation of preclinical, clinical, and toxicologic data by expert committees. Formal approval for use is made following the public deliberations of the expert committee, which, at that time, recommends approval or disapproval of a product. Without approval of a medicine, the product cannot be marketed in the US, and without approval of an indication, a company cannot promote the use of their product.

Since 1977, tamoxifen (Nolvadex) has been approved by the FDA for the treatment of advanced breast cancer in postmenopausal women. The product has been marketed in the US since then, and similar approvals have been obtained in 110 other countries. Tamoxifen has been used by millions of women worldwide and is currently the most frequently prescribed cancer drug.

During the past 25 years, additional approvals have been obtained from the FDA for other applications of tamoxifen. In 1985, tamoxifen was approved as an adjuvant therapy with chemotherapy in postmenopausal women with node-positive breast cancer. In 1986, approval was obtained for the use of adjuvant tamoxifen alone in the same group of postmenopausal women with node-positive breast cancer. In 1989, approval was obtained from the FDA for the use of tamoxifen in the treatment of premenopausal women with estrogen receptor-positive advanced breast cancer. In 1990, an indication as an adjuvant was approved for pre- and postmenopausal patients with node-negative, estrogen-receptor-positive breast cancer. And finally, now in 1998, tamoxifen has been approved for the reduction of the risk of breast cancer in high-risk pre- and postmenopausal women.

Tamoxifen has also been active in the treatment of male breast cancer, and in 1993, the FDA approved the use of tamoxifen to treat advanced breast cancer in men.

Overall, tamoxifen has repeatedly been shown to extend the survival of patients with breast cancer. Therefore, in 1994, the FDA approved the claim that tamoxifen prolonged the overall survival of the breast cancer patient.

Finally, based on the results from the National Cancer Institute-sponsored NSABP breast cancer prevention trial[1], the FDA approved tamoxifen for the reduction of breast cancer incidence in high-risk, well women. Similarly, based on the randomized adjuvant clinical trials,[2] tamoxifen is also approved for use in the reduction of contralateral breast cancer in women after a diagnosis of breast cancer.

The role of the FDA is to protect the general public from excessive claims of manufacturers of medicines. The system provides strict control of

Table I

Adjuvant Treatment for Patients with Lymph-Node-Negative Breast Cancer*

Patient Group	Minimal-Low Risk	Good Risk	High Risk
PREMENOPAUSAL			
ER positive	No adjuvant treatment vs tamoxifen†	**Tamoxifen** Oophorectomy†	**Chemotherapy** ± tamoxifen†
		Chemotherapy†	Oophorectomy†
		Gonadotropin-releasing hormone analogue†	Gonadotropin-releasing hormone analogue†
ER negative	Not applicable	Not applicable	**Chemotherapy**
POSTMENOPAUSAL			
ER positive	No adjuvant treatment vs tamoxifen†	**Tamoxifen**	**Tamoxifen** ± chemotherapy†
ER negative	Not applicable	Not applicable	**Chemotherapy** ± tamoxifen†
ELDERLY	No adjuvant treatment versus tamoxifen†	**Tamoxifen**	**Tamoxifen**; if ER negative: **chemotherapy** ± tamoxifen†

*Bold entries are treatments accepted for routine use or baseline in clinical trials.
†Treatments still being tested in randomized clinical trials
ER = estrogen receptor
From Goldhirsch, Wood, Senn, et al: *J Natl Cancer Inst* 87:1441-1445, 1995.

Table 2

Adjuvant Treatment for Patients with Lymph-Node-Positive Breast Cancer*

Patient Group	Treatment
PREMENOPAUSAL	
ER positive	**Chemotherapy** ± tamoxifen†
	Ovarian ablation ± tamoxifen†
	Gonadotropin-releasing hormone analogue†
	Chemotherapy ± ovarian ablation (gonadotropin releasing hormone analogue) ± tamoxifen†
ER negative	**Chemotherapy**
POSTMENOPAUSAL	
ER positive	**Tamoxifen** ± chemotherapy
ER negative	**Chemotherapy** ± tamoxifen†
ELDERLY	**Tamoxifen**; if ER negative: **chemotherapy** ± tamoxifen†

*Bold entries are treatments accepted for routine use or baseline in clinical trials.
†Treatments still being tested in randomized trials
ER = estrogen receptor
From Goldhirsch, Wood, Senn, et al: *J Natl Cancer Inst* 87:1441-1445, 1995.

manufacturers and what can be claimed in their advertising to physicians. The aim is to ensure that physicians are not misled into believing false claims for a medicine.

Outside the relationship between physicians and pharmaceutical advertising, a physician has the authority to prescribe medicines that he or she believes will aid the patient; physicians can also use medicines in the context of an approved clinical trial. In the latter case, the patient is expected to read and sign an informed consent form stating the potential benefits and side effects of the experimental approach. Clinical trials are strictly controlled and monitored to safeguard the patient. No clinical trial provides less than the accepted standards of care.

Periodically, physicians meet to provide guidelines for the profession about the suggested treatment approaches for patients with breast cancer. These are called "consensus conferences." The conclusions of the St. Gallen

(Switzerland) Breast Cancer Conference, for example, are published periodically in the *Journal of the National Cancer Institute*.

The recommendations offered in 1995 by the international clinical community are summarized in the two tables on the previous pages: adjuvant treatment for patients with lymph-node-negative breast cancer (Table 1) and lymph-node-positive breast cancer (Table 2). ■

References

1. Fisher B, Costantino JP, Wickerham DL, et al. Tamoxifen for prevention of breast cancer: Report of the National Surgical Adjuvant Breast and Bowel Project P-1 Study. *J Nat'l Cancer Inst* 90:1371-1388, 1998.

2. Early Breast Cancer Trialists' Collaborative Group. Tamoxifen for early breast cancer: An overview of the randomized trials. *Lancet* 351:1451-1467, 1998.

Chapter 4

Early Overviews of Adjuvant Tamoxifen Therapy

I. Craig Henderson, MD
Adjunct Professor of Medicine
University of California
San Francisco, California

An Overview Is a Meta-Analysis.

During the past 15 years, "overviews" (as the British prefer to call them) or meta-analyses, have been widely accepted as a powerful method for detecting small but clinically worthwhile treatment benefits. Most investigators consider a 10% survival advantage 10 years after treatment of cancer to be clinically worthwhile, especially if the toxicities of the treatment were modest. A benefit of that size, however, can only be reliably detected by a very large randomized trial. Although this is the preferred way to evaluate the effects of therapy, more frequently, multiple smaller trials are conducted because they are more easily administered and less costly to run. Unfortunately—even if there is a consistent trend—most trials of this nature do not demonstrate a statistically significant benefit.

Overviews can be used to circumvent the inadequate statistical power of small clinical trials by pooling the results of many smaller trials. In addition to detecting small but clinically worthwhile benefits, overviews provide greater statistical power, permitting evaluation of therapeutic effects in specific patient subsets.

Overviews of adjuvant tamoxifen (and adjuvant chemotherapy) trials were performed in 1985, 1990, and 1995. These clearly established that adjuvant tamoxifen could decrease breast cancer recurrence and mortality. Indirect comparisons of subsets within the overviews suggested that (1) longer durations of therapy were more effective than shorter treatment periods; (2) the effects of adjuvant tamoxifen were proportionally the same in all nodal subsets; and (3) patients whose tumors were estrogen receptor- (ER) positive derived greater benefit than those with few or no measurable estrogen receptors. Results of the 1985 and 1990 overviews have been published,[1-3] but the 1995 report was not available until 1998.

In the Beginning: 1984

The first overview of adjuvant systemic therapy for early breast cancer was performed by Drs. Richard Peto, Rory Collins, Richard Gray, and the team from the Clinical Trials Unit of Oxford University in 1984. At that time, three randomized trials had demonstrated that the use of adjuvant chemotherapy might prolong the lives of premenopausal women with breast cancer.[4-7] No survival advantage had been observed, however, for postmenopausal women. Based on those data, a US consensus conference concluded that adjuvant chemotherapy should be the standard for premenopausal women, but not postmenopausal women.[8]

Europeans were more reluctant to use adjuvant therapy in any group of women. They feared its toxicity and thought it plausible that the effects of such treatment in premenopausal women might be entirely due to chemically induced ovarian ablation. Instead, European investigators designed a series of adjuvant endocrine therapy trials, the first of which was conducted in Denmark.[9]

Americans, however, were skeptical about the likelihood that a cytostatic drug, such as tamoxifen, could destroy an adequate number of tumor cells to substantially and significantly prolong survival.[10] The first report, albeit only a brief letter to the editor of the *Lancet* by Baum et al,[11] stating that tamoxifen prolonged survival in patients with early breast cancer was published in 1983. During those years, most breast cancer conferences on either side of the Atlantic concluded with a debate between an American and a northern European, each espousing his or her particular perspective on this controversial subject.

By October of 1984, Dr. Peto had successfully obtained the cooperation of every principal investigator of an adjuvant therapy trial, as well as at least some data from almost every known randomized trial conducted anywhere in the world up to that time. He then organized a conference to review results. Although investigators had submitted their data to the Oxford unit for analysis, none of those attending the conference had yet seen the results of the overview when they gathered at Heathrow Airport.

On the first evening, Dr. Peto outlined the goals of the conference and carefully explained the methodology—which was largely unknown to most of the investigators. It was clear that the techniques used for the overview analyses were potentially quite powerful. The next morning, each trial was briefly presented. The tension and excitement mounted throughout the day until the results of the meta-analysis were presented in the afternoon. At the end of the presentation, there was no doubt in the minds of any but the most recalcitrant chemotherapy advocates that tamoxifen could not only prolong the recurrence-free survival of postmenopausal women with early breast cancer, but that it could prolong overall survival as well.

That evening at dinner, investigators placed small wagers on what the chemotherapy results would show the next day. Many of the Americans suspected that the overview was a British "trump card" that they would use to win the ongoing debate once and for all.

Overviews can be used to circumvent the inadequate statistical power of small clinical trials by pooling the results of many smaller trials.

On the second day, each of the chemotherapy trials was presented and discussed. At the end of the day, the overview demonstrated that chemotherapy also improved both disease-free survival and overall survival in postmenopausal women to about the same extent as tamoxifen.

During the course of the next year, these results were carefully checked and corrections were made. The analysis was again presented in Bethesda, Maryland in September 1985 at another National Cancer Institute Consensus Conference. After hearing and reviewing the data, the consensus panel concluded that adjuvant tamoxifen should be considered the standard treatment for postmenopausal women with positive axillary lymph nodes and estrogen receptor-positive tumors.[12] Thus, the 1985 Overview put an end to the debate about whether adjuvant therapy prolonged survival. The principle had been established. A new era had begun in which research could now focus on how to improve the efficacy of adjuvant treatment.

By the time the data were ready for publication, however, it was clear that the first overview had overestimated the benefits to be derived from the use of adjuvant chemotherapy for postmenopausal women. The preparation of an overview is a tedious, detail-oriented project. Data must be checked and rechecked. The first analyses are not always consistent with the final publication.

How Is an Overview Performed?

The term "meta-analysis" has been used to describe a multitude of approaches to pooling data.[1] Many ignore the fundamental principle of an overview, which is to compare "like with like." Quality overviews are based on randomized, case-control, and cohort studies. The size and direction (positive or negative) of the effects of treatment are determined independently for each of the trials included in an overview, and these effects or benefits are then summated. Patients in the treatment arm are only compared with the patients in the control arm of the same study—never with patients in the control arm of another study. Beyond this fundamental principle, however, there are many legitimate differences of opinion about how to best proceed.

Some overviews include only published data or give greater weight to published data because they have undergone a rigorous peer review and likely represent the highest quality studies. On the other hand, studies with negative or null results are less likely to be published, and the exclusion of unpublished data introduces a different kind of bias. Some investigators perform their own quality analysis of studies and give added weight to those trials that meet certain predefined standards. The breast cancer overviews utilize all available data, whether published or unpublished, and no adjustments are made on the basis of any factor, including perceived quality of the trial. As a consequence, the largest trials have substantially more weight in the final estimate of treatment effect than do smaller trials.

The first breast cancer overview, performed in 1984-1985, included all randomized clinical trials of adjuvant systemic therapy that were initiated prior to January 1, 1985. Printouts of data entered into the computers in Oxford were verified by each investigator. The validity of the randomization

Table I

Expression of Overview Results as "Ratio" Vs "Rate" Differences in Survival

| | No. of Deaths in Five Years | | Survival at Five Years | |
	Treated	Control	Treated	Control
Trial 1	30	40	70%	60%
Trial 2	6	8	94%	92%

| | Reduction In Mortality | |
	Ratio Difference	Rate Difference
Trial 1	25%	10%
Trial 2	25%	2%

In each of these two hypothetical trials, 100 patients were randomized to the control arm and 100 to the treated arm. Results at 5 years are presented. In the first of the two trials, 30 of the 100 patients randomized to the treated group and 40 of the 100 randomized to the control group died within the first 5 years of follow-up. Thus, at 5 years, 70% of the treated and 60% of the control patients were alive. This represents an absolute or rate difference of 10%. Another way to look at these data from the first trial focuses upon patients who died in the control group (N=40) or who might have died in the treated group. If treatment had no effect, it would be reasonable to expect 40 deaths in the treatment group. Only 30 deaths were actually observed. The 10 deaths that were prevented, divided by the 40 deaths expected gives a ratio difference of 25%.

Gelber RD and Goldhirsch A: The Concept of an Overview of Cancer Clinical Trials with Special Emphasis on Early Breast Cancer. *J Clin Oncol* 4: 1696-1703, 1986.

process in each trial was evaluated and any imbalances were investigated. In one instance, a trial was omitted because of questions about the validity of the results that emerged during a site visit.

The first report of the 1985 Overview was published in 1988.[2] A very detailed report providing substantially more data and great detail on the overview methodology was subsequently published as a monograph in 1990.[1] A secondary review was conducted in 1990 and published in 1992.[3] No additional trials were added to this overview, but data from all the trials included in the 1985 Overview were updated through 1990. A third overview, which included all patients in trials initiated prior to January 1, 1990, was completed in 1995 and presented to the contributing trialists at a meeting in Oxford in September, 1995.

1990 Overview

The 1990 tamoxifen Overview was based on 40 trials that enrolled 29,892 patients, 8,219 of whom had died at the time of the analysis. The preliminary presentation of the 1995 Overview included 58 tamoxifen trials that had enrolled 45,469 women, 15,257 of whom had died. Like a randomized trial, the real statistical power of an overview is derived from the number of events, such as recurrences or deaths, rather than from the number of patients enrolled. The number of events in these overviews far exceeded anything imaginable with one, or even two, large trials.

Expression of Results

The overview analyses are presented in one of two ways:[13]

1) As a reduction in the annual odds of recurrence or death. This is an expression of the proportional effect, or the ratio of the effect, of therapy in the treated group compared to the control group.

2) As an absolute difference. This is the difference in the disease-free or overall survival curves on a life table plot at a single point in time. It is also referred to as the "rate difference."

The difference between the ratio and rate differences can be most readily understood by a simple example:[13] In Trial 1 presented in Table 1, 30 of the 100 patients randomized to the treated group and 40 of the 100 randomized to the control group died in the first 5 years of follow-up. Thus, at 5 years, 70% of the treated and 60% of the control patients were alive. This represents an absolute or rate difference of 10%. This represents the benefit from treatment for *all* treated patients, including patients who might not have died without treatment. Another way to look at these data from Trial 1 focuses entirely upon patients who died in the control group (N = 40), or patients who might have died in the treated group. If treatment had no effect, it would be reasonable to expect 40 deaths in the treatment group. Only 30 deaths were actually observed. The 10 deaths that were prevented, divided by the 40 deaths expected, gives a ratio difference of 25%. This is not precisely the same as a calculation of the annual odds of death. Nevertheless, it is rough approximation and illustrates the difference between a proportional and an absolute survival benefit. (For a more complete explanation of this method, see Reference 2.)

Overall Results of the 1990 Overview

All worldwide trials in which patients had been randomized to tamoxifen or no tamoxifen were included in the 1990 Overview. In some of these trials,

---

Table 2

Comparative Reductions in Mortality (Proportional and Absolute), Chemotherapy Vs Tamoxifen

Therapy	Reduction ± S.D. In Odds Of	
	Recurrence	**Death**
Chemotherapy	21% ± 2	11% ± 2
Tamoxifen	25% ± 2	17% ± 2

Therapy	Absolute Difference ± S.D. At 10 Years For	
	Recurrence	**Death**
Chemotherapy	9.2% ± 1.2	6.3% ± 1.4
Tamoxifen	6.6% ± 0.9	6.2% ± 0.9

The effects of therapy described here are derived from overviews of all trials in which patients were randomized to either chemotherapy vs no chemotherapy (including trials in which patients were randomized to chemotherapy plus tamoxifen vs tamoxifen alone) or tamoxifen vs no tamoxifen (including trials in which patients were randomized to tamoxifen plus chemotherapy vs chemotherapy alone). All patients were included regardless of age or nodal status. The chemotherapy trials were limited to those that used at least several months of a drug combination; trials that employed a single agent and those that administered one course of chemotherapy (eg, perioperative trials) were not included. All tamoxifen studies, however, were included in the overview regardless of the duration of tamoxifen therapy or the receptor status of the patient. All differences are statistically significant with a p *at least* < 0.0001. Proportional = reduction in annual odds of death; absolute = difference in survival between the two groups at 10 years.

Early Breast Cancer Trialists' Collaborative Group, 1992: Systemic treatment of early breast cancer by hormonal, cytotoxic, or immune therapy: 133 randomized trials involving 31,000 recurrences and 24,000 deaths among 75,000 women. *Lancet* 339:1-15, 71-85, 1992.

women were randomized following mastectomy or lumpectomy plus radio-therapy to receive either tamoxifen alone or no adjuvant treatment of any type (Nil). There were other trials that compared tamoxifen plus some other therapy with the other therapy alone. Most often, these trials evaluated tamoxifen plus chemotherapy compared with chemotherapy alone. In general, the trial design was irrelevant. If there were a benefit from the comparison of tamoxifen versus Nil, there was usually a benefit from tamoxifen plus chemotherapy compared to chemotherapy alone. The size of the benefit might be different in the two types of trials, but the direction of the benefit (positive or negative) would be the same. The overall result included women from all age groups in trials that utilized a variety of different tamoxifen doses and durations of therapy.

The reduction in the annual odds of recurrence or death and the absolute difference in recurrence or death at 10 years of adjuvant tamoxifen therapy are shown in Table 2. For comparative purposes, the results of the chemo-therapy overview are also shown. No significant differences between the effects of adjuvant chemotherapy and adjuvant tamoxifen can be seen. (This is not necessarily true for all patient subsets, but that is beyond the scope of this discussion.)

ADJUVANT TAMOXIFEN: ANALYSES OF PATIENT SUBSETS

Age and Menopause

In the 1990 Overview, adjuvant tamoxifen was found to be less beneficial in younger women and premenopausal women (Table 3). Age appeared to be at least as important as the patient's menstrual status, since the effects of adjuvant tamoxifen were nearly the same in women aged 50 to 59, regardless of whether they were pre- or postmenopausal. The effect of adjuvant chemo-therapy in women younger than 50 was less than half as great as that of adjuvant tamoxifen, and again it made no difference whether these younger women were pre- or postmenopausal. Nevertheless, these results must be interpreted very cautiously. Most of the trials evaluating tamoxifen in women older than 50 years of age were designed as "tamoxifen versus Nil." For women younger than 50, the trials more often compared tamoxifen plus chemotherapy vs the same chemotherapy alone. It is possible, therefore, that the positive effects of tamoxifen in women under age 50 might be much greater than shown by these studies. In fact, this is quite plausible (see Chapters 5 and 6).

Adjuvant chemotherapy caused transient amenorrhea in almost all pre-menopausal patients and permanent amenorrhea in the vast majority. Thus,

Table 3

Effect of Adjuvant Tamoxifen on Annual Odds of Recurrence and Death, by Age and Menopause Status

Premenopausal	No. of Patients	Reduction ± S.D. in Annual Odds of	
		Recurrence	Death
AGE < 50	7905	12% ± 4	6% ± 5
50-59	1583	33% ± 7	23% ± 9
Postmenopausal			
AGE < 50	681	12% ± 15	(ZERO TREND)
50-59	7804	28% ± 3	19% ± 4
60-69	9452	29% ± 3	17% ± 4
70+	2656	28% ± 5	21% ± 6

This overview includes trials of tamoxifen vs no tamoxifen, including trials comparing tamoxifen vs no adjuvant therapy of any type, as well as those comparing tamoxifen plus chemotherapy alone in all age groups. Trials among older women were more often of the tamoxifen vs no adjuvant type, while among younger women, the trials were predominantly tamoxifen plus chemotherapy vs chemotherapy alone.

Early Breast Cancer Trialists' Collaborative Group, 1992: Systemic treatment of early breast cancer by hormonal, cytotoxic, or immune therapy: 133 randomized trials involving 31,000 recurrences and 24,000 deaths among 75,000 women. *Lancet* 339:1-15, 71-85, 1992.

it could be argued that the predominant effect of chemotherapy in younger women was a chemical oophorectomy. If this is the case, the combination of tamoxifen plus chemotherapy may really be a combination of two hormone therapies: tamoxifen plus oophorectomy!

A comparison of the benefits of tamoxifen plus chemotherapy vs chemotherapy alone in women under the age of 50 to the benefits of tamoxifen vs Nil in women over the age of 50 would be inappropriate. Although combination chemotherapy has been shown in many randomized trials to be superior to single-agent regimens, this is not true for endocrine combinations. In multiple randomized trials, it has been impossible to show an advantage for such combinations.[14]

Tumor Estrogen-Receptor Status

In patients with metastatic breast cancer, there was an excellent correlation between estrogen- and progesterone-receptor status and response to tamoxifen. This correlation would be expected to hold true in the adjuvant setting as well. An overview of all patients in all age groups, analyzed according to estrogen-receptor status, demonstrated that adjuvant tamoxifen conferred a significantly greater advantage on those patients with moderately elevated or high levels of estrogen receptor (Table 4).

It was surprising to find that the 1990 Overview showed a significant reduction in the annual odds of recurrence (13% ± 4), even in those patients who had estrogen receptor-poor tumors; the reduction in the annual odds of death (11%, ± 5) was marginally significant. In fact, in women aged 50 and older, the reduction in the annual odds of death was significant in both patients with receptor-poor and receptor-rich tumors (16% ± 5 and 36% ± 3, respectively). Furthermore, in the 1990 Overview, the effect of adjuvant tamoxifen in older women with receptor-poor tumors was greater than the effect of adjuvant chemotherapy in these women. This led many physicians to use tamoxifen in all older women, regardless of receptor status. However, the results of the more recent 1995 Overview, described later in this chapter, should be noted.

Axillary Lymph Node Status

The *mathematical* interactions used to describe the relationship between a therapy and specific patient subsets may be qualitative or quantitative. In

Table 4

Effect of Adjuvant Tamoxifen on Annual Odds of Recurrence or Death, by ER Level

Receptor Level	No. of Patients	Reduction ± S.D. in Annual Odds Of	
		Recurrence	Death
ER - Poor or absent	5366	13% ± 4	11% ± 5
ER - Moderately elevated	11,733	29% ± 3	19% ± 4
ER - Highest Level	3174	43% ± 5	29% ± 7
ER - Unknown	9554	22% ± 3	15% ± 3
Test for Trend		p < 0.00001	p = 0.006

This overview includes trials of tamoxifen vs no tamoxifen, including trials comparing tamoxifen vs no adjuvant therapy of any type, as well as those comparing tamoxifen plus chemotherapy alone for all ER levels. Levels were defined by each trial group submitting data.

Early Breast Cancer Trialists' Collaborative Group, 1992: Systemic treatment of early breast cancer by hormonal, cytotoxic, or immune therapy: 133 randomized trials involving 31,000 recurrences and 24,000 deaths among 75,000 women. *Lancet* 339:1-15, 71-85, 1992.

general, a qualitative interaction is one in which one group of patients derives benefit while another derives none. (It is important not to conceptualize "qualitative" and "quantitative" in terms of the nonmathematical relationship between therapy and a group of patients defined by pretreatment risk factors.)

We might have anticipated that the interaction between tamoxifen and estrogen-receptor status would be a qualitative interaction. However, qualitative interactions are quite rare in medicine. A quantitative interaction is one in which there is an effect of therapy in all patient subsets, but the size of the benefit varies from one group to another. This is the most common interaction seen in medicine, and the one that is applicable in most breast cancer analyses.

The quantitative effect of an interaction in two groups of patients with a different underlying risk of recurrence can be illustrated by a comparison of the two simple trials shown in Table 1. Patients in the second of these trials were clearly at a lower risk of recurrence: Only 6 of the 100 treated patients and 8 of the 100 control patients died in 5 years. This resulted in 94% and 92% survival rates at 5 years—an absolute rate difference of 2%. The ratio or proportional difference is determined by assuming that 8 of the treated patients would have died if therapy had no benefit. Only 6 patients died. The 2 deaths prevented by treatment divided by the 8 expected deaths results in a 25% proportional or ratio difference. The proportional reduction in mortality is identical in the two trials. The absolute difference is 5 times greater in Trial 1, as shown in Table 1.

Table 5

Effect of Adjuvant Tamoxifen on Annual Odds of Recurrence or Death, by Nodal Status

N 0/− refers to patients in whom no nodes were found at the time of either node clearance or sampling. N 1-3 and N 4+ refers to the number of lymph nodes found to have histological evidence of metastases from breast cancer at the time of either node clearance or sampling.

Nodal Group	No. of Patients	Reduction ± S.D. in Annual Odds of	
		Recurrence	Death
N 0/−	12,813	27% ± 4	17% ± 5
N 1-3	6053	33% ± 4	21% ± 5
N 4+	3941	26% ± 4	16% ± 5
Test For Trend		p > 0.1	p > 0.1

Early Breast Cancer Trialists' Collaborative Group, 1992: Systemic treatment of early breast cancer by hormonal, cytotoxic, or immune therapy: 133 randomized trials involving 31,000 recurrences and 24,000 deaths among 75,000 women. *Lancet* 339:1-15, 71-85, 1992.

The interaction between tamoxifen therapy and risk, defined by the number of positive lymph nodes, is almost identical to that illustrated in the example (Table 5). All patients regardless of age, receptor status, or duration of therapy were included in this overview. The reduction in annual odds of recurrence and death is not significantly different for those who had no lymph node involvement; 1 to 3 positive lymph nodes, or > 3 positive lymph nodes. The *P* value from a test for trend exceeds 0.1. The absolute benefits from the use of adjuvant tamoxifen, however, were greater in node-positive than in node-negative patients (Figure 1). Thus, the proportional effect of tamoxifen is the same in all nodal subsets while the absolute benefit is greatest among those with the greatest risk.

In clinical practice, which patient is more likely to receive a prescription for adjuvant tamoxifen: a postmenopausal woman with an estrogen receptor-positive tumor and no axillary lymph nodes? Or a similar patient with eight positive lymph nodes? Figure 1 may be utilized to determine which patient is likely to derive the greatest benefit from adjuvant tamoxifen.

Few, if any, studies are large enough to allow analysis such as that shown in Table 5. Only an overview provides sufficient numbers of events and statistical power to which the method can be applied. Even in the performance of an overview, statistical power is rapidly spent when subsets of subsets are evaluated, such as analyses based on menopausal status, receptor status, plus number of involved axillary lymph nodes, for example.

OPTIMAL USE OF TAMOXIFEN: INDIRECT COMPARISONS

Dose

The overview data cited thus far have been derived from trials that used a variety of doses and durations of treatment. This is justified because the interaction between these factors and the benefits from tamoxifen are likely to be quantitative rather than qualitative. In other words, while both 2 years and 5 years of adjuvant tamoxifen therapy are likely to be beneficial, 5 years may be more beneficial than 2 years. Because of the enhanced statistical power achieved by combining both sets of trials, we can be more certain that adjuvant tamoxifen has an impact on patient survival; but an overview that combines these trials may actually underestimate tamoxifen's maximal effect when it is used optimally. Of course, the best way to determine the optimal dose or duration of tamoxifen is to conduct a randomized trial comparing two doses or two durations of therapy. Such trials have taken place and the results were published in 1996. These data, however, were not available in 1985 and 1990.

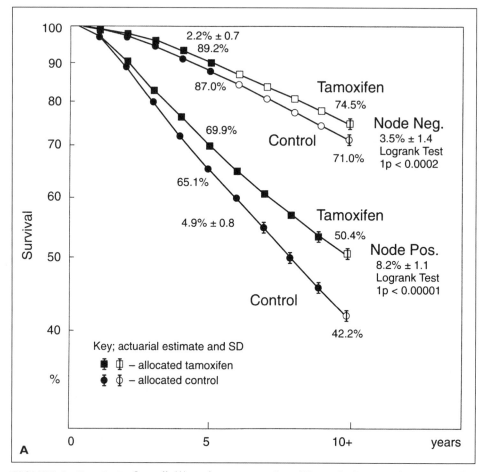

FIGURE I   Survival   Overall (A) and recurrence-free (B) survival curves from tamoxifen overviews performed among patients who were either node negative or node positive. All

When direct results from a randomized trial are unavailable, indirect comparisons may be made. For example, all of the trials that utilized 20 mg of tamoxifen per day might be compared with those that used either 30 mg or 40 mg per day. When this comparison was made for purposes of the overview, there was no discernible difference in the effect of tamoxifen, based on dose. Indirect comparisons of this type, however, are *never* as valid as direct randomized comparisons and should be interpreted with caution.

Ideally, indirect comparisons should only be used to generate hypotheses that can subsequently be evaluated in randomized clinical trials. Indirect comparisons that evaluated the optimal duration of adjuvant tamoxifen, performed in 1985 and 1990, have clearly had considerable impact on the use

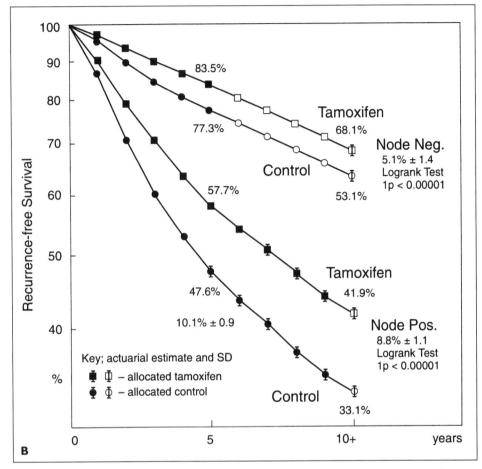

patients, regardless of age, receptor status, tamoxifen dose, or duration of tamoxifen therapy, were included in this overview. From: Early Breast Cancer Trialists' Collaborative Group.[3]

of adjuvant tamoxifen in clinical practice. (Unfortunately, warnings about the uncertainty of indirect comparisons that were included in the published reports of the Overview seem to have been largely unheeded by the medical community.)

Duration of Treatment

The first adjuvant tamoxifen trial, which was conducted by a group of Danish investigators in Copenhagen, administered the drug for 1 year.[9] Many subsequent trials also evaluated 1 year of adjuvant tamoxifen therapy. In the overview, these were grouped together as trials of "< 2 years." The first British trial, conducted by the NATO group, utilized 2 years of tamoxifen, which led to numerous similarly designed studies. These trials were grouped together in the "2-year duration of therapy" category.[11,15] A third group of trials, the first of which was the Scottish adjuvant therapy trial, utilized 5 years of therapy,[3] although one or two trials used only 3 years. These trials were grouped together and classified in an overview as "> 2 years." Practically, the overview on duration of adjuvant therapy was a comparison of trials that used 1 year, 2 years, and 5 years of adjuvant tamoxifen. At the time these overviews were conducted, no data were available from trials in which patients were treated with adjuvant tamoxifen for more than 5 years. When all of the patients were evaluated together without regard to patient age, there was an unequivocal trend towards greater benefit with greater duration of treatment (Table 6).

The optimal duration of treatment appears less certain when subsets defined by patient age were evaluated (Table 7). While significant reductions in the annual odds of recurrence and death were seen among older women with any duration of adjuvant tamoxifen, 2 years of treatment were better than 1 year. There was no evidence from these indirect comparisons that 5 years of treatment was associated with significantly better survival than 2 years.

In contrast, although no significant benefit from adjuvant tamoxifen was seen for younger women when 1 or 2 year(s) of therapy was/were given, a significant reduction in the annual odds of recurrence (43% ± 11), and a nearly

---

Table 6

Duration of Adjuvant Tamoxifen Therapy

The effects of adjuvant tamoxifen administered for 2 years, fewer than 2 years (mostly 1 year), and more than 2 years (mostly 5 years) were indirectly compared. This overview includes data on patients in all age groups and tumors from all ER categories.

Duration of Trials	Reduction ± S.D. in Annual Odds of	
	Recurrence	Death
< 2 Years	16% ± 3	11% ± 4
2 Years	28% ± 2	19% ± 3
> 2 Years	39% ± 4	24% ± 6
Test For Trend	1p < 0.00001	1p < 0.01

Early Breast Cancer Trialists' Collaborative Group, 1992: Systemic treatment of early breast cancer by hormonal, cytotoxic, or immune therapy: 133 randomized trials involving 31,000 recurrences and 24,000 deaths among 75,000 women. *Lancet* 339:1-15, 71-85, 1992.

Table 7

Duration of Adjuvant Tamoxifen Therapy, by Age

Patients were categorized as older or younger than 50 years of age and indirectly compared with respect to the effect of the duration of adjuvant tamoxifen therapy. As in Table 6, this analysis evaluated treatment for fewer than 2 years, 2 years, and more than 2 years.

Age and Trial Duration	No. of Patients	Reduction ± S.D. in Annual Odds of	
		Recurrence	Death
AGE 50+			
< 2 Years	5730	19% ± 4	13% ± 4
2 Years	10,443	33% ± 3	23% ± 3
> 2 Years	5039	38% ± 5	23% ± 6
AGE < 50			
< 2 Years	2475	5% ± 7	4% ± 8
2 Years	4789	10% ± 5	4% ± 6
> 2 Years	1254	43% ± 11	27% ± 17

Early Breast Cancer Trialists' Collaborative Group, 1992: Systemic treatment of early breast cancer by hormonal, cytotoxic, or immune therapy: 133 randomized trials involving 31,000 recurrences and 24,000 deaths among 75,000 women. *Lancet* 339:1-15, 71-85, 1992.

significant reduction in the annual odds of death (27% ± 17), were observed in the trials that utilized 5 years of tamoxifen. Once again, these comparisons in the value of tamoxifen for older vs younger women must be interpreted with caution, since the trials in older women were primarily of the type in which tamoxifen was compared with Nil; whereas those in younger women were predominantly of the type in which tamoxifen plus chemotherapy was compared with chemotherapy alone. Taken together, however, these data support an important hypothesis: The optimal duration of tamoxifen may be different for younger vs older women. Firm conclusions regarding the optimal duration of tamoxifen, therefore, should not be drawn until adequate data are available from randomized trials in each of these age groups, and ideally, from trials that compare tamoxifen with Nil.

Combining Tamoxifen With Chemotherapy

To achieve maximum statistical power, trials comparing tamoxifen to no adjuvant therapy and trials comparing tamoxifen plus chemotherapy with chemotherapy alone have been combined. Among women aged 50 and older, this combined analysis included 29,892 patients.

Reductions in the annual odds of recurrence and death were 29% ± 2 and 19% ± 2, respectively. The majority of these women (13,145) were in trials of tamoxifen vs Nil, and the reduction in the annual odds of recurrence and death were not much different than when the analysis was confined only to those randomized to tamoxifen vs Nil.

This was not true, however, for younger women. Only 8,612 women under the age of 50 were randomized in tamoxifen trials of any type; and the reductions in the annual odds of recurrence and death were 11% ± 4 and 8% ± 5, respectively. Of these women, only 2,266 participated in trials that compared tamoxifen with no adjuvant treatment. When this subset was evaluated, there was a greater benefit associated with adjuvant tamoxifen. Even then, though, the reduction in the annual odds of death (17% ± 10) among women aged 50 and younger did not reach levels usually considered statistically significant.

However, the 1992 trials, in which a combination of tamoxifen plus chemotherapy was compared with tamoxifen alone in women over the age of 50,

Table 8

Tamoxifen Vs Nil; Tamoxifen Plus Chemotherapy Vs Tamoxifen Or Chemotherapy by Age: Effect on Recurrence and Mortality

Direct comparisons of the overview comparing tamoxifen vs no adjuvant therapy of any type (Nil) and indirect comparison of the overviews of trials in which patients were randomized to a combination of tamoxifen plus chemotherapy vs tamoxifen alone or chemotherapy alone, analyzed by age. Too few data were collected on women younger than 50 in the tamoxifen vs chemotherapy trials. These results are included in parentheses. All patients were included regardless of estrogen receptor status, dose of tamoxifen, or duration of treatment.

Tamoxifen Vs Nil	No. of Patients	Reduction ± S.D. in Annual Odds of	
		Recurrence	Death
AGE < 50	2,266	27% ± 7	17% ± 10
AGE 50+	13,145	30% ± 2	19% ± 3

Tamoxifen Plus Chemotherapy Vs Tamoxifen or Chemotherapy

AGE < 50			
Tamoxifen Alone	383	(32% ± 16)	(−6% ± 23)
Chemotherapy Alone	6386	7% ± 4	3% ± 5
AGE 50+			
Tamoxifen Alone	3930	26% ± 5	10% ± 7
Chemotherapy Alone	8099	28% ± 3	20% ± 4

Early Breast Cancer Trialists' Collaborative Group, 1992: Systemic treatment of early breast cancer by hormonal, cytotoxic, or immune therapy: 133 randomized trials involving 31,000 recurrences and 24,000 deaths among 75,000 women. *Lancet* 339:1-15, 71-85, 1992.

demonstrated a highly significant reduction in the annual odds of recurrence (26% ± 5). The reduction in the annual odds of death (10% ± 7), however, did not reach levels that could be considered statistically significant (Table 8). Of course, there was a highly significant benefit from adding tamoxifen to chemotherapy. This is not surprising, since tamoxifen alone was superior to chemotherapy alone in this age group.

Worldwide, by 1985, only 386 women under age 50 had participated in randomized trials comparing tamoxifen plus chemotherapy with tamoxifen alone. This was too small a sample size to generate any meaningful results, however, and thus in Table 8, the data for these patients are shown in parentheses.

In the more than 6,000 women under age 50 who participated in trials that evaluated the value of adding tamoxifen to chemotherapy, tamoxifen added nothing in terms of either recurrence rate or overall survival (Table 8). Taken together, the early overview shows very little, if any, advantage for combining tamoxifen and chemotherapy in either age group, especially if the outcome of greatest interest is patient survival.

ADDITIONAL BENEFITS OF ADJUVANT TAMOXIFEN

Nonbreast Cancer Mortality

Although always referred to as an "antiestrogen," tamoxifen is really an attenuated estrogen. Tamoxifen has been shown, for example, to exert estrogenic effects on the uterus in some animal species, and it is well established that tamoxifen can reduce cholesterol levels in humans. Evaluating these effects in breast cancer patients, however, is difficult. For example, it is difficult to determine the effect of tamoxifen on cardiovascular mortality because the vast majority of patients—especially those who are node positive and make up the bulk of the early adjuvant studies—die of breast cancer before cardiovascular disease becomes an important risk in their lives. As more patients with a lower risk are treated with adjuvant tamoxifen, however, the issue of cardiovascular disease will become more important.

Similarly, the effects of tamoxifen on the incidence of uterine cancer are being studied. Nonetheless, even a 25-fold increase in uterine cancer mortality or incidence among patients using tamoxifen would still yield a small number in absolute terms. Meta-analysis may be potentially enlightening with regard to both the cardiovascular and uterine effects of tamoxifen, but the 1990 Overview confined itself to questions related to nonbreast cancer mortality and cardiovascular mortality. Endometrial cancer was not specifically addressed.

Table 9

Mortality from Causes Other Than Breast Cancer: Adjuvant Tamoxifen Vs Adjuvant Chemotherapy

Deaths from causes other than breast cancer (ie, myocardial infarction, stroke) among all patients who participated in adjuvant tamoxifen and chemotherapy trials were compared. All trials and patient subsets were included. Control group patients in the tamoxifen overview did not receive tamoxifen, whereas those in the chemotherapy trials did not receive chemotherapy but may have received tamoxifen. A total of 990 non-breast cancer related deaths were reported in the paper. p = 0.05. More deaths were reported for chemotherapy as well.

	Treatment	
	Tamoxifen	**Chemotherapy**
Number of deaths observed: T/C	429/450	154/137
% Reduction in NON-Breast Cancer Mortality	12% ± 6	–4% ± 12
p Value	0.05	NS

Early Breast Cancer Trialists' Collaborative Group, 1992: Systemic treatment of early breast cancer by hormonal, cytotoxic, or immune therapy: 133 randomized trials involving 31,000 recurrences and 24,000 deaths among 75,000 women. *Lancet* 339:1-15, 71-85, 1992.

NS = not significant, T = treatment group, C = control group.

Among the 29,892 patients included in the tamoxifen overviews, only 429 of those treated with tamoxifen and 450 of those randomized to the non-tamoxifen trial arms died of any cause other than breast cancer. The number dying of causes other than breast cancer in the chemotherapy trials was even smaller (Table 9), which probably reflects the tendency to place higher-risk patients on chemotherapy trials rather than tamoxifen trials. A statistically significant reduction in nonbreast cancer mortality was seen in the tamoxifen trials but not in the chemotherapy trials (Table 9). The reduction in mortality from vascular deaths (myocardial infarction and stroke) was more impressive: 25% ± 13 ($P = 0.06$). These data provide compelling evidence that tamoxifen has an estrogenic effect on cardiovascular mortality. This type of significant finding could not be demonstrated with a similar level of certainty by any single study.

Reduction in Contralateral Breast Cancer Incidence

When all of the tamoxifen trials were analyzed together, only 121 new cases of breast cancer in the contralateral breast occurred in women receiving adjuvant tamoxifen, compared with 184 contralateral breast cancers in

Table 10

Incidence of Contralateral Breast Cancer: Adjuvant Tamoxifen Vs Adjuvant Chemotherapy

The incidence of new breast cancers in the contralateral breast was assessed and compared among all patients in all adjuvant tamoxifen and chemotherapy trials. Control group patients in the tamoxifen trials did not receive tamoxifen, whereas those in the chemotherapy trials did not receive chemotherapy but may have received tamoxifen.

	Treatment	
	Tamoxifen	Chemotherapy
Number of contralateral breast cancers observed: T/C	122/184	40/42
% Reduction in incidence	39% ± 9	18% ± 20
p Value	< 0.00001	NS
% Reduction in incidence with durations of:		
< 2 Years	26% ± 21	—
2 Years	37% ± 13	—
> 2 Years	54% ± 16	—

Early Breast Cancer Trialists' Collaborative Group, 1992: Systemic treatment of early breast cancer by hormonal, cytotoxic, or immune therapy: 133 randomized trials involving 31,000 recurrences and 24,000 deaths among 75,000 women. *Lancet* 339:1-15, 71-85, 1992.

NS = not significant, T = treatment group, C = control group.

those randomized to no tamoxifen. This represents a 39% reduction in the incidence of contralateral breast cancer (Table 10). In addition, by the time of the 1990 Overview, it was evident that longer durations of tamoxifen treatment were associated with even greater reductions in incidence.

In contrast, a similar analysis of the chemotherapy trials revealed no reduction in the incidence of contralateral breast cancer. Unfortunately, the number of events was still too small at the time of the 1990 Overview to evaluate this outcome measure separately for subsets of younger and older women. Finally, it will never be possible to determine from this overview whether this reduced mortality *from the second breast cancer*. That would only be possible with a very large (> 20,000 person) randomized trial in which tamoxifen is used to prevent breast cancer in women at high risk (see Chapter 17).

Conclusions

Overviews of the early adjuvant tamoxifen trials have provided important insights regarding the benefits of this modality and its appropriate place in the cancer specialist's armamentarium. Prior to the overviews, many experts seriously doubted whether adjuvant tamoxifen could prolong the survival of any group of patients. Thanks to sophisticated overview techniques, however, it is now clear that adjuvant tamoxifen has a substantially greater impact on the survival of postmenopausal women and about the same impact on the survival of premenopausal women with receptor-positive tumors as that seen with chemotherapy. Findings such as these have a profound impact on the practice of oncology, as well as calling into question fundamental assumptions about the relative effects of chemotherapy vs endocrine therapy. These data suggest, for instance, that there may be very little difference in the cytostatic and/or cytocidal potential of these two modalities, indicating that the magnitude of their tumor cell kill is about the same.

Effects of adjuvant tamoxifen in postmenopausal women continue to be substantial and greater than those associated with chemotherapy.

The decision to initiate tamoxifen prevention trials in both the United States and Europe was predicated, in large measure, by evidence provided by the overviews that non-breast cancer mortality and the frequency of contralateral breast cancers might be reduced with adjuvant tamoxifen. The fact that the absolute increase in endometrial carcinoma is trivial should be reassuring to most patients and physicians. No other source of information regarding such risk would be considered quite as solid as the tamoxifen overview.

At the same time, the failure of the overview to show an advantage for adding tamoxifen to chemotherapy in premenopausal women demonstrates how these types of analyses can be used to avoid relatively ineffective treatments. ■

References

1. Early Breast Cancer Trialists' Collaborative Group: A systemic overview of all available randomized trials in early breast cancer of adjuvant endocrine and cytotoxic therapy. *Treatment of Early Breast Cancer, Volume 1: Worldwide Evidence 1985-1990,* p 207. Oxford, Oxford University Press, 1990.

2. Early Breast Cancer Trialists' Collaborative Group: The effects of adjuvant tamoxifen and of cytotoxic therapy on mortality in early breast cancer: An overview of 61 randomized trials among 28,896 women. *N Engl J Med* 319:1681-1692, 1988.

3. Early Breast Cancer Trialists' Collaborative Group, 1992: Systemic treatment of early breast cancer by hormonal, cytotoxic, or immune therapy: 133 randomised trials involving 31,000 recurrences and 24,000 deaths among 75,000 women. *Lancet* 339(8784):1-15; 339(8785):71-85,1992.

4. Valagussa P, Bonadonna G, Veronesi U: Patterns of relapse and survival in operable breast carcinoma with positive and negative axillary nodes. *Tumor* 64:241-258, 1978.

5. Bonadonna G, Valagussa P, Rossi A, et al: Are surgical adjuvant trials altering the course of breast cancer? *Semin Oncol* 5:450-464, 1978.

6. Bonadonna G, Rossi A, Valagussa P, et al: The CMF program for operable breast cancer with positive axillary nodes: Updated analysis on the disease-free interval, site of relapse, and drug tolerance. *Cancer* 39:2904-2915, 1977.

7. Fisher B: Adjuvant chemotherapy in breast cancer. *Int J Radiat Oncol Biol Phys* 4:295-298, 1978.

8. National Institutes of Health Consensus-Development Statement: Adjuvant chemotherapy of breast cancer. *N Engl J Med* 303:831-832, 1980.

9. Palshof T, Mouridsen HT, Daehnfeldt JL: Adjuvant endocrine therapy of primary operable breast cancer: Report on the Copenhagen breast cancer trials, in Mouridsen HT, Palshof T (eds): *Breast Cancer—Experimental and Clinical Aspects*, pp 183-187. Oxford, Pergamon, 1980.

10. Henderson IC, Canellos GP: Cancer of the breast: The past decade. *N Engl J Med* 302(1):17-30; 302(2):78-90, 1980.

11. Baum M, Brinkley DM, Dossett JA, et al: Controlled trial of tamoxifen as adjuvant agent in management of early breast cancer. *Lancet* 1:257-260, 1983.

12. Consensus Development Conference Report: Adjuvant chemotherapy for breast cancer. *J Am Med Assoc* 254:3461-3463, 1985.

13. Gelber RD, Goldhirsch A: The concept of an overview of cancer clinical trials with special emphasis on early breast cancer. *J Clin Oncol* 4:1696-1703, 1986.

14. Henderson IC: Endocrine therapy of metastatic breast cancer, in Harris JR, Hellman S, Henderson IC, et al (eds): *Breast Diseases, Second Edition*, pp 559-603. Philadelphia, J.B. Lippincott, 1991.

15. Baum M, Brinkley DM, Dossett JA, et al: Improved survival amongst patients treated with adjuvant tamoxifen after mastectomy for early breast cancer. *Lancet* 2:450, 1983.

16. Henderson IC: Adjuvant systemic therapy for early breast cancer. *Cancer* 47:401-409, 1994.

Chapter 5

Tamoxifen for Early Breast Cancer—1998

V. Craig Jordan, PhD, DSc

In the 1970s, three laboratory observations emerged that merited evaluation in clinical trial: 1) Tamoxifen blocks estrogen binding to the estrogen receptor (ER), meaning patients with ER-positive disease might be more likely to respond than those with ER-negative disease.[1,2] 2) Tamoxifen prevents mammary cancer in rats,[3,4] meaning the drug might prevent primary breast cancer, and 3) Longer adjuvant therapy with tamoxifen should be superior to short-term adjuvant therapy,[5] ie, 5 years of tamoxifen should be superior to 1 year of tamoxifen.

By the late 1980s, tamoxifen was shown in the laboratory to block estrogen-stimulated breast tumor growth, but to encourage the growth of human endometrial cancer implanted in the same athymic mouse.[6,7] The clinical question, therefore, became: "Are patients who are receiving long-term adjuvant tamoxifen therapy at risk for an increased incidence of endometrial cancer?"[7]

It is now possible to answer all four laboratory questions based on the worldwide evidence from the randomized clinical trials. Dr. I. Craig Henderson describes the methodology and evolution of the analytical technique in Chapter 4. The 1998 Oxford Overview Analysis[8] included any randomized trial that was started before 1990. The analysis included 55 trials of adjuvant tamoxifen vs no tamoxifen before recurrence. The study population was 37,000 women, thus comprising 87% of world evidence. Of these women, less than 8,000 had a very low or zero level of ER, and 18,000 were classified as ER positive. The ER status of the nearly 12,000 remaining women was unknown; it is estimated, however, that two thirds would be ER positive.

The published clinical trial database[8] can now be used to answer the questions posed by laboratory results and hypotheses. The process of evaluating the impact of translational research is important to establish what works and what does not. Indeed, it is the fundamental criterion of all effective clinical research that a clinical trial not be started without a strong hypothesis and the incorporation of the relevant scientific results. For convenience, the discussion in this chapter will be subdivided. The reader should appreciate, however, that the end points of duration of tamoxifen, menopausal status, and ER status interact so that the size of an effect can change independently. The reader should consult the original publication[8] for the description of the statistical analysis and the actual clinical trials used in the Oxford Overview Analysis process.

ER Status and the Duration of Tamoxifen

The analysis determined that the ER status of the patient was highly predictive of a treatment response to long-term tamoxifen therapy. The treatment effect based on receptor status is summarized in Table 1. The recurrence reductions produced by tamoxifen in ER-positive patients are all highly significant ($2P < 0.00001$); the trend between them is also highly significant ($\chi^2 = 45.5$, $2P < 0.00001$). By contrast, the effect on ER-negative patients was minimal. Additionally, the questions could be asked: "Does *more* ER give a better response to tamoxifen?" and "Does an additional progesterone receptor (PgR) assay help the results?" In the trials of about 5 years of tamoxifen, the proportional reductions of recurrence were $43 \pm 5\%$ and $60 \pm 6\%$ for trials with patients below or above 100 femtomoles/milligram cytosol protein. This translated to a reduction in mortality of $23 \pm 6\%$ and $36 \pm 7\%$, respectively. Clearly, one can conclude the ER is a powerful predictor of tamoxifen response—a conclusion consistent with a proven mechanism of action as an estrogen antagonist in breast cancer.[9] Concerning the PgR measurement, there was little additional value if the tumor was already ER positive.

Table 1

A comparison of the proportional risk reduction produced by adjuvant tamoxifen therapy, based on ER status. Nearly 8,000 patients are ER poor; 18,000 patients are ER positive.

a) Estrogen Receptor Poor	Duration of tamoxifen in years		
	1	2	5
Percent reduction in recurrence rates (± SD)	6 ± 8	13 ± 5	6 ± 11
Percent reduction in death rates (± SD)	6 ± 8	7 ± 5	-3 ± 11

b) Estrogen Receptor Positive	Duration of tamoxifen in years		
	1	2	5
Percent reduction in recurrence rates (± SD)	21 ± 5	28 ± 3	50 ± 4
Percent reduction in death rates (± SD)	14 ± 5	18 ± 4	28 ± 5

A comparison of inter-actions is shown in Table 2. Among the 2,000 women who had ER-negative and PgR-negative tumors, tamoxifen had no appar-ent effect on either the recurrence rates or mor-tality rates. The numbers were too few (602 women) to allow a meaningful pre-diction of the benefits of tamoxifen in patients who had an ER-negative but PgR-positive tumor.

Table 2

A comparison of the proportional risk reduction produced by adjuvant tamoxifen therapy, based on PgR status in populations of ER-positive patients.

	ER + PgR - (n = 2000)	ER + PgR + (n = 7000)
Percent reduction in recurrence rates (± SD)	32 ± 6	37 ± 3
Percent reduction in death rates (± SD)	18 ± 7	16 ± 4

The data from the Overview Analysis are also unequivocal proof of the laboratory principle that longer tamoxifen adjuvant tamoxifen therapy pro-vides more benefit. The strategy of a long duration of therapy is extremely important for the ER-positive, premenopausal woman whose large quantity of estrogen might rapidly reverse the effect of short-term tamoxifen treatment. The effect of the duration of tamoxifen treatment on the reduction of recur-rence rates and the reduction of death rates for estrogen receptor-positive premenopausal patients is shown in Figure 1. The duration of tamoxifen is clearly critical for the premenopausal patient, as an effect is virtually nonex-istent with 1 year of treatment compared with the clearcut benefit of 5 years of treatment. It is also important to point out that the reduction of death rates in women treated with 5 years of tamoxifen under 50 years of age and over 60 years of age is identical—at approximately 33%.

Table 3

Proportional risk reductions in 60- to 69-year-old women, when known ER-poor patients are excluded. The duration of tamoxifen is 1, 2, or 5 years.

	Duration of tamoxifen in years		
	1	2	5
Percent reduction in recurrence rates (± SD)	26 ± 6	33 ± 4	54 ± 5
Percent reduction in death rates (± SD)	12 ± 6	12 ± 5	33 ± 6

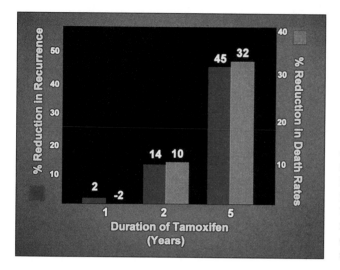

FIGURE 1 The relationship between the duration of adjuvant tamoxifen therapy in ER-positive, premenopausal patients and reduction in recurrence and death rate. Longer duration has a dramatic effect on patient survival. Adapted from [8].

By contrast, the effect of tamoxifen duration on women over the age of 60 is less dramatic because 1 year of tamoxifen is much more effective in postmenopausal women. These data are illustrated in Table 3; when tamoxifen's duration is increased from 1 to 5 years, its effectiveness is increased 2 to 3 times. Significantly, there is also a 20-fold increase in tamoxifen's effectiveness for premenopausal women with an increased duration of 1 to 5 years (Figure 1).

Contralateral Breast Cancer

Independent of age, tamoxifen consistently reduced the risk of contralateral breast cancer. The analysis determined that women had a proportional risk reduction that was 27 + 11% or 31 + 7% if they were below or above the age of 50, respectively. It is clear that "longer is better" for the reduction of risk for contralateral breast cancer with adjuvant tamoxifen therapy. Five years was better than 2 years which was better then 1 year of therapy with tamoxifen (Figure 2). In fact, 1 year of adjuvant tamoxifen was not significantly different from control because the standard deviation was so large ($13 \pm 13\%$) reduction compared to control).

It is interesting to note that a quarter of the women allocated to the trials were Japanese, where the annual incidence of contralateral breast cancer in controls is 2 per 1,000 compared with 6 per 1,000 elsewhere in the world. Therefore, if 5 years of tamoxifen can halve the incidence of contralateral breast cancer, then the absolute benefit for Japanese women would be 1 per 1,000 and 3 per 1,000 elsewhere for both young and old women. Finally, the proportional reduction in contralateral breast cancer appeared to be similar in

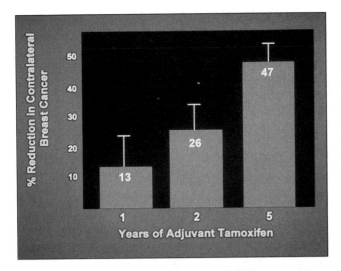

FIGURE 2 The relationship between the duration of adjuvant tamoxifen and the reduction in contralateral breast cancer. Longer duration is clearly superior; the 5-year result that produces a 47% reduction in contralateral breast cancer is equivalent to the result observed in the tamoxifen prevention trial presented in Figure 4. Adapted from [8].

women with ER-poor tumors (29 ± 15%) compared with the rest of the study population (30 ± 6%). This is an important result for the potential application of tamoxifen for the reduction of contralateral breast cancer in the woman with a primary breast cancer that is unequivocally ER negative.

Endometrial Cancer

The analysis concluded that the overall increase in the incidence of endometrial cancer was 2- to 3-fold. There was no association with dose, ie, 20 mg and 30 mg to 40 mg daily produced ratios of 2.7 and 2.4, respectively. However, there was a suggestion that 1 and 2 years of tamoxifen doubled the incidence of endometrial cancer and 5 years quadrupled incidence. Unfortunately (or fortunately from the patients' point of view!), the side effect is so rare (ie, the numbers are too small) to make firm statistical conclusions. These data are too weak to make the ratios significantly different for each duration of tamoxifen. It is, however, important to state that the absolute increase in endometrial cancer was only half as big as the absolute decrease in contralateral breast cancer.

The Overview Analysis was able to identify 3,673 women who took 5 years of adjuvant tamoxifen. There were 7 endometrial cancer deaths during 26,400 women years of follow-up before breast cancer recurrence. During the whole first decade, it was estimated the cumulative risk was 2 deaths per 1,000 women.

Conclusions

Tamoxifen has been extensively tested in clinical trials of adjuvant therapy for 20 years. The Overview showed that the proportional mortality reductions

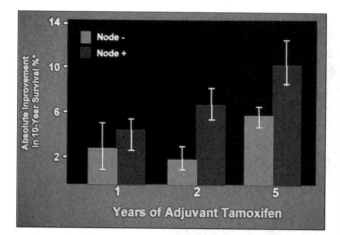

FIGURE 3 The absolute improvement in 10-year survival of node-negative and node-positive breast cancer patients with different durations of adjuvant tamoxifen. All known ER-negative patients were excluded. Adapted from [8].

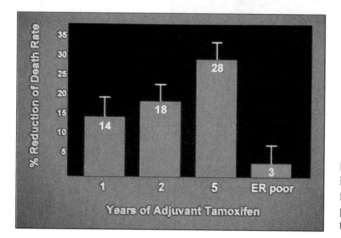

FIGURE 4 The increase in the reduction of death rate for ER-positive patients compared with ER-negative patients. Adapted from [8].

were similar for women with node-positive or node-negative disease. However, absolute reductions in mortality were much greater in node-positive than node-negative disease. This result is illustrated in Figure 3. Additionally, patients with ER-positive disease had an increased reduction in death rate with longer duration of tamoxifen treatment, whereas ER-negative patients did not (Figure 4).

The value of a long duration of treatment is most important for the premenopausal patient (Figure 1). This latter finding is new, as the results for premenopausal women could not be made with certainty in earlier overviews (see Chapter 4). There is now much more secure data on premenopausal women.

Clearly, the Oxford Overview Analysis has established the veracity of the laboratory concepts that tamoxifen would be most effective in ER-positive disease, longer duration would be more beneficial, and tamoxifen would prevent primary breast cancer, in this case, contralateral disease. Overall, the absolute improvement in recurrence was greater during the first 5 years following surgery; but improvement in survival increased steadily throughout the first 10 years. This is an important finding because the patient is clearly benefiting from tamoxifen despite therapy cessation. In other words, long-term benefits accrue despite the fact that therapy is not being taken. There is an accumulation of the tumoristatic/tumoricidal actions for at least the first 5 years of treatment; but the benefit continues after therapy has stopped. This is also true for the reduction in contralateral breast cancer; the breast seems to be protected so the value remains after therapy stops. This observation is extremely important for the application of tamoxifen as a preventive because a 5-year pulse of tamoxifen appears to protect a woman from breast cancer for many years afterwards (see Chapter 4).

Finally, it can be stated that the risk/benefit of tamoxifen therapy can fit strongly into the benefit category. The risk of endometrial cancer—a concept derived from laboratory studies[7]—is a concern, but the benefits clearly outweigh the risks. In contrast, early concerns about the carcinogenic potential of tamoxifen in the rat liver[10] *did not* translate to the clinic as there was no evidence from the overview analysis of an increase in either liver or colorectal cancer in patients taking tamoxifen.[8] ■

References

1. Jordan VC, Koerner S: Tamoxifen and the human carcinoma 8S oestrogen receptor. *Eur J Cancer* 11:205-206, 1975.

2. Jordan VC, Jaspan T: Tamoxifen as an antitumour agent: Oestrogen bindings as a predictive test for tumor response. *J Endocrinol* 68:453-460, 1976.

3. Jordan VC: Antitumor activity of the antioestrogen ICI 46,474 (tamoxifen) in the dimethylbenzanthracene- (DMBA) induced rat mammary carcinoma model. *J Steroid Biochem* 5:354, 1974.

4. Jordan VC: Effect of tamoxifen (ICI 46,474) on initiation and growth of DMBA-induced rat mammary carcinomata. *Eur J Cancer* 12:419-425, 1976.

5. Jordan VC, Dix CJ, Allen KE: The effectiveness of long-term treatment on a laboratory model for adjuvant therapy of breast cancer, in Salmon SE, Jones, SE (eds): *Adjuvant Therapy of Cancer II*, pp 19-24. New York, Grune and Stratton, 1979.

6. Satyaswaroop PG, Zaino RJ, Mortel R: Estrogen-like effects of tamoxifen on human endometrial carcinoma transplanted in nude mice. *Cancer Res* 44:4006-4010, 1984.

7. Gottardis MM, Robinson SP, Satyaswaroop PG, et al: Contrasting actions of tamoxifen on endometrial and breast tumor growth in the athymic mouse. *Cancer Res* 48:812-815, 1988.

8. Early Breast Cancer Trialists' Collaborative Group: Tamoxifen for early breast cancer: An overview of the randomized trials. *Lancet* 351:1451-1467, 1998.

9. MacGregor JI, Jordan VC: Basic guides to the mechanisms of antiestrogen action. *Pharm Rev* 50:1-46, 1998.

10. Greaves P, Goonetilleke R, Nunn G, et al: Two-year carcinogenicity study of tamoxifen in Alderley Park Wistar–derived rats. *Cancer Res* 53:3919-3924, 1993.

Chapter 6

Tamoxifen for Adjuvant Therapy and for the Treatment of Advanced Disease in Premenopausal Breast Cancer Patients

Peter M. Ravdin, MD, PhD
Associate Professor of Medicine/Oncology
The University of Texas Health Science Center
San Antonio, Texas

The last decade has seen a resurgence of interest in the use of endocrine therapy for breast cancer. New endocrine agents have been developed for the treatment of advanced disease, and the role of endocrine therapy in the adjuvant setting has been supported by new clinical trial evidence. An example of this increased interest in the use of endocrine therapy can be seen in the evolution of recommendations that have emerged from the St. Gallen conferences over the last decade.[1-3]

In 1988, a summary of recommendations for adjuvant therapy by the international adjuvant therapy meeting at St. Gallen (Table 1) did not identify any subgroup of premenopausal patients for whom adjuvant endocrine therapy would definitively be the standard of care. This situation radically changed by 1995, however, when endocrine therapy was included as the standard of care or worthy of clinical investigation for several subsets of premenopausal patients.

This chapter will address current views about the use of tamoxifen in premenopausal breast cancer patients.

Impact of the Adjuvant Therapy Overview Analyses

A role for tamoxifen as endocrine adjuvant therapy for premenopausal patients was not supported by the Overview analysis of 1985[4] (Table 2). Overall, the risk of death among premenopausal patients receiving adjuvant tamoxifen did not appear to be reduced. This result was not accepted as definitive, however, since some data still suggested that premenopausal patients who received adjuvant tamoxifen without receiving additional adju-

Table 1

Changes in St. Gallen Consensus Panel Recommendations for Adjuvant Therapy in Premenopausal Breast Cancer Patients

		March 1988		March 1992		March 1995	
		ER+	ER–	ER+	ER–	ER+	ER–
Axillary Node Negative	Low Risk	**None vs T**	NA	**None vs T**	NA	None vs T	NA
	Good Risk	ND	ND	**T**	NA	**T** C Ooph, LHRH-A	NA
	High Risk	**C**	**C**	**C ± T**	**C**	**C ± T** Ooph LHRH-A	**C**
Axillary Node Positive	Any	**C**	**C**	**C ± T**	**C**	**C ± T** **Ooph** ± T LHRH-A	**C**

Bold entries are treatments accepted for routine use or baseline in clinical trials.

ER = estrogen receptor, T = tamoxifen, C = polychemotherapy, Ooph = oophorectomy or ovarian ablation, LHRH-A = gonadotropin-releasing hormone analogue, NA = not applicable, ND = not defined.

Table 2

Proportional Risk Reductions in Overall Mortality Afforded by Adjuvant Tamoxifen – 1985

Subgroup	Patient Age	Number of Patients	% Reduction (Standard Error)
All Trials	< 50	3,418	–1% (8)
	≥ 50	10,465	**20% (3)**
No Concurrent Chemotherapy	< 50	NG	21% (14)
	≥ 50	NG	**19% (4)**
With Concurrent Chemotherapy	< 50	NG	–9% (9)
	≥ 50	NG	**22% (6)**

Data from the 1985 Overview Analysis.

Bold entries are statistically significant.

NG = not given.

Table 3

**Proportional Risk Reductions in Overall Mortality
Afforded by Adjuvant Tamoxifen – 1990**

Subgroup	Patient Age	Number of Patients	% Reduction (Standard Error)
All Trials	< 50	8,612	6% (5)
	≥ 50	21,280	**20% (2)**
No Concurrent Chemotherapy	< 50	2,226	17% (10)
	≥ 50	13,145	**19% (3)**
With Concurrent Chemotherapy	< 50	6,386	3% (5)
	≥ 50	8,135	**20% (4)**

Data from the 1990 Overview Analysis.
Bold entries are statistically significant.

vant chemotherapy did indeed derive benefit. Another recognized important limitation of this early overview was that most patients had received fewer than 2 years of adjuvant tamoxifen treatment.

The second overview analysis in 1990[5] was somewhat more supportive of a role for adjuvant tamoxifen (Table 3). Again, premenopausal patients in unselected trials did not experience a net benefit with adjuvant tamoxifen therapy. In trials not confounded by the addition of chemotherapy, however, a trend for benefit with adjuvant tamoxifen was again noted. Although this trend did not reach statistical significance for survival, it was statistically significant for reducing risk of recurrence. Again, most of these patients were treated for 2 years or less with adjuvant tamoxifen. The notion that this duration of treatment might have been suboptimal was suggested by an analysis (Table 4) that indicated that the duration of adjuvant tamoxifen appeared to be important.

Oophorectomy Trials

A second line of evidence that appeared in the 1990 Overview supporting the efficacy of prolonged endocrine therapy in premenopausal patients was the unexpected degree of benefit associated with oophorectomy. Individually, these relatively small trials had not appeared to strongly support the efficacy of adjuvant oophorectomy. Such trials were small by their very nature and were designed to detect only very large effects. Nevertheless, when analyzed together in the meta-analysis, it became evident that the proportional risk

Table 4

Effect of Duration of Adjuvant Tamoxifen Treatment on the Proportional Risk Reductions in Overall Mortality

Subgroup	Patient Age	Number of Patients	% Reduction (Standard Error)
Tamoxifen ≤ I Year	< 50	2,478	4% (8)
	≥ 50	5,735	**13% (4)**
Tamoxifen 2 Years	< 50	4,794	4% (6)
	≥ 50	10,496	**23% (3)**
Tamoxifen > 2 Years	< 50	1,311	27% (17)
	≥ 50	5,087	**23% (6)**

Data from the 1990 Overview Analysis.
Bold entries are statistically significant.

reduction afforded by oophorectomy in women younger than 50 years old was 30% for recurrence and 28% for death. This benefit was comparable to the 36% and 24% risk reductions for recurrence and death, respectively, that could be achieved by polychemotherapy in this group. This result was made all the more provocative by the fact that the oophorectomy trials were carried out in an era in which the estrogen-receptor (ER) status of patients was not routinely assessed. These trials could be expected to have included, therefore, substantial numbers of patients who probably could not benefit from therapy. Using estrogen-receptor status to select patients for these trials might have resulted in even higher proportional risk reductions.

Scottish investigators reported just such a result in a trial comparing adjuvant cyclophosphamide with methotrexate, and fluorouracil (CMF) to ovarian ablation.[6] Although the two arms in that Scottish trial had the same overall efficacy, a subset analysis showed that oophorectomy was the superior treatment for ER-positive patients, whereas CMF polychemotherapy was superior for ER-negative patients.

The 1985 and 1990 Overview analyses of adjuvant trials thus show that endocrine therapy may have an important role in the adjuvant treatment of breast cancer in premenopausal women.

Duration of Therapy

The significance of the duration of tamoxifen treatment is supported by the excellent efficacy of oophorectomy, which, by its very nature, is a

Table 5

Proportional Risk Reductions in Overall Mortality Afforded by Adjuvant Oophorectomy

Subgroup	Patient Age	Number of Patients	% Reduction (Standard Error)
All Trials	< 50	1,817	**25% (7)**
No Concurrent Chemotherapy	< 50	878	**28% (9)**
With Concurrent Chemotherapy	< 50	939	19% (11)

Data from the 1990 Overview Analysis.

Bold entries are statistically significant.

prolonged endocrine therapy. Nevertheless, the numbers of premenopausal women who received more than 2 years of tamoxifen as adjuvant endocrine therapy were too small to define with narrow confidence, thus limiting the proportional risk reduction afforded by such therapy. Unfortunately, some of the most important studies addressing this issue included mostly, or only, postmenopausal patients, leaving the question of optimal duration of tamoxifen use in premenopausal patients largely unanswered. The 2 vs 5 years of adjuvant tamoxifen trial conducted by the Swedish Breast Cancer Cooperative Group, for example (which showed a significantly improved efficacy of 5 years of tamoxifen over 2 years), did not include premenopausal patients.[7] Likewise, the NSABP trial comparing 5 vs 10 years of adjuvant tamoxifen included primarily postmenopausal patients, and to date, has not been analyzed by menopausal status.[8]

Confounding Effects of Adjuvant Chemotherapy

Another important issue in the adjuvant use of tamoxifen is whether the effects of the drug are less evident in patients who also receive adjuvant chemotherapy. The overview analyses from tamoxifen and oophorectomy trials suggest that this may indeed be the case in premenopausal patients. Therefore, combined chemoendocrine therapy would not seem to be a preferred approach for premenopausal patients. This simple conclusion, while perhaps true overall, may depend on the type of chemotherapy given, the duration of tamoxifen, and selection of patients. Some of the ongoing clinical trials may further clarify this issue. However, the recent NSABP trial of tamoxifen and chemotherapy in ER-positive women showed a greater benefit for adding chemotherapy in premenopausal patients.[9]

Therapies for Low-Risk Patients

The value and limitations of adjuvant tamoxifen were suggested by the Intergroup adjuvant therapy trial for low-risk, ER-positive, premenopausal women, which randomized women to tamoxifen alone or tamoxifen plus oophorectomy. Given that this population had an excellent prognosis (most were cured by surgery), the average potential benefit from any therapy, in terms of increased average life expectancy, was expected to be modest. Therefore, only a low-toxicity regimen, such as an endocrine therapy, was justified. However, in situations where the patient has a high risk of recurrence and death, current proportional risk reductions of < 50% are clearly very unsatisfactory, and more aggressive, even toxic, approaches are justified. This is why most ongoing clinical trials for patients at high risk for recurrence are focused on new treatment modalities and new chemotherapeutic regimens, and not on what are expected to be only modest improvements with endocrine therapy.

Tamoxifen in the Treatment of Metastatic Disease in Premenopausal Women

One of the early concerns about the use of tamoxifen was that it might act on the hypothalamus and pituitary to block the negative feedback regulation of estrogens, which could result in supra-physiologic levels of estradiol. These high levels of estradiol might, in turn, overcome the antiestrogenic effects of tamoxifen. Indeed, supra-physiologic levels of estradiol have been noted in normal women taking tamoxifen,[10] and in breast cancer patients during and after adjuvant therapy.[11] Total estrogen levels can rise to 2 to 5 times those that normally occur in nonpregnant premenopausal women. Because tamoxifen is thought to exert much, if not all, of its antineoplastic effect by reversible binding to the estrogen receptor, there is obvious reason for concern about whether high levels of estradiol might interfere with its action.

There has been conflicting evidence about whether tamoxifen is less effective in premenopausal patients with metastatic breast cancer than in postmenopausal patients. In a large cooperative group trial examining predictors of response to tamoxifen in patients with ER-positive metastatic breast cancer (SWOG 8228), response rates were significantly lower in premenopausal women (24%) compared with postmenopausal women (57%).[12] Multivariate analysis in that trial showed that premenopausal status was an independent predictor of lower response rate, shortened time to treatment failure, and lower objective response rate. This trial, which included 342 patients, was the largest prospective study to address predictors of response to tamoxifen. Nevertheless, since only 37 of those patients were premenopausal, and the confidence interval for response rate to tamoxifen was quite broad, the authors felt that their conclusion—namely, that response rates to tamoxifen were lower in premenopausal patients—needed independent validation.

Overall, tamoxifen is an effective agent for the treatment of patients with ER-positive metastatic breast cancer.

Tamoxifen and oophorectomy were associated with similar response rates (24% and 21%, respectively) in a trial randomizing 122 premenopausal patients to tamoxifen or surgical oophorectomy,[13] with no significant differences in time to treatment failure or overall survival. This finding in itself would seem to argue against the idea that tamoxifen is an inferior endocrine therapy in premenopausal women. A similar study of 53 patients randomized to tamoxifen or surgical oophorectomy also found no significant differences in response rate or survival between the two arms.[14]

If the elevated estradiol levels seen in premenopausal women treated with tamoxifen blocked or interfered with the drug's benefits, then one might expect an ovarian ablative regimen to be particularly effective in combination with tamoxifen. The concept of inducing total endocrine blockade by combining oophorectomy or an ovarian ablating treatment with tamoxifen is an interesting one. In general, however, studies have not shown major improvements in efficacy with such an approach.[15] Indeed, results of randomized trials suggest that no major benefit can be gained by adding tamoxifen to an ovarian ablation over that which can be achieved with ovarian ablation alone.[16,17]

Overall, tamoxifen is an effective agent for the treatment of patients with ER-positive metastatic breast cancer. There is conflicting evidence as to whether tamoxifen is somewhat less effective in premenopausal women than in postmenopausal women, but if such a difference exists, it is relatively modest. Therefore, before cytotoxic therapy is initiated in an ER-positive premenopausal woman with metastatic disease, a trial of an endocrine therapy, such as tamoxifen, is nearly always indicated.

Safety of Tamoxifen in Premenopausal Women

In general, the side effects of tamoxifen are tolerated as well by premenopausal women as by postmenopausal women. Some of the best data in this regard (unconfounded by events due to cancer) emerged from the Royal Marsden Hospital pilot tamoxifen chemoprevention trial. These investigators reported that, relative to placebo, tamoxifen was associated with increased rates of hot flashes (36% vs 17%), vaginal discharge (13% vs 3%), and menstrual irregularities (22% vs 13%), but was not associated with increased rates of nausea, headache, or mood change in premenopausal women.[18]

Special considerations may be necessary when using tamoxifen in premenopausal women. For example, ultrasonographic studies have suggested than many premenopausal women develop ovarian cysts while on tamoxifen.[18,19] However, these cysts are generally asymptomatic, many are not clinically detected, and they often resolve after cessation of tamoxifen therapy.[20] Long-term use of tamoxifen by premenopausal women also seems to be associated with an increased incidence of uterine fibroids,[18] but again, these rarely become clinically significant.

In contrast, some of the beneficial effects of tamoxifen may be less apparent in premenopausal women. For example, the presumably favorable effects of tamoxifen on serum lipids are more pronounced in postmenopausal women than in premenopausal women.[20] Also, although the use of tamoxifen seems to be associated with increased bone mineral density in postmenopausal women, paradoxically, it is associated with a *loss* of bone mineral density in premenopausal women.[21]

Overall, however, tamoxifen is well tolerated by premenopausal women, with few patients developing toxicities that would require therapy cessation.*

Summary

Tamoxifen is the best single agent for the treatment of breast cancer in premenopausal women who are likely to be responsive to endocrine therapy. It has a favorable toxicity profile, as well as high levels of activity in selected subsets of patients, both in the adjuvant setting and in the setting of metastatic disease. Its use may be optimized further by ongoing clinical and basic research designed to answer questions about which patients are likely to respond, what is the optimal duration of treatment, how to optimize use of tamoxifen in combination with chemotherapy in the adjuvant setting, and how to delay or prevent the onset of clinical drug resistance. ∎

*Editor's note: See Chapter 5 for additional information about adjuvant therapy in premenopausal patients. See Chapter 16 for a comparison of toxicities in well women who are pre- or postmenopausal.

References

1. Glick JH: Meeting highlights: Adjuvant therapy for breast cancer. *J Natl Cancer Inst* 80:471-475, 1988.

2. Glick JH, Gelber RD, Goldhirsch A: Meeting highlights: Adjuvant therapy for primary breast cancer. *J Natl Cancer Inst* 84(19):1479-1485, 1992.

3. Goldhirsch A, Wood WC, Senn HJ: Meeting highlights: International consensus panel on the treatment of primary breast cancer. *J Natl Cancer Inst* 87(19):1441-1445, 1995.

4. Early Breast Cancer Trialists' Collaborative Group: Effects of adjuvant tamoxifen and of cytotoxic therapy in early breast cancer: An overview of 61 randomized trials among 28,896 women. *N Engl J Med* 319:1681-1692, 1988.

5. Early Breast Cancer Trialists' Collaborative Group: Systemic treatment of early breast cancer by hormonal, cytotoxic, or immune therapy. *Lancet* 339:1-15, 71-85, 1992.

6. Anonymous: Adjuvant ovarian ablation versus CMF chemotherapy in premenopausal women with pathological stage II breast carcinoma: The Scottish trial. *Lancet* 341(8856):1293-1298, 1993.

7. Swedish Breast Cancer Cooperative Group: Randomized trial of 2 versus 5 years of adjuvant tamoxifen in postmenopausal early-stage breast cancer. *J Natl Cancer Inst* 88:1543-1549, 1996.

8. Fisher B, Digman J, Bryant J, et al: Five versus more than five years of tamoxifen therapy for breast cancer patients with negative lymph nodes and estrogen receptor-positive tumors. *J Natl Cancer Inst* 88:1529-1542, 1996.

9. Fisher B, Dignam J, Wolmark N, et al: Tamoxifen and chemotherapy for lymph node-negative estrogen receptor-positive breast cancer. *J Natl Cancer Inst* 89:1673-1682, 1997.

10. Groom GV, Grilliths K: Effect of the anti-oestrogen tamoxifen on plasma levels of luteinizing hormone, follicle-stimulating hormone, prolactin, oestradiol and progesterone in normal premenopausal women. *J Endocrinol* 70(3):421-428, 1976.

11. Ravdin PM, Fritz NF, Tormey DC, et al: Endocrine status of premenopausal node-positive breast cancer patients following adjuvant chemotherapy and long-term tamoxifen. *Cancer Res* 48(4):1026-1029, 1988.

12. Ravdin PM, Green S, Dorr TM, et al: Prognostic significance of progesterone receptor levels in estrogen receptor-positive patients with metastatic breast cancer treated with tamoxifen: Results of a prospective Southwest Oncology Group study. *J Clin Oncol* 10(8):1284-1291, 1992.

13. Buchanan RB, Blamey RW, Durrant KR, et al: A randomized comparison of tamoxifen with surgical oophorectomy in premenopausal patients with advanced breast cancer. *J Clin Oncol* 4(9):1326-1330, 1986.

14. Ingle JN, Krook JE, Green SJ, et al: Randomized trial of bilateral oophorectomy versus tamoxifen in premenopausal women with metastatic breast cancer. *J Clin Oncol* 4(2):178-185, 1986.

15. Buzzoni R, Biganzoli L, Bajena E, et al: Combination goserelin and tamoxifen therapy in premenopausal advanced breast cancer: A multicentre study by the ITMO group. Italian Trials in Medical Oncology. *Br J Cancer* 71(5):1111-1114, 1995.

16. Jonat W, Kaufmann M, Blamey RW, et al: A randomised study to compare the effect of the luteinising hormone releasing hormone (LHRH) analogue goserelin with or without tamoxifen in pre- and perimenopausal patients with advanced breast cancer. *Eur J Cancer* 31A(2):137-142, 1995.

17. Boccardo F, Rubagotti A, Perrotta A, et al: Ovarian ablation versus goserelin with or without tamoxifen in pre- and perimenopausal patients with advanced breast cancer: Results of a multicentric Italian study. *Ann Oncol* 5(4):337-342, 1994.

18. Powles TJ, Jones AL, Ashley SE, et al: The Royal Marsden Hospital pilot tamoxifen chemoprevention trial. *Breast Cancer Res Treat* 31(1):73-82, 1994.

19. Cohen L, Rosen DJ, Altaras M, et al: Tamoxifen treatment in premenopausal breast cancer patients may be associated with ovarian overstimulation, cystic formations and fibroid overgrowth [letter]. *Br J Cancer* 69(3):620-621, 1994.

20. Shushan A, Peretz T, Uziely B, et al: Ovarian cysts in premenopausal and postmenopausal tamoxifen-treated women with breast cancer. *Am J Obstet Gynecol* 174(1):141-144, 1996.

21. Ilanchezhian S, Thangaraju M, Sachdanandam P: Plasma lipids and lipoprotein alterations in tamoxifen-treated breast cancer women in relation to the menopausal status. *Cancer Biochem Biophys* 15(2):83-90, 1995.

22. Powles TJ, Hickish T, Kanis JA, et al: Effect of tamoxifen on bone mineral density measured by dual-energy x-ray absorptiometry in healthy premenopausal and postmenopausal women. *J Clin Oncol* 14(1):78-84, 1996.

Chapter 7

Additional Benefits of Tamoxifen for Postmenopausal Patients

Malcolm M. Bilimoria, MD
Fellow in Surgical Oncology
M. D. Anderson Cancer Center
The University of Texas
Houston, Texas

Monica Morrow, MD
Director
Lynn Sage Comprehensive Breast Program
Department of Surgery
Northwestern University Medical School
Chicago, Illinois

V. Craig Jordan, PhD, DSc

The benefits of tamoxifen therapy for patients with breast cancer have been established and confirmed. Results from the overview analyses show that postmenopausal women receive greater benefits from tamoxifen therapy with respect to disease-free and overall survival than premenopausal women.[1] In addition, tamoxifen causes a reduction in contralateral breast cancers—a finding that has led to prevention trials both in the United States and abroad. Tamoxifen has also been shown to maintain bone density and decrease morbidity and mortality from cardiac disease. These effects are a further rationale for the use of the drug in postmenopausal breast cancer patients who are not routinely given hormone replacement therapy (HRT).

A definition of the magnitude of benefit is essential in guiding physicians towards the proper duration of tamoxifen therapy. Previously, we have noted that results from several large clinical trials were needed to determine whether 5 years of therapy or longer was the best therapeutic regimen.[2] Based on the modest clinical database, we concluded that the proven length of therapy would largely depend on the amount and degree of tamoxifen resistance

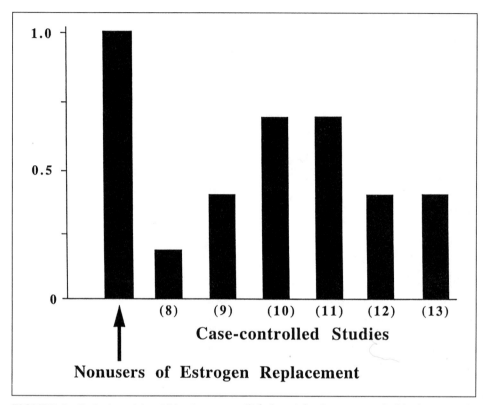

FIGURE I   Relative risk of hip fracture   Relative risk of osteoporotic hip fractures in postmenopausal women who are nonusers of estrogen replacement (relative risk 1.0), compared with the relative risk in women on estrogen replacement therapy in 6 case-controlled studies.[8-13]

within the heterogeneous clinical sample. Currently, tamoxifen trials in the United Kingdom are addressing whether 5 years of therapy or longer is the ideal treatment regimen. (These trials are discussed in detail in Chapter 11). In the meantime, each physician must weigh the benefits and risks of extending therapy beyond 5 years for each individual patient.

This chapter will highlight the degree of benefit in preserving bone density and reducing cardiac disease in women at risk that can be expected from tamoxifen therapy. In addition, we will analyze the extent of the reduction in contralateral breast cancers.

Menopause and Its Effects on Osteoporosis and Coronary Heart Disease

The majority of patients with early stage breast cancer can expect to be cured of their disease. Approximately 30% of patients with T1 and T2 node-negative disease will die as a result of their cancer, and only 10% of patients with tumors 1 cm or less in size will develop metastatic disease. Many of these women will be at risk of death from diseases associated with meno-pause, since a diagnosis of breast cancer usually prevents a woman from receiving HRT. Rosen et al[3] demonstrated that patients with node-negative tumors less than 1 cm had a greater risk of dying from cardiac disease than breast cancer between 10 and 20 years post-diagnosis.

Osteoporosis is another major source of morbidity and mortality for post-menopausal women. Women begin to lose bone mass at about age 30; however, a significant acceleration of this loss (up to 5% per year) is noted after menopause.[4] It has been estimated that women can lose up to 35% of cortical bone mass and up to 50% of trabecular bone mass over their life-time.[5] Population-based studies from the United States indicate that the lifetime risks of hip and vertebral fractures in postmenopausal, white females may be as high as 16% and 32%, respectively.[6]

Estrogen replacement therapy (ERT) has been shown to greatly reduce the degree of osteoporosis in postmenopausal women. An overview of hip fractures in current estrogen users showed that the relative risk is reduced to a range of 0.2 to 0.7 (Figure 1).[7-13] Although osteoporosis is a long-term concern for postmenopausal women after a diagnosis of breast cancer, a

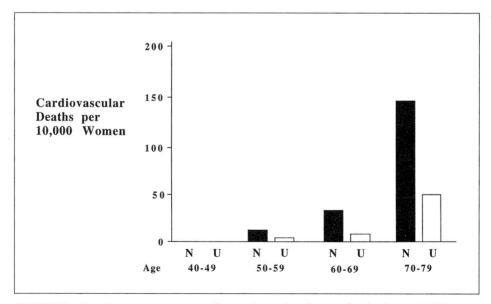

FIGURE 2 Cardiovascular deaths Comparison of cardiovascular deaths per 10,000 wom-en in nonusers (N) and users (U) of estrogen replacement therapy for four different age groups. Adapted from Bush et al: *Circulation* 75:1102-1109, 1987.

Table I

Effects of Tamoxifen on Bone Resorption

Study	Duration of Tamoxifen (Years)	Area Studied	Study Design	Control	Tamoxifen Treated Group	Statistical Significance
Gotfredsen	1	Distal radius	% change in BMC (g/cm)	−2.5%	−3.2%	NS
Fornander	2	Proximal radius	BMD (g/cm²)	1.04	.99	NS
	2	Distal radius	BMD (g/cm²)	.74	.70	NS
	5	Proximal radius	BMD (g/cm²)	1.05	1.06	NS
	5	Distal radius	BMD (g/cm²)	.74	.78	NS
Fentiman	0.5	Femur	gHA/cm²	.81	.81	NS
	0.5	Lumbar spine	gHA/cm²	.95	.94	NS
Love	2	Lumbar spine	%/year change in BMD	−1.0%	.6%	p < .0001
	2	Radius	%/year change in BMD	1.29%	.88%	NS
Cuzick	6	Lumbar spine	BMD (g/cm²)	.97	1.08	NS
	6	Trochanter	BMD (g/cm²)	.75	.81	NS
Ward	1	Lumbar spine	%/year change in BMD	−2.3%	.09%	p = .04
	1	Trochanter	%/year change in BMD	−1.8%	1.4%	p = .03
Neal	5	Lumbar spine	BMD (g/cm²)	1.028	1.059	NS
	5	Femur	BMD (g/cm²)	.838	.894	NS
Turken	1	Lumbar spine	%/year change in BMD	−2.7%	2.4%	p < .003
Kristensen	2	Lumbar spine	% change in BMD	−4.3%*	2.5%*	p = .00074
	2	Distal radius	% change in BMD	−6.3%*	−2.0%*	p = .024

Adapted from Bilimoria et al: *Cancer J Sci Amer* 2:140-150, 1996, with permission.

NS = Not statistically significant, BMC = Bone mineral content, BMD = Bone mineral density, gHA = grams of hydroxyapatite.

*Percentages extrapolated from data graphs.

more immediate problem is the risk of dying from coronary heart disease.

It is estimated that, over her lifetime, a 50-year-old white female has a 46% chance of developing coronary artery disease and a 31% chance of dying from heart disease.[7] Sullivan et al[14] found estrogen use reduced the relative risk (RR) of angiography-detected coronary artery disease to 0.44, while Bush et al[15] found decreased rates of cardiovascular death for estrogen replacement users in nearly all age groups studied (Figure 2).

Beneficial Effects of Tamoxifen on Bone

Initially, it was feared that the antiestrogenic effects of tamoxifen would actually accelerate bone resorption and increase the risk of developing osteoporosis. However, in vitro and in vivo studies have demonstrated quite the opposite. In one study, bone organ cultures pretreated with tamoxifen showed inhibition of bone absorption.[16] Ovariectomized rats treated with tamoxifen also showed a significant decrease in bone resorption compared to controls.[17]

The effects in patients on tamoxifen therapy have been equally impressive. Nine studies[2] examining the effects of tamoxifen on bone resorption are summarized in Table 1. Fornander et al[18] used a single-photon

Table 2

Effects of Tamoxifen on Lipoproteins

Study	Total Cholesterol (mg/dl)			LDL Cholesterol (mg/dl)			HDL Cholesterol (mg/dl)		
	control (# of patients)	TT (# of patients)	% change	control	TT	% change	control	TT	% change
Rossner	302(10)	258(11)	−15%	201	156	−22%	87	75	NS
Bruning	220(46)	205(46)	−7%	151	124	−18%	43	50	NS
Bertelli	254(36)	213(55)	−16%	180	127	−29%	55	56	NS
Bagdade	193(8)	204(8)	NS	122	115	−6%	45	49	NS
Love	216(70)	190(70)	−12%	138	110	−20%	57	53	NS
Ingram	259(47)	234(13)	−9%	193	171	−10%	66	61	NS
Cusick	256(47)	225(14)	−12%	186	145	−22%	50	43	−14%
Dnistria	244(13)	203(24)	−17%	169	123	−27%	55	56	NS
Thangaraju	224(45)	190(39)	−15%	149	132	−17%	54	58	7%
Saarto	237(26)	210(26)	−11%	154	122	−21%	63	60	NS
Average	249	214	**−13%**	165	134	**−19%**	57	52	NS

Adapted from Bilimoria et al. *Cancer J Sci Amer* 2:140-150, 1996, with permission.

TT = Tamoxifen treated group, NS = Not statistically significant.

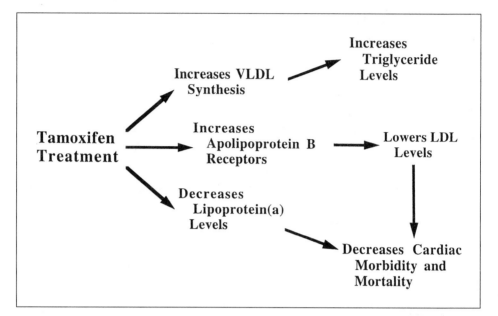

FIGURE 3   Lipoproteins   Effects of tamoxifen treatment on very low-density lipoproteins (VLDL), apoliprotein B, and lipoprotein(a).

absorptiometry technique to measure bone mineral density at the distal forearm in 75 postmenopausal breast cancer patients, and observed no increase in bone loss in patients taking tamoxifen for 2 to 5 years. Since then, several studies have utilized the more sensitive dual-photon absorptiometry technique to study tamoxifen's effects on bone density. Love et al[19] utilized this technique as part of a randomized, placebo-controlled trial of 140 postmenopausal breast cancer patients. Patients treated for 2 years with tamoxifen had a statistically significant increase in the bone mineral density of their lumbar spine when compared to patients receiving placebo. The 5-year analysis of this same study supported the maintenance of bone density by tamoxifen therapy.[20] Seven other studies on both pre- and postmenopausal patients treated with tamoxifen confirmed that bone mineral density was preserved or increased with respect to controls (Table 1). Three of these studies also noted preservation of trabecular bone at the femoral neck—a common site of postmenopausal osteoporotic fractures.

Beneficial Effects of Tamoxifen on Serum Lipids

When tamoxifen emerged as a proven therapy for breast cancer, there were genuine concerns that treating women with an antiestrogen would adversely effect their lipid profile and lead to an increased risk of heart disease. Since then, several studies have shown that, much like tamoxifen's estrogenic effects on bone, tamoxifen also has estrogenic effects on serum lipid profiles. Analysis of 9 separate studies revealed an average decrease in total cholesterol of 13% and an average decrease in low-density lipoproteins (LDL) of 19% (Table 2).[2,21]

In a randomized, double-blind study of tamoxifen vs placebo, Love et al[22] noted increased synthesis of very low-density lipoproteins (VLDL), leading to increased triglyceride levels and increased apolipoprotein B receptors, which resulted in lower LDL levels (Figure 3). Analysis at 5 years supported the maintenance of decreased LDL and total cholesterol.[23] Others have noted that tamoxifen interfered with cholesterol synthesis by inhibiting the conver-

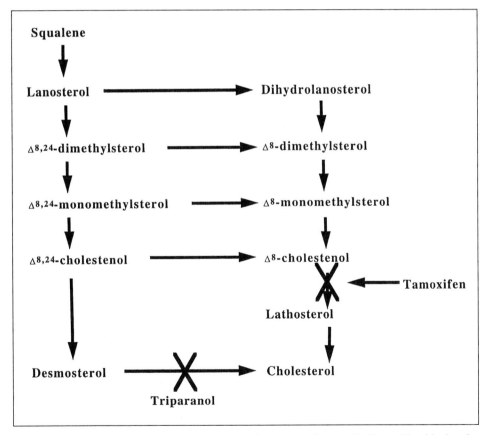

FIGURE 4 Schematic of squalene conversion to cholesterol Tamoxifen blocks the conversion of Δ8-cholestenol to lathosterol, thus decreasing cholesterol production. It is important to note that tamoxifen does not cause a significant increase in circulating desmosterol. In the 1960s, a drug called triparanol was withdrawn from the market because it caused cataracts in patients after a few months of therapy. The drug blocked the conversion of desmosterol to cholesterol.

Table 3

Incidence of Contralateral Breast Tumors

Clinical Trial	Menopausal Status	Median Follow-Up, (Months)	Tamoxifen Treated Patients		Controls	
			Number of Patients	Number of Cancers	Number of Patients	Number of Cancers
NATO	pre & post	66	564	15	567	17
BCTC	pre & post	47	661	9	651	12
Rutqvist	post	53	931	18	915	32
Palshof	pre & post	78	164	3	153	4
Pritchard	post	70	198	3	202	3
Cummings	post	55	91	1	90	3
Fisher	pre & post	59	1419	23	1428	32
CRC	pre & post	40	947	7	965	18
Andersson	post	96	864	10	846	8
Ryden	post	108	239	11	236	15
Mason	NG	NG	367	4	1980	57
Total			6445	104	8033	201
				1.6%		2.5%

Adapted from Bilimoria et al: *Cancer J Sci Amer* 2:140-150, 1996, with permission.

NATO = Nolvadex Adjuvant Trial Organization, BCTC = Breast Cancer Trials Committee
CRC = Cancer Research Campaign, NG = not given.

sion of Δ8-cholestenol to lanosterol (Figure 4).[24] These metabolic changes are consistent with an estrogenic effect on lipid metabolism. Interestingly enough, high-density lipoprotein (HDL) levels, which are usually increased by estrogen therapy, appear to be unaffected by tamoxifen therapy.

Beneficial Effects of Tamoxifen on Coronary Heart Disease

Tamoxifen's ability to lower serum lipids translates to a significant reduction in clinical cardiac disease. In 1991, McDonald and Stewart,[25] in a retrospective review of a randomized trial of tamoxifen vs placebo, noted that 10 of 200 women in the tamoxifen-treated arm had died of myocardial infarction, while 25 of 251 had died of the same disease in the control group.

An update of their patient data in 1995 showed that women in the tamoxifen-treated arm of the study had a rate of 14 myocardial infarctions per 1,000 years at risk compared to 23 myocardial infarctions per 1,000 years of risk for the control group.[26] Others have also found that longer durations of tamoxifen have a greater benefit in regard to cardiovascular disease. Rutqvist et al,[27] upon analysis of the Stockholm randomized trial, found that hospital admissions for cardiac disease were statistically lower for women taking 5 years of tamoxifen as opposed to women on only 2 years of the therapy.

Tamoxifen's ability to lower serum lipids translates to a significant reduction in clinical cardiac disease.

The reduction in cardiovascular risk obtained from tamoxifen use appears to be mediated through the lowering of cholesterol levels mentioned earlier. It has been suggested that a 1% decrease in serum cholesterol results in a 2% decrease in the incidence of coronary heart disease.[28] Another possible mechanism for the cardioprotective effects of tamoxifen lies in the finding that tamoxifen-treated patients have a statistically significant reduction in serum lipoprotein(a) levels (Figure 3).[21] Several epidemiologic and clinical studies have shown that increased lipoprotein(a) levels were an independent risk factor for coronary heart disease.[29,30]

Given that the majority of women with breast cancer are postmenopausal and that the number one cause of death in postmenopausal women (without a history of breast cancer) is cardiovascular disease, the lipid-lowering properties of tamoxifen become clinically significant. However, to date, no trials of tamoxifen in women at high risk for coronary heart disease have been undertaken to prove efficacy.

Beneficial Effects of Tamoxifen
in Regard to Contralateral Breast Cancer

Women with a previous diagnosis of breast cancer have a 3-fold increased risk of developing a contralateral breast cancer when compared to age-matched women without breast cancer.[31] An analysis of 11 separate trials in a total of nearly 15,000 women revealed that the incidence of contralateral breast tumors in women on tamoxifen therapy was reduced by 36% (Table 3).[2] In the 6,445 pre- and postmenopausal women who received adjuvant tamoxifen, there were 104 (1.6%) contralateral breast cancers; while in the 8,033 patients randomly assigned to placebo or observation, contralateral breast cancers were present in 201 (2.5%). Though the trial patients varied with respect to stage of disease and menopausal status, as well as duration and dose of tamoxifen therapy, the chemosuppressive and chemopreventive effects of tamoxifen were evident in all of these studies (see Chapters 5 and 16). ■

References

1. Early Breast Cancer Trialists' Collaborative Group: Systemic treatment of early breast cancer by hormonal, cytotoxic, or immune therapy. *Lancet* 339:1-15,71-85, 1992.

2. Bilimoria MM, Assikis VJ, Jordan VC: Should adjuvant tamoxifen therapy be stopped at 5 years? *Cancer J Sci Am* 2:140-150, 1996.

3. Rosen PP, Groshen S, Kinne DW: Factors influencing prognosis in node-negative breast carcinoma: Analysis of 767 T1N0M0/T2N0M0 patients with long-term follow-up. *J Clin Oncol* 11:2090-2100, 1993.

4. Cohn SH, Vaswani A, Zanzi I, et al: Effect of aging on bone mass in adult women. *Am J Physiol* 230:143-147, 1976.

5. Lobo RA, Pickar JH, Wild RA, et al:Metabolic impact of adding medroxyprogesterone acetate to conjugated estrogen therapy in postmenopausal women. *Obstet Gynecol* 84:987-995, 1994.

6. Cummings SR, Black DM, Rubin SM: Lifetime risks of hip, Collesi or vertebral fractures and coronary heart disease among white postmenopausal women. *Ann Int Med* 149:2445-2450, 1989.

7. Grady D, Rubin SM, Pettiti DB, et al: Hormone therapy to prevent disease and prolong life in postmenopausal women. *Ann Int Med* 117:1016-1037, 1992.

8. Hutchinson TA, Polansky SM, Feinstein AR: Postmenopausal oestrogens protect against fractures of hip and distal radius: A case-control study. *Lancet* 2:705-709, 1979.

9. Weiss NS, Ure CL, Ballard JH: Decreased risk of fractures of the hip and lower forearm with postmenopausal use of estrogen. *N Engl J Med* 303:1195-1198, 1980.

10. Johnson RE, Specht EE: The risk of hip fracture in postmenopausal females with and without estrogen drug exposure. *Am J Public Health* 71:138-144, 1981.

11. Paganini-Hill A, Ross RK, Gerkins VR, et al: Menopausal estrogen therapy and hip fractures. *Ann Intern Med* 95:28-31, 1981.

12. Kreiger N, Kelsey JL, Holford TR: An epidemiologic study of hip fracture in postmenopausal women. *Am J Epidemiol* 116:141-148, 1982.

13. Williams AR, Weiss NS, Ure CL: Effect of weight, smoking, and estrogen use on the risk of hip and forearm fractures in postmenopausal women. *Obstet Gynecol* 60:695-699, 1982.

14. Sullivan JM, VanderZwaag R, Lemp UF: Postmenopausal estrogen use and coronary atherosclerosis. *Ann Int Med* 108:358-363, 1988.

15. Bush TL, Barrett-Connor E, Cowan LD, et al: Cardiovascular mortality and noncontraceptive use of estrogen in women: Results from the Lipid Research Clinics Program Follow-up Study. *Circulation* 75:1102-1109, 1987.

16. Stewart PJ, Stern PH: Effects of antiestrogens, tamoxifen, and clomiphene on bone resorption in vitro. *Endocrinology* 118:125-131, 1986.

17. Jordan VC, Phelps E, Lindgren UJ: Effects of antiestrogens on bone in castrated and intact female rats. *Breast Cancer Res Treat* 10:31-35, 1987.

18. Fornander T, Rutqvist LE, Sjoberg HE, et al: Long-term adjuvant tamoxifen in early breast cancer: Effect on bone mineral density in postmenopausal women. *J Clin Oncol* 8:1019-1024, 1990.

19. Love RR, Mazess RB, Barden HS, et al: Effects of tamoxifen on bone mineral density in postmenopausal women with breast cancer. *N Engl J Med* 326:852-856, 1992.

20. Love RR, Barden HS, Mazess RB: Effect of tamoxifen on lumbar spine bone mineral density in postmenopausal women after 5 years. *Arch Int Med* 154:2585-2588, 1994.

21. Saarto T, Blomqvist C, Ehnholm C: Antiatherogenic effects of adjuvant antiestrogens: A randomized trial comparing the effects of tamoxifen and toremifene on plasma lipid levels in postmenopausal women with node-positive breast cancer. *J Clin Oncol* 14:429-433, 1996.

22. Love RR, Wiebe D, Newcomb P, et al: Effects of tamoxifen on cardiovascular risk factors in postmenopausal women. *Ann Intern Med* 115:860-864, 1991.

23. Love RR, Wiebe DA, Feyzi JM: Effects of tamoxifen on cardiovascular risk factors in postmenopausal women after 5 years of treatment. *J Natl Cancer Inst* 86:1534-1539, 1994.

24. Gylling H, Pyrhonen S, Mantyla E: Tamoxifen and toremifene lower serum cholesterol by inhibition of delta 8-cholestenol conversion to lathosterol in women with breast cancer. *J Clin Oncol* 13:2900-2905, 1995.

25. McDonald CC, Stewart HJ: Fatal myocardial infarctions in the Scottish adjuvant tamoxifen trial. *Br Med J* 303:435-437, 1991.

26. McDonald CC, Alexander FE, Whyte BW, et al: Cardiac and vascular morbidity in women receiving adjuvant tamoxifen for breast cancer in a randomised trial. *Br Med J* 311:977-980, 1995.

27. Rutqvist LE, Mattsson A: Cardiac and thromboembolic morbidity among postmenopausal women with early stage breast cancer in a randomized trial of adjuvant tamoxifen. *J Natl Cancer Inst* 85:1398-1406, 1993.

28. Castelli WP: Cholesterol and lipids in the risk of coronary artery disease—the Framingham Heart Study. *Canad J Card* 4:5A-10A, 1988.

29. Loscalzo J: Lipoprotein (a): A unique risk factor for atherothrombotic disease. *Arteriosclerosis* 10:672-679, 1990.

30. Utermann G: Lipoprotein (a): A genetic risk factor for premature coronary heart disease. *Curr Opin Lipidol* 1:404-410, 1990.

31. Boring C, Squire T, Tong T, et al: Cancer Statistics. *CA Cancer J Clin* 44:7-26, 1994.

Chapter 8

Endometrial Cancer and Tamoxifen

Richard R. Barakat, MD
Associate Attending Surgeon
Gynecology Division
Memorial Sloan-Kettering Cancer Center
New York, New York

Tamoxifen, a nonsteroidal antiestrogen, was first approved by the US Food and Drug Administration for the treatment of patients with breast cancer in 1978. Large clinical trials involving over 75,000 patients have demonstrated an improved recurrence-free and overall survival benefit in both pre- and postmenopausal women. Long-term adjuvant tamoxifen is the hormonal treatment of choice for selected patients with breast cancer, and large-scale trials are continuing to evaluate its role as a chemopreventive agent in healthy women at risk for breast cancer (see Chapter 16).

One of the most significant potential complications of long-term tamoxifen use is the development of endometrial cancer. Tamoxifen is believed to exert its main effect by blocking the binding of estrogen to the estrogen receptor (ER). Although primarily an antiestrogen, tamoxifen also exhibits some mild estrogenic actions. Following the initial report by Killackey et al[1] suggesting a possible link between tamoxifen use and the development of endometrial carcinoma in 3 patients, approximately 250 additional cases of tamoxifen-associated uterine cancer have been reported.[2] Recently, the results of the National Surgical Adjuvant Breast and Bowel Project (NSABP) B-14 trial were published.[3] This randomized trial of tamoxifen vs placebo in women with estrogen receptor-positive breast cancer confined to the breast with negative axillary nodes revealed a 7.5-fold increase in the risk of developing endometrial cancer in the tamoxifen-treated group.

The indications for tamoxifen use have broadened to include long-term adjuvant therapy as well as preventive therapy for selected high-risk women. Consequently, a large number of individuals, including healthy young women with no history of cancer, will be subjected to the long-term effects of tamoxifen.

The purpose of this chapter is to review the literature regarding endometrial cancer in breast cancer patients being treated with tamoxifen, and to explore the role of screening for endometrial cancer in these patients.

Endometrial Cancer and Tamoxifen

Despite the overwhelming benefit of tamoxifen for prevention of breast cancer recurrence, many patients worry about the possibility of developing endometrial cancer. Risk of developing endometrial cancer among tamoxifen-treated patients has been defined by results of the NSABP trial B-14. Data on the rates of endometrial and other cancers were analyzed for 2,843 patients with node-negative, ER-positive, invasive breast cancer randomly assigned to placebo or tamoxifen (20 mg/day), as well as for 1,220 tamoxifen-treated patients registered on NSABP B-14 subsequent to randomization.

Two of the 1,424 patients assigned to receive placebo developed endometrial cancer; both of these patients, however, had subsequently received tamoxifen for treatment of breast cancer recurrence. Fifteen patients randomized to tamoxifen treatment developed endometrial cancer, although one of these patients never actually accepted therapy. Eight additional cases of uterine cancer occurred among the 1,220 tamoxifen-treated patients, 76% of which were in women 60 years of age or older. The mean duration on tamoxifen therapy was 35 months. Thirty-six percent of the endometrial cancers developed within 2 years of beginning therapy and 6 cases occurred less than 9 months after treatment was initiated, suggesting that some of the cancers may have been present prior to the commencement of tamoxifen therapy.

The average annual risk of developing endometrial cancer in the placebo group was 0.2/1,000 compared with 1.6/1,000 for the randomized tamoxifen-treated group. This is an important figure that clinicians may pass on to their patients. Physicians should inform patients on tamoxifen that their annual risk of developing endometrial cancer is approximately 2/1,000 or 0.2%. Furthermore, any discussion regarding the risk of endometrial cancer with tamoxifen treatment must also take into account tamoxifen's beneficial ability to reduce both breast cancer recurrence and new contralateral breast cancers, and tamoxifen's preventive effects in high-risk women. In the B-14 trial, the cumulative rate/1,000 of breast cancer relapse was 227.8 in the placebo group compared to 123.5 in the tamoxifen-treated group. In addition, the cumulative rate of contralateral breast cancer was reduced from 40.5 to 23.5, respectively, in the two groups. There was also a 38% reduction in the 5-year cumulative risk of cancer recurrence in the tamoxifen-treated group. Many patients are reassured by these data.

The Role of Screening

Published data appears to support an association between tamoxifen and the development of both benign and malignant endometrial neoplasia. The increased risk of endometrial cancer associated with tamoxifen use increases morbidity in breast cancer patients, but does not outweigh the significant advantage that tamoxifen confers by controlling breast cancer. This issue is clear for the patient with a diagnosis of breast cancer (see Appendix 6). Of greater concern, however, are the implications for healthy, albeit high-risk, women considering tamoxifen because of family histories of breast cancer. Large-scale trials of tamoxifen as a chemopreventive agent are now underway in England and the US. Whether the postulated reduction in breast cancer outweighs the risk of endometrial cancer in this population remains to be determined. The issue of endometrial incidence in well women who use tamoxifen as a chemopreventive is addressed in Chapter 11.

Endometrial Biopsy

What, if any, recommendations can be made at this point regarding screening for endometrial cancer in breast cancer patients on tamoxifen? First, as defined by the B-14 trial, the expected annual risk of endometrial cancer is approximately 2/1,000. A screening program may detect premalignant endometrial precursors, such as atypical hyperplasia or benign endometrial conditions including polyps, the incidence of which will be higher than 2/1,000.

The best method for screening remains to be determined. Some have proposed annual endometrial sampling; however, this procedure has proven to be difficult. In one study, investigators were unable to perform office endometrial biopsies with a Novak curette in 44% of 89 postmenopausal patients due to atrophic changes.[4] Clinicians who recommend office endometrial biopsies to their patients must be prepared for the possibility of being unable to access the endometrial cavity. Should these patients then be subjected to the inherent morbidity of a fractional dilatation and curettage (D&C) under general anesthesia? Barakat et al[5] presented the preliminary results of a prospective endometrial screening study in tamoxifen-treated breast cancer patients at the 1995 Annual Meeting of the American Society of Clinical Oncology. The study consisted of 126 patients with a mean age of 51 years; 6 (4.8%) could not undergo the biopsy procedure due to a stenotic cervix. Of the remaining 120 patients, 7 (5.8%) were noncompliant, 4 were removed from the study due to progression of breast cancer, 4 discontinued use of tamoxifen, and 4 were considered protocol violators. The remaining

101 evaluable patients underwent a total of 296 biopsies (mean, 3), utilizing a Pipelle endometrial biopsy device (Unimar; Wilmington, Conn.), with a median surveillance time of 16.2 months. Four (4%) biopsies were abnormal, including two complex hyperplasias, one atypical hyperplasia, and one with an abnormal amount of histiocytes. All abnormal biopsies were confirmed by fractional D&C. Six (6%) additional patients required D&C for persistent bleeding despite benign biopsies. The findings at D&C included polyps (3), benign endometrium (2), and pseudodecidualization (a benign effect due to progesterone therapy) in 1 patient. Three patients underwent hysterectomy. The first developed complex atypical hyperplasia following 12 months of tamoxifen. The second underwent a hysterectomy for a pelvic mass—which, on final pathology, revealed a high-grade leiomyosarcoma—following 15 months of tamoxifen. A third patient underwent hysterectomy for complex hyperplasia with extensive mucinous change after 13 months of tamoxifen.

The authors concluded that office endometrial biopsies can be used to monitor the endometrium in the majority (95%) of breast cancer patients on tamoxifen. Six percent of patients may require D&C for persistent bleeding. Significant pathology was detected by endometrial biopsy in two (2%) patients, and by close surveillance in a third. However, longer follow-up will be required to determine the value of routine endometrial biopsies in tamoxifen-treated breast cancer patients.

Transvaginal Sonography

Transvaginal sonography provides a noninvasive means of screening for endometrial pathology in tamoxifen-treated breast cancer patients. The definition of an abnormal endometrial stripe in the case of a tamoxifen-treated woman remains to be defined. As reported by Lahti et al[6], if a cutoff of > 5 mm was used to define an abnormal endometrial echo, 22 (51.2%) patients had no abnormal endometrial pathology. Kedar et al[7] reported a predictive value of 100% (16/16) for atypical hyperplasia or polyps with an endometrial stripe of > 8 mm. These findings suggest that premalignant changes can be detected with transvaginal sonography and that the use of ultrasound and/or endometrial sampling to screen for endometrial neoplasia needs to be evaluated in large prospective trials before recommendations for screening can be made.

Care must be taken, however, to avoid over-interpretation of ultrasonographic findings of the endometrium in tamoxifen-treated patients. Goldstein[8] recently reported 5 postmenopausal, tamoxifen-treated patients who, on routine surveillance with vaginal probe ultrasonography, were described as having heterogeneous, bizarre-appearing endometria with multiple sonolucent areas suggestive of a polyp. Because of concerns regarding tamoxifen use and endometrial neoplasia, the first patient was referred for a curettage and hysteroscopy. Minimal tissue was obtained, and hysteroscopic evaluation revealed a smooth atrophic endometrium. When the abnormal sonographic appearance persisted, the patient underwent a sonohysterogram, which involved the instillation of 3 mL to 10 mL of saline at the time of sonography. The fluid enhancement revealed that the changes originally interpreted as endometrial were actually subendometrial in origin. Four additional patients with similar abnormal sonographic findings were actually found to have subendometrial abnormalities on sonohysterogram. To date, it is unclear what these abnormal areas represent as none of the patients has undergone hysterectomy. Some have speculated that they may represent adenomyomatous-like changes. Further studies regarding the sonographic appearance of the endometrium in tamoxifen-treated patients are warranted.

Screening Issues

Many patients with breast cancer who are taking tamoxifen worry a great deal about the possibility of developing a different cancer. Clinicians who care for these patients sense this anxiety, and, in an effort to help, may attempt to screen for endometrial cancer. Although the chance of detecting endometrial cancer is very low, the patient may benefit from the reassurance that a negative test provides. The ultimate goal of any screening study is to detect cancer at an earlier stage and thereby improve outcome. To date, there is still no evidence that any form of screening for endometrial cancer in tamoxifen-treated patients will accomplish this.

Table I

Recommendations for Women Taking Tamoxifen

- Annual gynecologic examination including Pap smear, bimanual, and rectovaginal examination

- Patient counseling regarding the risk of endometrial cancer and reporting of symptoms (bloody discharge, spotting, abnormal bleeding)

- Prompt endometrial sampling for any abnormal bleeding

- Dilatation and curettage for biopsy which reveals endometrial hyperplasia to rule out a more significant lesion

- If tamoxifen must be continued, hysterectomy should be considered for atypical hyperplasia

- Tamoxifen can be continued following hysterectomy for atypical hyperplasia or carcinoma following discussion with the physician responsible for the patient's breast care

---

First, the majority of tamoxifen-associated endometrial cancers appears to have a similar stage, grade, histology, and prognosis as those endometrial cancers occurring in the general population.[9] Since their prognosis is generally good, early detection will probably not improve outcome. Furthermore, the treatment for preinvasive cancer (atypical endometrial hyperplasia) is still hysterectomy; therefore, the patient will not gain any benefit by undergoing a less radical procedure. Approximately 80,000 of the 182,000 women diagnosed with breast cancer annually will be started on tamoxifen. In addition, approximately 500,000 women are currently on tamoxifen for the treatment of breast cancer. If one were to assume a 30% prior hysterectomy rate, this would leave 30% of 580,000, or 406,000 women, at risk for endometrial cancer by the end of the year. If the annual risk of developing endometrial cancer, according to the B-14 trial, is 2/1,000, this would result in approximately 812 cases (2/1,000 · 406,000) of endometrial cancers. A review of the published cases of tamoxifen-associated endometrial cancers revealed that approximately 15% of these patients will actually die from endometrial cancer.[10] If screening were able to detect endometrial cancer earlier and thus prevent deaths, potentially 15% of these 812 cases, or 122 deaths, could potentially be prevented—if one assumes a 100% efficacy for the screening method used. The cost of screening 406,000 women with either endometrial biopsy, transvaginal sonography, or both would, however, be extremely high.

Current Screening Recommendations

How then should clinicians follow their breast cancer patients on tamoxifen (Table 1)? According to a recent Committee Opinion of the American College of Obstetricians and Gynecologists (ACOG), women with breast cancer who take tamoxifen should undergo annual gynecologic evaluations, including Pap tests and pelvic exams.[11] Any abnormal bleeding, including bloody discharge, spotting, or other symptoms, should be thoroughly evaluated by an endometrial biopsy. No distinction should be made based on the amount, color, or frequency of bleeding. In a review from Memorial Sloan-Kettering Cancer Center, Gibson et al[12] reported that all cases of endometrial carcinoma detected by D&C in tamoxifen-treated breast cancer patients presented with abnormal bleeding. ACOG further recommends that practitioners be alert to the increased incidence of endometrial malignancy, and screening procedures be employed at the discretion of the individual gynecologist. No comment, however, is made as to what these screening procedures should be.

If atypical endometrial hyperplasia or carcinoma is detected, the patient should undergo a hysterectomy; however, tamoxifen can be reinstituted immediately afterwards. Although progestins are used to reduce the risk of endometrial hyperplasia and cancer in women on estrogen replacement therapy, ACOG does not advocate this practice in breast cancer patients as the impact of progestins on the course of breast cancer is still not known.

Perhaps the most important task that clinicians can perform is to educate and counsel their patients. All postmenopausal women taking tamoxifen need to know that the annual risk of endometrial cancer is 2/1,000. Furthermore, they should be informed that the majority of any cancers that develop have a low stage and grade, and are usually curable by hysterectomy. Moreover, they need to be informed that despite the increased risk of endometrial cancer, the overwhelming benefit is in favor of taking tamoxifen as shown by the results of the NSABP B-14 trial, which demonstrated a 38% reduction in the 5-year cumulative risk of cancer recurrence in the tamoxifen-treated group.

As more information is obtained about the effect of tamoxifen on the endometrium, and as more studies determine the sensitivity and specificity of various tests used to screen for endometrial cancer, more definite recommendations for following this group of patients can be made. For now, all women, whether or not they are receiving tamoxifen, should be encouraged to undergo annual gynecologic evaluation, which should include endometrial sampling in the presence of abnormal vaginal bleeding. ■

References

1. Killackey MA, Hakes TB, Pierce VK: Endometrial adenocarcinoma in breast cancer patients receiving antiestrogens. *Cancer Treat Rep* 69:237-238, 1985.

2. Assikis VJ, Jordan VC: Gynecologic effects of tamoxifen and the association with endometrial carcinoma. *Int J Gynecol Obstet* 49:241-257, 1995.

3. Fisher B, Costantino JP, Redmond CK, et al: Endometrial cancer in tamoxifen-treated breast cancer patients: Findings from the National Surgical Adjuvant Breast and Bowel Project (NSABP) B-14. *J Natl Cancer Inst* 86:527-537, 1994.

4. Gal D, Kopel S, Bashevkin M, et al: Oncologic potential of tamoxifen on endometria of postmenopausal women with breast cancer: Preliminary report. *Gynecol Oncol* 42:120-123, 1991.

5. Barakat RR, Gilewski TA, Saigo PE, et al: The effect of adjuvant tamoxifen on the endometrium in women with breast cancer: An interim analysis of a prospective study (abstract). *Proc Am Soc Clin Oncol* 779, 1995.

6. Lahti E, Blanco G, Kauppila A, et al: Endometrial changes in postmenopausal breast cancer patients receiving tamoxifen. *Obstet Gynecol* 81:660-664, 1993.

7. Kedar RP, Bourne TH, Powles TJ, et al: Effects of tamoxifen on uterus and ovaries of postmenopausal women in a randomised breast cancer prevention 13 trial. *Lancet* 343:1318-1321, 1994.

8. Goldstein SR: Unusual ultrasonographic appearance of the uterus in patients receiving tamoxifen. *Am J Obstet Gynecol* 170:447-451, 1994.

9. Barakat RR, Wong G, Curtin JP, et al: Tamoxifen use in breast cancer patients who subsequently develop corpus cancer is not associated with a higher incidence of adverse histologic features. *Gynecol Oncol* 55:164-168, 1994.

10. Barakat RR: The effect of tamoxifen on the endometrium. *Oncology* 9:129-139, 1995.

11. American College of Obstetricians and Gynecologists: ACOG Committee Opinion: Tamoxifen and endometrial cancer, page 169, 1996.

12. Gibson LE, Barakat RR, Venkatraman ES, et al: Endometrial pathology at dilatation and curettage in breast cancer patients: Comparison of tamoxifen users and nonusers. *Cancer J Sci Am* 2:35-38, 1996.

Chapter 9

Tamoxifen and Endometrial Cancer: The Worldwide Clinical Database

Vasileios J. Assikis, MD
Resident in Medicine
Department of Medicine
Cook County Hospital
Chicago, Illinois

V. Craig Jordan, PhD, DSc

The World Health Organization (WHO) lists tamoxifen as an essential medicine for the treatment of breast cancer. However, in 1996, the International Agency for Research on Cancer (IARC) declared tamoxifen to be a carcinogen based on laboratory studies in rats and the detection of endometrial cancers in women. Nevertheless, the benefits of tamoxifen to aid the survival of patients with breast cancer exceed any risks (see Appendix 6). The Agency further stated that their findings should not be used for regulatory purposes nor should any woman be denied tamoxifen based on concerns about the risks from the detection of endometrial cancer.

In this chapter, we will place the concerns about a link between tamoxifen and endometrial cancer into perspective. Key issues of the study designs conducted earlier are: a) studies that have not prescreened women for endometrial cancer, or b) studies that have only screened tamoxifen-treated patients.

Endometrial Cancer Epidemiology

Endometrial cancer is the most common gynecologic malignancy. In 1996, 32,800 new cases were diagnosed and 5,900 cancer deaths occurred. Women with elevated endogenous estrogens (early menarche, obesity, Stein-Leventhal syndrome, estrogen-secreting ovarian tumors) or exogenous unopposed estrogens (estrogen replacement therapy) are typically at increased risk for endometrial cancer. In this group of patients, the development of endometrial carcinoma is usually preceded by a benign precursor—endometrial hyperplasia—that slowly develops with increasing degrees of cytologic atypia over time. Typically, small segments of the tumor outgrow their blood supply during the early exophytic growth phase, resulting in focal necrosis, which, in turn, gives rise to the symptom of postmenopausal bleeding. These early symptoms prompt women to seek medical attention at a time when the tumor is usually still confined to the uterus. Indeed, the Surveillance, Epidemiology, and End Results Program (SEER) data[1] showed that the majority of endometrial cancers were of low stage (stage I = 74%) and that the overall 5-year survival rates were high (83%).

In the SEER data, there was, however, a minority of endometrial carcinomas that demonstrated a different clinical behavior. These tumors were of aggressive histologic types (serous carcinoma, papillary carcinoma, clear cell carcinoma), and usually occurred in women who had endometrial atrophy and lacked the risk factors described earlier for estrogen-dependent endometrial disease. In addition, although tumors of mesenchymal origin, namely sarcomas, comprised only a small percentage of uterine tumors, they exhibited quite aggressive clinical behavior. Typically, these tumors were associated with a history of pelvic radiation exposure, while there was also evidence of a possible link with stimulation by high estrogen levels.

The mean age of patients diagnosed with endometrial cancer was 59 years; age seemed to play a role in the pattern of tumors detected. Elderly patients had an increased incidence of endometrial cancer and a tendency towards more virulent histologic types that resulted in invasive, aggressive disease.[2] The increased virulence of endometrial cancer in the elderly may be related to the tumors' independence from hormonal factors.

Tamoxifen and Endometrial Cancer

In the past decade, there have been a number of reports regarding the interaction of tamoxifen with the female reproductive tract. While endometrial cancer had been the main focus, tamoxifen had also been associated with minor changes in gonadotrophin levels; amenorrhea; oligomenorrhea; ovarian hyperstimulation in premenopausal women that occasionally led to ovarian cysts; exacerbation or regression of endometriosis; promotion of the growth of uterine leiomyomas; and endometrial polyps. There were even isolated case reports of women who developed ovarian or fallopian tube tumors who had a history of tamoxifen intake.[3]

In general, the gynecologic concerns were mainly anecdotal. Estrogenic effects of tamoxifen have been demonstrated in the vaginal epithelium and increased endometrial proliferation has been observed in about one third of treated postmenopausal women.[3] In 1998, however, the major clinical problem is still the inability to predict which women will respond to tamoxifen as an estrogen-like substance and which will not.

Since 1985, a number of reports linking tamoxifen to endometrial cancer have appeared in the world literature. Many of these cases represented noncontrolled case reports and most were collected retrospectively. In addition, a number of double-blind, randomized trials have documented an increased frequency of endometrial cancer in tamoxifen-treated patients. These trials, however, were not designed to specifically answer the question of an association between tamoxifen and endometrial cancer. A number of biases may have thus confounded the results of these studies.[4]

The benefits of tamoxifen on overall survival of patients with breast cancer exceed any risks.

In none of these trials did the patients have a baseline endometrial screening for any existing lesions before commencing tamoxifen, nor were they randomized in respect to major risk factors for the development of endometrial cancer. It can, therefore, not be excluded that a significant number of these women already had an undetected endometrial malignancy. In support of this notion are the findings of a large series of autopsies that showed the incidence of occult endometrial cancer to be 5 times higher than the reported rate for the same geographical area and the same period of time.[5]

Worldwide, there are now more than 10 million women-years of experience with tamoxifen treatment. Since uterine toxicity is the most prominent adverse effect associated with tamoxifen treatment, there has been intense interest in reporting cases regarding endometrial abnormalities—both benign and malignant. In the past decade, a number of reports have linked tamoxifen with the detection of endometrial cancer. Previously, we have reviewed the literature and found a total of only 349 endometrial carcinomas reported in tamoxifen-treated patients (Table 1).[3,4] A number of sarcomas and mixed Müllerian tumors (MMT) (listed separately) were also reported in association with tamoxifen treatment. Contrary to recent concerns expressed in regard to the potentially detrimental endometrial effects of tamoxifen in premenopausal women,[6] the vast majority of the reported endometrial cancers occurred in postmenopausal women. Although the duration of tamoxifen therapy was not reported for all cases, it still appears that both short-term (≤ 2 years) and long-term therapy (> 2 years) are implicated in the higher frequency of endometrial tumors. The daily dose of tamoxifen administered to these patients varied among the different reports, with 20 mg as the prevailing dosage. Some investigators have suggested that doses higher than the current standard (20 mg/day) may lead to an increase in the detection of endometrial cancer; however, in 1998, our database at Northwestern University still provides no clearcut evidence of such a relationship (see Chapter 5).

Is Tamoxifen Related to a More Aggressive Endometrial Cancer?

In 1993, a case-control study from Yale was published in the *Journal of Clinical Oncology*.[7] The authors conducted a retrospective search of the Yale/New Haven tumor registry for the 1980 to 1990 decade.

After screening 3,457 records, they identified 53 breast cancer patients who later developed uterine tumor. Fifteen of these patients had taken 40 mg/day of tamoxifen for an average of 4.2 years. Ten of these tumors (67%) were of an aggressive histologic type (high-grade endometrioid carcinoma, MMT, clear-cell carcinoma, papillary serous carcinoma); one third of the patients died of endometrial cancer. The authors concluded that ". . . women receiving tamoxifen are at risk for high-grade endometrial cancers that have a poor prognosis. . . ."

This report created a lot of concern among clinicians as it challenged the longstanding belief that endometrial tumors arising in tamoxifen-treated patients had a favorable outcome, as did endometrial tumors in patients with a history of estrogen replacement therapy (ERT).

Table I

Detection and Distribution of Uterine Malignancies in Patients Exposed to Tamoxifen

Endometrial carcinomas	349
Mixed Müllerian Tumors	18
Sarcomas	9
Patients	
Postmenopausal	200
Premenopausal	2
Duration of tamoxifen therapy	
≤ 2 years	91
> 2 years	108

Information derived from Assikis et al[4] with permission.

To address this issue, we have gathered all the available data in the published literature on stage and grade of endometrial carcinomas occurring in tamoxifen-treated patients.[4] Stage was reported for 234 of these patients and grade was reported for 225 of them. In Table 2, we compared the stage of endometrial tumors as reported in the Yale study[7] with the data from our literature review,[4] as well as the SEER data.[1]

There is general agreement that endometrial cancer detected in tamoxifen-treated women is typically confined to the uterus. Comparing the same three

Table 2

Distribution of the Stage of Endometrial Cancer in the Yale Study[7], a Review of the International Literature[4] and the SEER Database[1]

	Yale		Review		SEER
Stage I	7/9	78%	184/234	79%	74%
Stage II-IV	2/9	22%	50/234	21%	26%

data sources, we depicted the data on grade in Figure 1. As the figure shows, there is a significant discrepancy among the three data sources.

Contrary to the Yale data, which showed a predominance of high-grade tumors, our review showed that, similar to the SEER data, endometrial cancer in patients treated with tamoxifen is of low (grade 1) or intermediate (grade 2) grade.

Past and present, no other clinical study supports the Yale study.

Endometrial Cancer and the Duration of Tamoxifen

The first large-scale prospective clinical trial that offered evidence of a possible association between tamoxifen and endometrial cancer was the

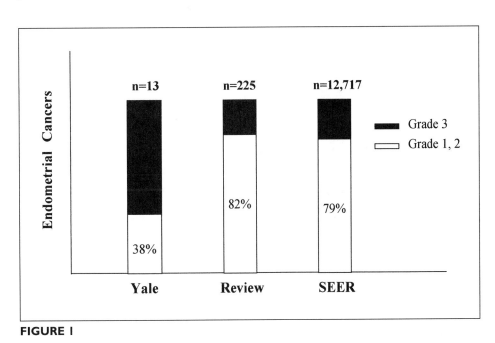

FIGURE I

Stockholm trial in 1989.[8] A total of 1,846 patients were randomized to receive either 40 mg of tamoxifen or placebo for 2 years. Patients who were initially randomized to take tamoxifen for 2 years were offered the option to be re-randomized to receive tamoxifen for another 3 years, for a total of 5 years.

Although tamoxifen proved beneficial in controlling second primary breast cancer, there was an increase in the incidence of endometrial cancer. This increase was reported to be higher for the long-term tamoxifen therapy (> 2 years) group than the short-term (≤ 2 years) group, and led the authors to conclude that ". . . the cumulative frequency of endometrial cancers was significantly greater in patients who continued on tamoxifen, than in those who stopped at 2 years. . . ."

Four years later, the same group published an update of their findings, detailing the individual characteristics of all patients afflicted with endometrial cancer.[9] Seventeen endometrial cancers were diagnosed in the tamoxifen-treated group and 5 in the control group.

Interestingly, however, plotting the actual data (Figure 2) leads to a conclusion different than the one reported by the Stockholm group. From Figure 2,

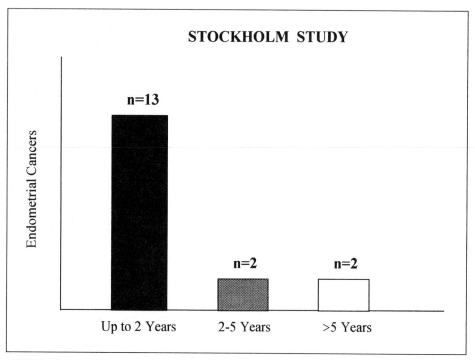

FIGURE 2

it is clear that the majority of endometrial cancer cases (13/17) occurred in patients who were treated with tamoxifen for 2 years or less.[10] Furthermore, the results of the NSABP B-14 trial[11] showed that most tumors were of low grade and stage, and that, over time, the rate of detection of endometrial cancer was constant. Significantly, clinical trials, concerning both short-term (Christie Hospital trial) and long-term therapies (Scottish trial), have failed to detect an increase in the frequency of endometrial cancer in association with tamoxifen treatment.[3]

It is imperative that patients with breast cancer not be denied the benefits of tamoxifen.

Thousands of women have taken or are currently receiving tamoxifen. Should the effect of tamoxifen be as detrimental to the endometrium as some investigators have suggested, there would have been an "epidemic" of endometrial malignancies by now.[12] Clearly, this is not the case. Based on the findings of the world's literature and those of randomized clinical trials, we believe that tamoxifen treatment confers a 2- to 3-fold increase in the detection of preexisting endometrial cancer.[3,11]

Conclusions

The development of tamoxifen is one of the few success stories in the treatment of breast cancer. Tamoxifen is now the adjuvant treatment of choice for all stages of hormonal-responsive breast cancer. Its success as an antineoplastic agent has much to do with its low toxicity profile, despite the fact that the most significant side effect has been a modest increase in the detection of endometrial malignancies. Estrogenic properties of the drug are believed to account for this growth-promoting effect on the uterus. In 1998, however, evidence still suggests that tamoxifen's effect on the uterine tissues is more complicated than those typically seen with ERT.[13,14]

In the past decade, a great number of investigators have looked into the association of tamoxifen and endometrial growth. Although the exact mechanisms by which tamoxifen exerts its growth-promoting effects in some patients and growth-inhibiting effects in others are yet to be identified, there is evidence of an association between tamoxifen therapy and an increase in the detection of endometrial malignancies.

However, the existing findings point more towards a stimulation of an already initiated uncontrolled endometrial growth rather than a carcinogenic insult. In support of this notion is the fact that no DNA adducts have been reported from human uterine samples.[15]

We have reviewed the world's literature and found that endometrial cancer detected in tamoxifen-treated women is not an aggressive malignancy. More so, it usually produces symptoms at early stages and can, therefore, be dealt with quite effectively. Taking into account the frequency of endometrial cancer reported in prospective trials, in conjunction with the findings of case-controlled studies, we conclude that tamoxifen produces a 2/1,000 women-years annual relative risk for endometrial cancer. The concern is mainly confined to postmenopausal women. The dose of the drug does not seem to play a role.

The choice of monitoring techniques aimed at the earliest detection of potential gynecological pathology was discussed in the preceding chapter. Aggressive screening of tamoxifen-treated women carries the risk of identifying patients with benign endometrial changes that might alarm patients and clinicians, but cannot be justified on the basis of cost effectiveness. It is of utmost importance that physicians caring for tamoxifen-treated women be well aware of these effects. It is of utmost importance that they do not consider stopping tamoxifen prematurely out of fear of an overestimated risk of secondary malignancies

Tamoxifen's benefit in the treatment of all stages of breast cancer has been proven. It has been shown to prolong disease-free and overall survival while maintaining a uniquely low toxicity profile.[16] It is clear that the benefits of tamoxifen in the treatment of breast cancer far outweigh any adverse gynecological effects. It is imperative that patients with breast cancer not be denied the benefits of tamoxifen. The risk of dying from endometrial cancer is far less than the risk of dying from recurrence of breast cancer.[17]

The International Agency for Research on Cancer (an agency of the World Health Organization) has evaluated all the available data concerning the carcinogenic risk from tamoxifen. Their conclusions are published in an extensive report,[18] but a press release (*IARC Evaluates Carcinogenic Risk Associated With Tamoxifen* located at hhttp://www.iarc.fr/preleases/111e.htm) summarized the findings of the committee. This report is reproduced in full in Appendix 5. ■

References

1. National Cancer Institute: SEER Cancer Statistics Review 1973-1990, Document 932789. Bethesda, NM:NCI, 1993.

2. Hoffman K, Nekhlyudov L, Deligdisch L: Endometrial carcinoma in elderly women. *Gynecol Oncol* 58:198-201, 1995.

3. Assikis VJ, Jordan VC: Gynecologic effects of tamoxifen and the association with endometrial carcinoma. *Int J Gynecol Obstet* 49:241-257, 1995.

4. Assikis VJ, Neven P, Jordan VC, et al: A realistic clinical perspective of tamoxifen and endometrial carcinogenesis. *Eur J Cancer* 32A:1464-1476, 1996.

5. Horwitz RI, Feinstein AR, Horwitz SM, et al: Necropsy diagnosis of endometrial cancer and detection-bias in case/control studies. *Lancet* 2:66-68, 1981.

6. Sasco AJ: Tamoxifen and menopausal status: Risks and benefits. *Lancet* 347:761, 1996.

7. Magriples U, Naftolin F, Schwartz PE, et al: High-grade endometrial carcinoma in tamoxifen-treated breast cancer patients. *J Clin Oncol* 11:485-490, 1993.

8. Fornander T, Rutqvist LE, Cedermark B, et al: Adjuvant tamoxifen in early breast cancer: Occurrence of new primary cancers. *Lancet* 1:117-120, 1989.

9. Fornander T, Helistrom AC, Moberger B: Descriptive clinicopathologic study of 17 patients with endometrial cancer during or after adjuvant tamoxifen in early breast cancer. *J Natl Cancer Inst* 85:1850-1855, 1993.

10. Jordan VC, Morrow M: Should clinicians be concerned about the carcinogenic potential of tamoxifen? *B Eur J Cancer* 30A:1714-1721, 1994.

11. Fisher B, Costantino JP, Redmond CK, et al: Endometrial cancer in tamoxifen-treated breast cancer patients: Findings from the National Surgical Adjuvant Breast and Bowel Project (NSABP) B-14. *J Natl Cancer Inst* 186:527-537, 1994.

12. DeGregorio MW, Maenpaa JU, Wiebe VJ: Tamoxifen for the prevention of breast cancer, in DeVita VT, Hellman S, Rosenberg SA (eds): *Important Advances in Oncology.* pp 175-186, Philadelphia, JB Lippincott, 1995.

13. Decensi A, Fontana V, Bruno S, et al: Effect of tamoxifen on endometrial proliferation. *J Clin Oncol* 14:434-440, 1996.

14. Goldstein SR: Unusual ultrasonographic appearance of the uterus in patients receiving tamoxifen. *Am J Obstet Gynecol* 170:447-451, 1994.

15. Carmichael PL, Ugwumadu AHN, Neven P, et al: Lack of genotoxicity of tamoxifen in human endometrium. *Cancer Res* 56:1475-1479, 1996.

16. Early Breast Cancer Trialists' Collaborative Group: Systemic treatment of early breast cancer by hormonal, cytotoxic, or immune therapy: 133 randomized trials involving 31,000 recurrences and 24,000 deaths in 75,000 women. *Lancet* 339:1-15, 71-85, 1992.

17. Early Breast Cancer Trialists' Collaborative Group: Tamoxifen for early breast cancer: An overview of the randomized trial. *Lancet* 351:1451-1467, 1998.

18. International Agency for Research in Cancer (IARC): Tamoxifen. *IARC Monographs* 66:274-365, 1996.

Chapter 10

Controversies on the Duration of Tamoxifen Administration in an Adjuvant Setting

Norman Wolmark, MD
Chairman
National Surgical Adjuvant Breast and Bowel Project (NSABP)

Chairman and Professor
Department of Human Oncology
Allegheny University of the Health Sciences
Pittsburgh, Pennsylvania

Over the past two decades, an accumulating database has demonstrated that tamoxifen used in the adjuvant setting for stage I and II breast cancer resulted in an unequivocal prolongation of disease-free survival and overall survival. What was considerably less apparent was the optimal duration for the administration of tamoxifen. On November 30, 1995, the National Cancer Institute issued a clinical announcement,[1] based largely on data from the National Surgical Adjuvant Breast and Bowel Project (NSABP) protocol B-14. In it, it was concluded that there was no advantage for continuation of tamoxifen beyond 5 years in women with node-negative, estrogen receptor- (ER) positive breast cancers.

The casual observer with an interest in breast cancer, who is not directly involved in clinical trials, might appropriately ask why it took 20 years to address a question as basic as the duration of treatment for the most commonly used agent in the management of breast cancer. In an effort to respond to this hypothetical question, it might be of interest to review the sequence of NSABP protocols in the adjuvant setting, since invariably, this sequence was reflective of the rationale and beliefs that were then extant outside the context of clinical trials.

This exercise provides a historical perspective and a partial explanation for the rather convoluted approach that evolved to determine the optimum duration of tamoxifen therapy.

The first NSABP randomized prospective clinical trial addressing the value of adjuvant therapy in breast cancer was initiated in 1972. The initial series of trials all assessed various chemotherapeutic regimens administered with the rationale that chemotherapy, given in the postoperative setting, would eradicate established micro-metastases and prolong survival. Since it was hypothesized that patients with histologically positive nodes were more likely to harbor micro-metastases at the time of operation, the first generation of NSABP trials was limited to women with histologically positive nodes.

When it became apparent that adjuvant chemotherapy was of benefit in this patient population, it was elevated to the status of standard therapy, and consequently, adjuvant chemotherapy became the baseline against which the efficacy of tamoxifen would be measured. As a direct result of this event, when the NSABP initiated its first clinical trial assessing the utility of tamoxifen in the adjuvant setting in 1978, protocol B-09, it was carried out in an environment where all patients received chemotherapy—the standard of the day. At that time, the NSABP chemotherapeutic regimen consisted of L-PAM and 5-FU given for a period of 2 years.[2] The duration of tamoxifen administration was empirically chosen to coincide with the period of chemotherapy administration. Patients with histologically positive nodes were randomized to receive either chemotherapy alone or chemotherapy together with 2 years of tamoxifen; an analysis of the results after 12 years of follow-up indicated that "tamoxifen-responsive" patients—a group largely comprised of women > 49 years of age—had a highly significant prolongation in disease-free survival and survival as a result of the addition of tamoxifen.

While NSABP protocol B-09 was accruing patients, it was already appreciated that the 2-year period selected for tamoxifen administration might not represent the optimal regimen. Accordingly, following the closure of patient accession in 1980, an additional group of patients with similar tamoxifen-responsive characteristics were all treated with L-PAM, 5-FU, and tamoxifen. However, in this latter patient population, tamoxifen was given for a total period of 3 years. Thus, there was an opportunity, albeit an indirect one, to compare the effects of 2 years of tamoxifen to 3 years of tamoxifen when added to a chemotherapy baseline in patients with positive nodes.[3]

The results from this study indicated that at 8 years of follow-up, there was a disease-free survival and overall survival advantage for the group receiving 3 years of tamoxifen; this advantage became attenuated, however, by the 10th year of follow-up and was no longer statistically significant.

By the early 1980s, after the first decade of clinical trials assessing adjuvant therapy in stage II breast cancer had elapsed, it was believed that women < 50 years of age sustained the greatest benefit from adjuvant chemotherapy, and that women > 49 years of age benefited from tamoxifen-containing regimens. Preliminary evidence also suggested that 3 years of tamoxifen added to chemotherapy was superior to 2 years and that, perhaps, the longer duration of treatment would be translated into further incremental gains. It became increasingly apparent that in tamoxifen-responsive women with histologically positive nodes the role of tamoxifen, used alone without chemotherapy, had not yet been determined. At that time, it was argued that the benefits attributable to L-PAM and 5-FU in women > 49 years of age were, at best, modest. It was further postulated that the advantages obtained by the combination of L-PAM, 5-FU, and tamoxifen might have been achieved by the administration of tamoxifen alone without chemotherapy. Accordingly, the NSABP made the decision to retrace its steps: A study was introduced that compared the combination of chemotherapy plus tamoxifen to tamoxifen alone in women > 49 years age with histologically positive nodes.

Initially, the duration of tamoxifen administration was empirically chosen to coincide with the period of chemotherapy administration.

Protocol B-16 was initiated in October of 1984, and approximately 1,300 patients were randomized to receive one of three treatment options:[4]

- Tamoxifen alone
- Adriamycin, cyclophosphamide, and tamoxifen, or
- L-PAM, 5-FU (with or without Adriamycin) together with tamoxifen.

A pair-wise comparison between the group receiving tamoxifen alone and patients receiving the combination of Adriamycin/cyclophosphamide plus tamoxifen indicated that tamoxifen in combination with chemotherapy was significantly superior to tamoxifen alone relative to disease-free survival and overall survival at 7 years of follow-up. This study was one of the first to demonstrate an unequivocal benefit for chemotherapy when used in a population of women > 49 years of age; furthermore, it demonstrated that the concomitant addition of tamoxifen to chemotherapy was superior to tamoxifen alone in this population.

As a result of these findings, Adriamycin/cyclophosphamide and tamoxifen became the NSABP standard for this patient cohort in subsequent trials. At the study's beginning in 1984, the duration of tamoxifen administration was established at 5 years—a determination based more upon empiricism than fact. The definitive test for assessing the optimal duration of tamoxifen administration would be conducted in a setting where tamoxifen could be used as a single agent in node-negative patients.

Because of the prevalent belief during the 1970s that the risk of chemotherapy prohibited its investigation in node-negative patients with alleged good prognoses, it was not until 1981, despite several prior attempts, that the

NSABP was able to initiate two clinical trials evaluating adjuvant therapy in patients with negative nodes: NSABP protocols B-13 and B-14.

NSABP protocol B-13 was restricted to node-negative patients whose tumors were receptor negative; 760 patients were randomized to receive no chemotherapy or sequential methotrexate and 5-FU.[5] This regimen was selected because it was considered inappropriate to use an alkylating agent with a putative leukemogenic potential in a good risk population—a conclusion that subsequently could not be substantiated. Results through 7 years of follow-up showed a significant disease-free survival benefit for women < 50 years of age as well as those > 49 years.

Concomitant with the start of protocol B-13, protocol B-14 was commenced in women with histologically negative nodes whose tumors were receptor positive (≥ 10 fmol). Patients were randomized to receive either tamoxifen or a placebo and a potential setting was finally provided where a definitive assessment of duration of tamoxifen administration could be carried out.

At the start of this study in January of 1982, however, the question of tamoxifen duration was not addressed. Originally, tamoxifen was to have been administered for 2 years, but as the proponents of prolonged tamoxifen administration became more numerous and outspoken (unencumbered by data), the trial was modified so that tamoxifen would be given for a period of 5 years.

It was not until 1986 that the decision was made to modify protocol B-14 in order to compare 5 years of tamoxifen with 10 years of tamoxifen.

Because the NCI-generated clinical announcement on the duration of tamoxifen therapy[1] relied heavily on data from NSABP protocol B-14, it would seem appropriate to review this trial in some detail.

NSABP Protocol B-14: Study Rationale and Conduct

This study was limited to patients with primary breast cancer and histologically negative axillary nodes whose tumor estrogen receptors were positive (≥ 10 fmol). Following either mastectomy or lumpectomy, patients were randomized to receive either 5 years of tamoxifen or 5 years of placebo. Patients who were initially treated with lumpectomy received postoperative radiotherapy to the ipsilateral breast together with tamoxifen or placebo administration. There were two basic components associated with this trial: The first and principal component ("principal randomization") was formulated to determine whether patients who received tamoxifen had a superior disease-free survival and overall survival compared with those patients who were randomized to receive a placebo (Figure 1). This part of the study was initiated in January of 1982. Randomization was closed in January of 1988 after 2,818 eligible patients had been entered.

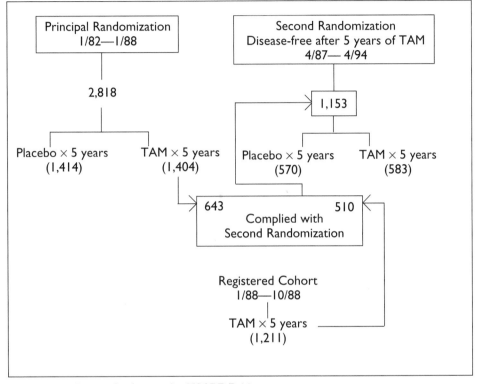

FIGURE 1 Protocol schemas for NSABP B-14

The "second randomization" was initiated in 1987, after the decision had been made to modify the trial to address the tamoxifen duration question. This latter part of the study, therefore, was designed to compare the efficacy of 5 years of tamoxifen treatment with 10 years of tamoxifen treatment.

Patients eligible for this second randomization were derived from two patient populations. Firstly, those women who had initially been randomized into protocol B-14, who had completed the assigned 5 years of tamoxifen treatment, remained free of breast cancer recurrence, and who agreed to participate, were re-randomized to either an additional 5 years of tamoxifen or 5 years of placebo in a double-blinded fashion. Patients who had been randomized to a placebo in the initial component of this trial were not eligible for the second randomization.

Secondly, to achieve sufficient power to answer the duration question, it became evident that additional patients who had all received 5 years of tamoxifen needed to be recruited. For this reason, between January of 1988 and October of 1988, an additional 1,211 eligible patients who fulfilled the above criteria were registered to receive 5 years of tamoxifen ("registered cohort"). Patients in this cohort who were free of cancer recurrence at 5 years were offered the second randomization to an additional 5 years of tamoxifen or an additional 5 years of placebo. Thus, between 1987 and 1994, there were 1,153 eligible patients who were disease free after 5 years of tamoxifen and who agreed to be re-randomized; 55% of this population was derived from the original tamoxifen patient population, and 45% entered the second randomization as part of the registered cohort. Patient characteristics were similar among all subjects. In all components of the study, those patients who were randomized to receive tamoxifen were treated with 10 mg bid. Of these 1,153 patients, approximately 57% were treated with total mastectomy and 43% with a breast-preserving procedure followed by radiotherapy.

The results from both components of protocol B-14 were published in the latter part of 1996.[6]

Results: Tamoxifen Vs Placebo—Principal Randomization

It is important not to confuse the results from the second randomization comparing 5 vs 10 years of tamoxifen with those from the first component of the trial addressing the principal aim, namely, whether tamoxifen is superior to placebo in node-negative, receptor-positive patients (principal randomization).

Four-year results comparing tamoxifen to placebo were first reported in 1989[7], at which time, there was a significant disease-free survival and a borderline survival advantage in favor of tamoxifen-treated patients. The results at 10 years confirmed and extended the conclusions of the initial analyses performed at 4 years (Table 1). The tamoxifen group included those patients who stopped treatment after 5 years as well as those who continued tamoxifen as part of the second randomization. There was a highly significant prolongation in disease-free survival (69% vs 57%) in favor of the tamoxifen-treated group ($P < 0.0001$). This difference in disease-free survival was reflected in a similar advantage in distant disease-free survival, 76% vs 67% ($P < 0.0001$), and overall survival, 80% vs 76% ($P = 0.02$). This analysis was limited to the patients randomized to tamoxifen or placebo between 1982 and 1988 (Table 1).

At 10 years, the incidence of tumor recurrence within the ipsilateral breast was 10.3% for the placebo-treated patients compared with 3.4% for

Table I

Principal Randomization: Tamoxifen vs Placebo

	Tamoxifen	Placebo	P
DFS	69%	57%	< 0.0001
DDFS	76%	67%	< 0.0001
S	80%	76%	0.02

DFS = disease-free survival, DDFS = distant disease-free survival, S = survival.

those treated with tamoxifen. That the benefits of tamoxifen therapy were not limited to local and regional disease was clearly demonstrated by the highly significant differences in distant disease-free survival and overall survival. The reduction in the occurrence of contralateral breast cancer attributable to tamoxifen in the original report of the data was apparent at 10 years. The cumulative incidence of contralateral breast tumor occurrence at 10 years was 3.8% in tamoxifen-treated patients and 6.1% for patients randomized to the placebo arm (56 vs 82 events). The advantage associated with tamoxifen was not related to the age of the patient; patients who were < 50 years of age derived a benefit at least as great as those > 49 years.

Hot flashes, vaginal discharge, and irregular menses were more frequent in women who were treated with tamoxifen.

Adverse Effects and Endometrial Cancer (Principal Randomization)

Hot flashes, vaginal discharge, and irregular menses were more frequent in women who were treated with tamoxifen, whereas fluid retention and weight gain were similar in the placebo and tamoxifen-treated groups. Thromboembolic phenomena were higher in the tamoxifen-treated group (1.3% vs 0.4%), and 2 patients in the tamoxifen-treated group died of pulmonary emboli.

There was an increased incidence of endometrial carcinoma in women who were randomized to receive tamoxifen. There were 21 endometrial carcinomas that occurred as first events in the tamoxifen-treated population (1.5%) compared with 3 in the placebo group. The estimated annual incidence of endometrial carcinoma was 1.9/1,000 women.

The incidence of other second primary tumors, excluding endometrial cancers, was not significantly different in the two groups.

Five Years of Tamoxifen Vs Ten Years of Tamoxifen (Second Randomization)

The average time on study for this second randomization was 48 months. All study treatment was terminated in December of 1995 when it became apparent that there was no additional advantage in prolonging the administration of tamoxifen beyond 5 years. Thus, for the second randomization, patients assigned to additional tamoxifen received an average of 4 additional years (9 years in total) instead of the protocol-mandated period of 5 years (10 years in total).

Data from the 1,153 eligible patients indicated that there was a significant disease-free survival advantage in favor of patients who stopped tamoxifen

Table 2

**Second Randomization: 5 Years
of Tamoxifen vs 10 Years**

	5 Yrs Tam	10 Yrs Tam	P
DFS	92%	86%	0.003
DDFS	96%	90%	0.01
S	96%	94%	0.08

Tam = tamoxifen, DFS = disease-free survival,
DDFS = distant disease-free survival, S = survival.

after 5 years compared to those randomized to receive 10 years of tamoxifen, 92% vs 86% (P = 0.003 [Table 2]). Similarly, distant, disease-free survival differences were in favor of the 5-year group compared to 10 years of tamoxifen—96% vs 90% (P = 0.01). Although the survival differences only approached statistical significance, they too favored the group that stopped tamoxifen at 5 years, with overall survival being 96% for the 5-year group and 94% for the group randomized to 10 years P = 0.08).

These differences were also reflected in a greater number of events occurring in the group randomized to 10 years of tamoxifen, 66 vs 36. These events were not limited to nonlife-threatening sites; there was an increased number of distant failures (16 vs 7) in the group randomized to 10 years of tamoxifen.

For patients in the second randomization, there continued to be an increased number of endometrial cancers in the group receiving 10 years of tamoxifen. Although the numbers were small, there were 6 endometrial carcinomas in the group receiving 10 years of tamoxifen, compared to 3 in those receiving 5 years of tamoxifen. Moreover, there did not appear to be a continued benefit in the reduction of ipsilateral breast cancer occurrence following 5 years of treatment. This lack of further benefit appeared true for the contralateral breast as well.

Deaths without evidence of disease were not reduced in the 10-year tamoxifen cohort: There were 9 such deaths in the 10-year group compared to 5 in patients receiving 5 years of tamoxifen. This information is relevant when assessing the potential reduction in fatal cardiac events attributable to prolonged tamoxifen administration.

Thus, clearly, there is no advantage to prolonging tamoxifen beyond 5 years; if anything, there is a small, but significant, diminution in disease-free survival and distant disease-free survival.

In the second randomization, as was the case in the first randomization, there were no differences related to age; results in women younger than 50 years of age and women older than 49 years were similar. Other characteristics, such as tumor size and progesterone receptors, showed no interaction with duration of tamoxifen treatment.

Commentary

It is essential that conclusions based on results from protocol B-14 be kept in perspective. Although, clearly, 10 years of tamoxifen is not superior to 5 years, this finding should not be confused with the overall observation derived from the initial and principal randomization: When tamoxifen is compared to placebo (eg, those patients who never received tamoxifen), there continues to be a highly significant benefit in disease-free survival, distant disease-free survival, and overall survival in favor of tamoxifen. The data are incontrovertible in confirming that tamoxifen is a highly effective and relatively nontoxic therapy in women with stage I breast cancer.

The data are incontrovertible in confirming that tamoxifen is a highly effective and relatively nontoxic therapy in women with stage I breast cancer.

In the past several years, a great deal has been written about the increased incidence of endometrial carcinoma associated with tamoxifen. The estimated annual incidence of endometrial carcinoma in the B-14 patient cohort was 1.9 per 1,000 women. This is certainly no greater than the incidence of endometrial carcinoma associated with the use of estrogen replacement therapy (ERT) in postmenopausal women. While the increased incidence of endometrial carcinoma associated with tamoxifen must be viewed with utmost concern, it seems inexplicable that ERT is prescribed in a seemingly perfunctory manner to healthy patients, whereas a similar risk of endometrial cancer associated with tamoxifen has resulted in a host of regulatory interventions both in the treatment of women with breast cancer, as well as in those women at high risk for developing breast cancer who previously participated in tamoxifen-related prevention trials.

One of the most important and often overlooked benefits associated with tamoxifen is the dramatic reduction in the incidence of ipsilateral breast tumor recurrence in those women treated with breast-preserving operations and postoperative radiotherapy. The 3-fold reduction in ipsilateral breast tumor recurrence is of considerable relevance to quality of life and the cost of healthcare delivery. The rationale for a breast-preserving operation is obviously to preserve the breast. In the B-14 protocol, 10% of the placebo group developed a local breast tumor recurrence at 10 years compared to 3.4% in the tamoxifen group. Women who developed a tumor recurrence in the ipsilateral breast were generally treated with a mastectomy. Since breast-preserving procedures are being performed with greater frequency, the number of patients who are able to preserve their breast as a result of tamoxifen therapy is cumulatively increasing. Because ipsilateral breast tumor recurrences were included as events in the analysis of disease-free survival, and since only 38% of the initial patient population (principal randomization) was treated with breast-preserving operations, the benefits in disease-free survival for the overall population tend to underestimate the results that would have been achieved in a population limited to patients treated with lumpectomy.

At the initiation of the principal randomization in early 1982, it was thought that tamoxifen might prolong survival by reducing fatal cardiac events. Some still contend that tamoxifen in the adjuvant setting cannot be measured simply by its effects in controlling breast cancer recurrence. However, potential reduction in cardiac events, osteoporosis and major fractures, and the potential delay in the onset of organic brain syndrome, must also be taken into account when assessing the overall benefit of tamoxifen.

It has become abundantly clear that such ancillary end points, at least in the stage I breast cancer setting, will not influence outcome. It has become equally clear that the breast cancer setting is not the appropriate model in which to determine the cardiac and bone effects of tamoxifen. In patients treated with prolonged tamoxifen, there was no reduction in the overall number of patients dying without evidence of disease; indeed, any potential reduction in fatal cardiac events would have been detected in this cohort. These ancillary end points are, however, being addressed in the Breast Cancer Prevention Trial (BCPT), NSABP protocol P-1, where women at high risk for the development of breast cancer were randomized to receive a placebo or 5 years of tamoxifen treatment (see Chapter 16).

The fact that women < 50 years of age—those thought for many years not to be responsive to tamoxifen—demonstrated at least the same benefit as women older than 49 should probably stimulate a reassessment of the use of tamoxifen together with chemotherapy in women with histologically positive nodes. It would be surprising, although certainly not impossible, that women with histologically positive nodes would demonstrate a different response to tamoxifen by age when it has been clearly shown that women with node-negative disease benefit uniformly, regardless of age.

The results obtained with the second randomization (where patients receiving 5 years of tamoxifen were compared with those who were randomized to receive 10 years of tamoxifen) are as counterintuitive as they are perplexing. The arduous quest to determine the optimal duration of tamoxifen administration has been punctuated by a number of phases; the preliminary trials initiated in the 1970s disclosed a cautious and circumspective approach exemplified by tamoxifen being given for 1 or 2 years. In keeping with the belief that tamoxifen was cytostatic and in light of preliminary demonstrations that 3 years were better than 2 years of tamoxifen, a more cavalier approach began to emerge: Many serious and well-informed clinical investigators believed that tamoxifen should be given indefinitely. Data from the 5- vs 10-year second randomization have certainly brought this era to a convincing and abrupt halt.

Although these findings are limited to patients with histologically negative nodes, the results from this study still provide the most compelling biological information relative to duration of treatment. While it is recognized that it is not justifiable to reflexly transpose this information to women with histologically positive nodes, it is apparent that the proponents of giving tamoxifen beyond 5 years to women with histologically positive nodes are now compelled to demonstrate the merit of such an approach in controlled clinical trials.

The arduous quest to determine the optimal duration of tamoxifen administration has been punctuated by a number of phases.

Until such a demonstration is forthcoming, the NSABP has limited tamoxifen therapy in all its protocols—node negative and node positive—to a period of 5 years.

The findings from a trial carried out by the Scottish Cancer Trials Breast Group,[8] where patients who were free of disease after 5 years of tamoxifen treatment were re-randomized to no additional therapy or prolonged tamoxifen, also demonstrated that treatment beyond 5 years does not improve upon the results obtained at 5 years. Although the number of patients in this study was small (173 patients on prolonged tamoxifen, 169 receiving 5 years), approximately 25% were node positive. There appeared, therefore, to be no interaction between duration of treatment and nodal status.

Not only do patients who receive more than 5 years of tamoxifen (an average of 9 years) not fare better than patients receiving 5 years of tamoxifen, but they actually have a significantly decreased disease-free survival and distant disease-free survival. This finding should lead to a number of new hypotheses that could be tested in the preclinical setting. Numerous theories have been promulgated to explain the seemingly detrimental effect of prolonging tamoxifen beyond 5 years in patients with histologically negative nodes. The most prevalent hypothesis suggests that long-term tamoxifen administration results in the development of resistance in persistent micrometastatic foci.[9] This, of course, would explain an increased incidence of breast tumor recurrence in the group receiving tamoxifen for a longer duration.

A second and more plausible hypothesis suggests that after a given period of time, tamoxifen functions as an agonist and stimulates residual foci of micrometastatic disease. Whereas this hypothesis would explain the increased failure rate in the group randomized to receive 10 years of treatment, there were some findings from these analyses that were not immediately supportive of the agonist thesis. The annual failure rate per 1,000 patients in the principal randomization was 56.6 for placebo and 37.6 for tamoxifen, with a mean time on study of 10 years. The rates at 5 years were similar. The group receiving prolonged tamoxifen in the second randomization seemed to have an identical annual failure rate compared to those patients randomized to tamoxifen in the initial randomization—namely, 35.4. Although this represents an indirect comparison, there appears to be no evidence of a stimulatory effect when tamoxifen was prolonged beyond 5 years. The dramatic difference seems to be derived from those women who stopped tamoxifen after 5 years, where the annual failure rate per 1,000 patients fell to 19.3.

It has been suggested, therefore, that the withdrawal of tamoxifen has an inhibitory effect that may not be related to an agonist phenomenon. Based on these findings, one might postulate that the administration of tamoxifen on an intermittent schedule be seriously explored. Regardless of the hypothetical mechanism of action, however, the findings are unequivocal; an important question has been answered relative to the most commonly used therapeutic intervention in the management of primary breast cancer: Tamoxifen should not be given beyond 5 years for women with node-negative disease. ■

References

1. NSABP halts B-14 trial: No benefit seen beyond 5 years of tamoxifen use. *J Natl Cancer Inst* 87:1829, 1995.

2. Fisher B, Redmond C, Brown A., et al: Adjuvant chemotherapy with and without tamoxifen in the treatment of primary breast cancer: Five-year results from the NSABP trial. *J Clin Oncol* 4:459-471, 1986.

3. Fisher B, Brown A, Wolmark N, et al: Prolonged tamoxifen therapy for primary breast cancer. Findings from an NSABP clinical trial. *Ann Intern Med* 106:649-654, 1987.

4. Fisher B, Redmond C, Legault-Poisson S, et al: Postoperative chemotherapy and tamoxifen compared with tamoxifen alone in the treatment of positive-node breast cancer patients aged 50 years and older with tumors responsive to tamoxifen: Results from the National Surgical Adjuvant Breast and Bowel Project B-16. *J Clin Oncol* 8:1005-1018, 1990.

5. Fisher B, Redmond C, Dimitrov NV, et al: A randomized clinical trial evaluating sequential methotrexate and fluorouracil in the treatment of patients with node-negative breast cancer who have estrogen receptor-negative tumors. *N Engl J Med* 320:473-478, 1989.

6. Fisher B, Dignam J, Bryant J, et al: The worth of 5 versus more than 5 years of tamoxifen therapy for breast cancer patients with negative nodes and estrogen receptor-positive tumors: An update of NSABP B-14. *J Natl Cancer Inst* 88:1529-1542, 1996.

7. Fisher B, Costantino J, Redmond C, et al: A randomized clinical trial evaluating tamoxifen in the treatment of patients with node-negative breast cancer who have estrogen receptor-positive tumors. *N Engl J Med* 320:479- 484, 1989.

8. Scottish Cancer Trials Breast Group, Edinburgh: Randomised comparison of five years of adjuvant tamoxifen with continuous therapy for operable breast cancer. *Br J Cancer* 74:297-299, 1996.

9. Tonetti D, Jordan VC: Possible mechanisms in the emergence of tamoxifen-resistant breast cancer. *Anticancer Drugs* 9:498-507, 1995.

Chapter 11
The Duration of Tamoxifen

V. Craig Jordan, PhD, DSc

The argument has been made[1] that the statistical power of the node-negative trial of 5 or more years of tamoxifen[2] is too weak to define the optimal duration of tamoxifen therapy as *precisely* 5 years. Indeed, a small randomized trial performed by the Eastern Cooperative Oncology Group (ECOG)[3] showed that estrogen receptor- (ER) positive, node-positive women benefited from extending tamoxifen therapy beyond 5 years. Additionally, it can be argued that since 5 years of tamoxifen is clearly superior to 2 years of tamoxifen in the Overview Analysis (see Chapter 5), there is a need to establish whether the optimal duration of tamoxifen is 6, 7, or more years. Only large clinical trials, with many events, will define the precise optimal duration of tamoxifen. A positive result, even if only a 5% or 10% advantage, translates into hundreds of lives saved—if, that is, new guidelines are adopted.

Part of the difficulty in achieving a precise result in clinical trials is the heterogeneity of breast cancer and the competing, but shifting, balance of multiple mechanisms of drug resistance. The effectiveness of tamoxifen—even after treatment cessation—is also a major factor in determining whether "longer is better" or "how long is long enough."[4]

Even after tamoxifen is stopped, it is clear that the patient continues to benefit from the antitumor action of prior tamoxifen treatment. Dr. I. Craig Henderson best exemplifies this in Chapter 4, where it is shown that survival curves continued to widen for 5 years after tamoxifen was stopped. Based on these data, a long-term view must be taken, ie, What will the curves look like 20 years after the diagnosis of breast cancer if a woman has taken 5 or 10 years of adjuvant tamoxifen? In other words, in the analysis of an appropriate clinical study, a huge number of events is necessary to avoid an aberrant result based on only a few events that occur at an early analysis. The latter effect, obtained by the play of chance, will confound the ultimate benefit that might be demonstrated 10 or 20 years later.

Figure 1 illustrates the ultimate effects of extending tamoxifen therapy. The diagram shows the extremes that could be obtained from a single large trial of 5 vs 10 years of adjuvant tamoxifen.

To address the issue of tamoxifen duration, two large clinical trials are in place in the United Kingdom. The first trial, referred to as: Does "adjuvant

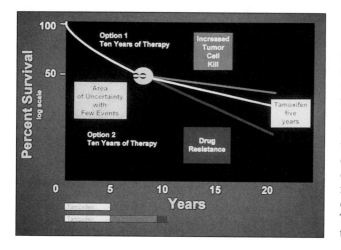

FIGURE I The effect of the duration of tamoxifen therapy on the ultimate survival of a large node-positive, ER-positive patient population if either significant additional benefit accrues with extending tamoxifen therapy, or if drug resistance in the form of tamoxifen-stimulated or -resistant growth occurs. The comparison is made with the current 5-year data.

Tamoxifen Treatment offer more?" (aTTom) is headquartered in Birmingham, England. It was organized by the United Kingdom Coordinating Committee on Cancer Research and funded by the Cancer Research Campaign, the Imperial Cancer Research Fund, and the Medical Research Council. The trial was started in 1993 when an aTTom questionnaire clearly demonstrated that British physicians had major concerns and uncertainties over the optimal duration of tamoxifen treatment. At the time, the controversy was whether 5 years was superior to 2 years of adjuvant tamoxifen. This has now been resolved, and therefore, the new issue for the trial has become: Is more than 5 years superior to 5 years of tamoxifen?

The second study is the Adjuvant Tamoxifen Longer Against Shorter (ATLAS) trial headquartered at the Clinical Trials Service Unit, Radcliffe Infirmary, Oxford, England. The recruitment of patients is worldwide with an overall goal of 20,000 women. If large-scale recruitment occurs before the year 2000, preliminary findings might be available in the year 2005; furthermore, a reliable finding for the duration of tamoxifen therapy might be obtained by 2010.

The aTTom Trial

The aTTom trial in the United Kingdom is a simple randomized study to assess, much more reliably, the balance of benefits and risks of prolonging adjuvant tamoxifen treatment in early breast cancer. The eligibility criteria for randomization into the study are wide: any woman with histologically proven breast cancer which has been completely excised and who is clinically relapse-free; any woman who has been taking tamoxifen for at least 2 years; and any woman who is still taking tamoxifen.

The trial design (Figure 2) is pragmatic with randomization taking place at the point when the woman and the clinician become substantially uncertain whether to stop or to continue tamoxifen treatment for at least 5 extra years. The primary end point of the aTTom trial is overall survival, with secondary end points of breast cancer mortality, second primary cancers (in particular endometrial cancer), and breast cancer recurrence.

A total of 2,830 patients have now been randomized into the aTTom trial by 175 physicians from 95 centers. Women who are potential candidates for aTTom in the United Kingdom can be initially registered if they are not yet ready to be randomized. A total of 2,012 registered patients are continuing tamoxifen and remain eligible for randomization.

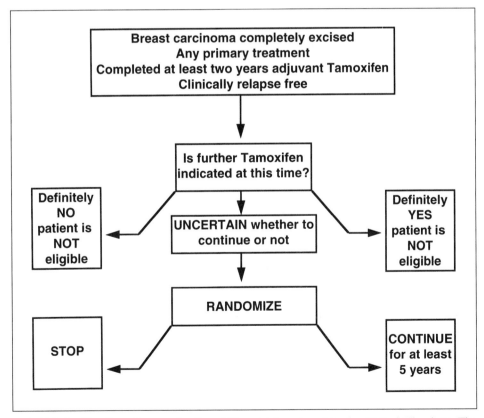

FIGURE 2 The flow diagram for the aTTom trial centered in the United Kingdom. The design is essentially the same as the worldwide ATLAS trial centered at Oxford, England.

The ATLAS Trial

Tamoxifen is free for participants of the ATLAS trial. The required features for eligibility are patients currently on tamoxifen who are uncertain whether to stop or continue, and patients who are disease free of breast cancer. To be effective, the trial is simple: A patient can be either pre- or postmenopausal, with any type of node-positive or node-negative breast cancer. A patient can be categorized as ER positive or unknown, but she *will not* be randomized if she has a tumor that is ER poor. The patient can have had any type of surgery or other adjuvant therapy. Eligible women are randomized to either stop tamoxifen or continue for another 5 years.

More than 3,200 patients have been recruited (Dr. Christina Davis, September 11, 1998 personal communication) from more than 200 centers worldwide.

Conclusions

The issue of the appropriate duration of adjuvant tamoxifen therapy has proved to be a fascinating question in translational research.[5] Laboratory results from homogeneous animal models clearly showed that longer proved better to control recurrence of breast cancer. The concept has proved its worth in clinical disease treatment, as 5 years is clearly of benefit compared to 1 or 2 years.[6] Yet the goal of determining how long will be long enough requires a long duration for evaluation and large numbers of enrolled patients to clinical trials. The worldwide ATLAS trial will provide the opportunity to answer that question.

If you would like to join ATLAS, contact: ATLAS Office, Clinical Trial Service Unit, Radcliffe Infirmary Oxford, 0X2 6HE, England, telephone 44-1865-794569, fax telephone 44-1865-31616; email atlas@ctsu.ox.ac.uk. ∎

References

1. Peto R: Five years of tamoxifen—or more? *J Natl Cancer Inst* 88:1791-1793, 1996.

2. Fisher B, Dignam J, Bryant J, et al: The worth of five versus more than five years of tamoxifen therapy for breast cancer patients with negative lymph nodes and estrogen receptor-positive tumors. *J Natl Cancer Inst* 88:1529-1542, 1996.

3. Tormey DC, Gray R, Falkson HC (for the Eastern Cooperative Oncology Group): Postchemotherapy adjuvant tamoxifen therapy beyond five years in patients with lymph-node positive breast cancer. *J Natl Cancer Inst* 88:1828-1833, 1996.

4. Tormey DC: Long-term adjuvant therapy with tamoxifen in breast cancer: How long is long? *Ann Int Med* 106:762-763, 1987.

5. Jordan VC: Laboratory studies to develop general principles for the adjuvant treatment of breast cancer with antiestrogens: Problems and potential for future clinical applications. *Breast Cancer Res Treat* 3 (suppl):73-86, 1983.

6. Early breast Cancer Clinical Trials' Group: Tamoxifen for early breast cancer: An overview of the randomized trials. *Lancet* 351:1451-1467, 1998.

Chapter 12

What To Do After Tamoxifen?

V. Craig Jordan, PhD, DSc

Tamoxifen is used for the treatment of breast cancer in pre- and postmenopausal women with all stages of breast cancer. However, tamoxifen may only be effective for a limited period of time and other treatment options must then be considered by the physician.

Resistance to tamoxifen therapy is complex. It may occur at the physiologic level, or drug insensitivity may be a property of the tumor. Unfortunately, the molecular events of resistance to tamoxifen are imprecisely understood;[1] however, several general principles have emerged through the translation of laboratory concepts to clinical medicine.

In this chapter, the potential forms of drug resistance will be considered and the rationale for the use of a therapeutic option will be presented. The concepts will be discussed in the form of a clinical scenario.

DRUG RESISTANCE

There are three potential mechanisms to explain the eventual failure of tamoxifen treatment:

1) Reversal of the effects of the antiestrogen with high estrogen levels

2) Tamoxifen-stimulated growth

3) The loss of the estrogen receptor (ER) and the loss of hormone-dependent growth

Reversal of the Effects of the Antiestrogen With High Estrogen Levels

Tamoxifen is an effective antitumor agent in premenopausal patients; however as pointed out in Chapter 6, tamoxifen can cause an increase in the circulatory levels of estrogens at all times in the menstrual cycle.[2] Estrogen levels can increase by 3 to 10 times, depending upon the time in the cycle when a comparison is made. Although the rise in estrogen may suggest that the antitumor actions of tamoxifen are being reversed, because it is a competitive inhibitor of estrogen action, there is no evidence that this occurs in the absence of clearcut information about disease recurrence. Indeed, it may be tempting to discontinue tamoxifen in the belief that the high level of circulating estrogen is a disadvantage to the patient, but there is no justification for the position that a premenopausal woman will benefit without tamoxifen to block the action of her own estrogen in the tumor.

Clinical trials are currently evaluating the value of adjuvant tamoxifen with luteinizing-hormone-releasing-hormone (LHRH) superagonists, eg, goserelin (Zoladex). Goserelin is currently FDA approved and available as a treatment for the premenopausal patient with ER-positive advanced breast cancer.[3] It acts initially to hyperstimulate and ultimately desensitize the pituitary gland from releasing the gonadotropins luteinizing and follicle-stimulating hormones that control steroidogenesis in the ovaries. Without gonadotropins, the ovary becomes quiescent and stops producing estrogens (Figure 1). The rapid fall in estrogen during the first month of treatment is equivalent to an oophorectomy, as the circulating estrogen levels are now in the postmenopausal range. However, the action of goserelin is reversible. The drug is

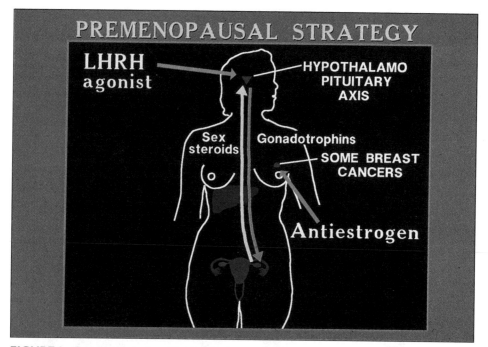

FIGURE I Potential strategy for the treatment of the premenopausal patient with ER-positive breast cancer Tamoxifen is an acceptable therapeutic intervention despite an increase in circulating estradiol from the ovaries. Although tamoxifen is proven effective as an anti-breast cancer agent, there is evidence that premenopausal patients who first respond to tamoxifen and then fail, can again respond to ovarian ablation. The LHRH agonists are able to switch off the secretion of gonadotropins from the pituitary gland, which, in turn, stops ovarian steroidogenesis. The administration of sustained-release preparations of LHRH superagonists represents a medical oophorectomy that is reversible once therapy is discontinued.

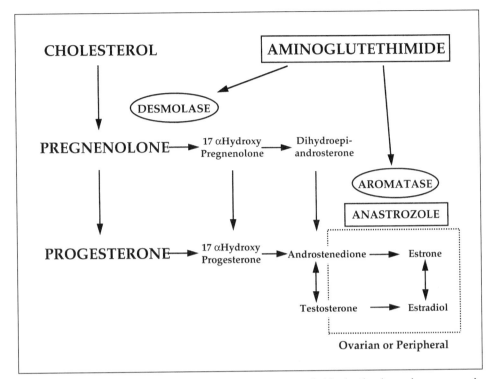

FIGURE 2   Aminoglutethimide exerts a dual action   It blocks the desmolase enzyme in the adrenal, as well as blocking peripheral aromatization enzyme systems. Anastrozole is targeted only to peripheral aromatase and is currently used for the treatment of advanced breast cancer after tamoxifen in postmenopausal women.

administered as a once-monthly subcutaneous injection of a sustained-release formulation in a rice grain-sized pellet. If the injections are discontinued, ovarian activity returns within 2 to 3 weeks.

Studies in premenopausal patients who receive tamoxifen to treat advanced breast cancer have shown that 30% to 50% of those who initially benefit from the antiestrogen can subsequently benefit from ovarian ablation following the failure of tamoxifen treatment. The inference is that tamoxifen can eventually be reversed by high circulating levels of estrogen in ER-positive disease—but only after tamoxifen has been initially successful. The sustained-release preparation of goserelin (Zoladex) could be used as a medical oophorectomy in selected patients under these circumstances. Similarly, the premenopausal, ER-positive, node-negative patient who has a recurrence after 3 to 5 years of adjuvant tamoxifen therapy could receive benefits from Zoladex when tamoxifen is stopped. The strategy is illustrated in Figure 1.

Tamoxifen-Stimulated Growth

Laboratory studies using athymic mice have shown that long-term tamoxifen treatment can eventually cause the growth of ER-positive, MCF-7 breast cancer cells into tumors. The cells are clonally selected so that either estrogen or tamoxifen can become the growth stimulus.[4] Tamoxifen-stimulated advanced breast cancer has been documented in postmenopausal patients who exhibit a withdrawal response when treatment is stopped.[5] However, tumor growth can become restimulated by the small, but adequate, levels of circulating estrogen in postmenopausal women.

Postmenopausal women make estrogen by the peripheral aromatization of the adrenal steroids, androstenedione and testosterone (Figure 2). Estrogen production is related to weight and is associated with the aromatase enzyme located in fatty tissue. Thus, nonestrogenic steroids secreted by the adrenals are converted to estradiol and estrone by peripheral aromatase enzyme systems; these estrogens ultimately activate the ER in metastatic breast cancers.

This knowledge provides an explanation for the success of adrenal ablation in the 1950s and 60s to treat postmenopausal patients with advanced breast cancer. However, a chance observation with the drug, aminoglutethimide, (unsuccessfully used as an antiseizure medicine in children) showed that adrenal insufficiency occurred. Aminoglutethimide works in the adrenal by blocking the enzyme desmolase so all steroid synthesis stops. Regrettably, aminoglutethimide's action also stops the glucocorticoid synthesis that is essential for the ubiquitous control of metabolism. There is a feedback loop to the pituitary gland that ensures constant production of glucocorticoids through the pituitary hormone adrenal corticotropic hormone (ACTH); if glucocorticoid levels fall, ACTH increases to cause more adrenal production of the appropriate steroids. Unfortunately, the decrease in glucocorticoids produced by aminoglutethimide causes a reflex rise in pituitary ACTH that signals the adrenals to produce more steroids in general. Trials in breast cancer showed activity, but hydrocortisone has to be coadministered to maintain the drug's effectiveness.[6] The addition of hydrocortisone to the treatment with aminoglutethimide maintains a low level of ACTH and maintains the block on adrenal steroidogenesis.

Although an aminoglutethimide/hydrocortisone combination has been shown to be of value for the treatment of postmenopausal breast cancer, the toxicity and side effects of the therapy have precluded general use as a standard therapy. Fortunately, aminoglutethimide also acts as an inhibitor of the peripheral aromatase enzyme system (Figure 2). This provided the first clues that drugs could be targeted to the aromatase enzyme and avoid the adrenal target. This new strategy avoids the toxicities and complication of hydrocortisone coadministration.

The first specifically active aromatase enzyme blocker was 4-hydroxyandrostenedione, which acts as a suicide inhibitor of the enzyme. Dr. Angela Brodie first described the activities and antitumor properties of the compound at the Worcester Foundation for Experimental Biology in 1974-78.[7] Animal studies using the DMBA-induced rat mammary carcinoma model were started in 1974. They subsequently advocated clinical testing of the drug that is now approved and available for the treatment of advanced breast cancer in some countries. This discovery opened the door for the investigation of numerous, more specific, nonsteroidal compounds by the pharmaceutical industry. A range of drugs has been tested,[8] but one compound, anastrozole (Arimidex) (Figure 3), is available in the US for the treatment of ER-positive postmenopausal breast cancer after the failure of tamoxifen.[9] The principle is to deny a woman's own estrogen to the estrogen-receptor growth system by blocking synthesis of the hormone.

Another approach currently being explored is the development of compounds that block and destroy the ER in the tumor. Destruction of this essential transcription factor will prevent tumor cell replication and again deny estrogen access to its growth mechanism. The compounds should not exhibit any estrogen-like properties.[10] These compounds, referred to as pure antiestrogens, were first described by Dr. Alan Wakeling at Zeneca

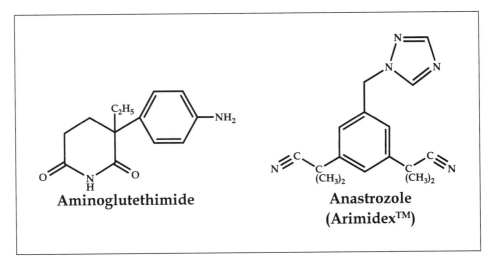

FIGURE 3 Compounds available as inhibitors of the aromatase enzyme system and for the treatment of postmenopausal women with advanced breast cancer.

Pharmaceuticals in the mid 1980s. The compounds inhibit tamoxifen-stimu- lated tumor growth in laboratory models of human breast and endometrial cancer; preliminary clinical trials in England have demonstrated activity in postmenopausal patients who eventually fail tamoxifen therapy.[12,13]

No pure antiestrogens are currently available for general usage outside the context of a clinical trial.

The Loss of the ER and the Loss of Hormone-Dependent Growth

Clinicians usually exhaust the options of different endocrine therapies after a prolonged successful response to tamoxifen. However, the loss of the ER mechanism (determined by immunocytochemistry in a tissue biopsy) indicates only a low (< 10%) probability of a response to hormonal therapies. Nevertheless, combination chemotherapy with the most active agents can still produce objective long-term responses in advanced breast cancer.

In summary, tamoxifen's proven effectiveness and established safety pro- file have made it the endocrine therapy of choice for all stages of breast cancer. Nevertheless, once treatment with tamoxifen fails, a range of other endocrine strategies is available to provide palliation for the patient with advanced disease before combination chemotherapy becomes the only option. ■

References

1. Tonetti D, Jordan VC: Possible mechanisms in the emergence of tamoxifen- resistant breast cancer. *Anticancer Drugs* 9:498-507, 1995.

2. Jordan VC, Fritz NF, Langan-Fahey S, et al: Alteration of endocrine parameters in premenopausal women with breast cancer during long-term adjuvant therapy with tamoxifen as a single agent. *J Natl Can Inst* 83:1488-1491, 1991.

3. Dixon AR, Jackson L, Nicholson RI, et al: The use of goserelin (Zoladex) in premenopausal advanced breast cancer. *Br J Cancer* 62:32, 1990.

4. Gottardis MM, Jordan VC: Development of tamoxifen- stimulated growth of MCF- 7 tumors in athymic mice after long-term antiestrogen administration. *Cancer Res* 48:5183-5187, 1988.

5. Howell A, Dodwell DJ, Anderson H, et al: Response after withdrawal of tamoxifen and progestogens in advanced breast cancer. *Ann Oncol* 3:611-617, 1992.

6. Santen RJ, Manni A, Harvey HA, et al: Endocrine treatment of breast cancer in women. *Endocrine Rev* 11:221-265, 1990.

7. Brodie AM, Wing LY, Coombes RC, et al: Inhibitors of the aromatase enzyme system: Basic and clinical studies with 4-hydroxyandrostenedione, in Jordan VC (ed): *Estrogen/Antiestrogen Action and Breast Cancer Therapy,* pp 221-234. Madison, Univer- sity of Wisconsin Press, 1986.

8. Goss PE, Gwyn KMEH: Current perspectives on aromatase inhibitors in breast cancer. *J Clin Oncol* 12:2460-2470, 1994.

9. Plourde PV, Dyroff M, Dukes M: Arimidex: A potent and selective fourth generation aromatase inhibitor. *Breast Cancer Res Treat* 30:95-102, 1994.

10. Jordan VC: The only true antiestrogen is no estrogen. *Mol Cell Endocr* 74:91-95, 1990.

11. Wakeling AE: A new approach to breast cancer therapy—total estrogen ablation with pure antiestrogens, in Jordan VC (ed): *Long-Term Tamoxifen Treatment for Breast Cancer,* pp 219-234. Madison, University of Wisconsin Press, 1994.

12. Howell A, DeFriend D, Robertson J, et al: Response to a specific antioestrogen (ICI 182,780) in tamoxifen-resistant breast cancer. *Lancet* 345:29-30, 1995.

13. Howell A, DeFriend D, Robertson J, et al: Pharmacokinetics, pharmacological and antitumour efforts of the specific antioestrogen ICI 182, 780 in women with breast cancer. *Br J Cancer* 74:300-308, 1996.

Chapter 13

Talking With the Breast Cancer Patient About Tamoxifen

Amy S. Langer, MBA
Executive Director
National Alliance of Breast Cancer Organizations
(NABCO)
New York, New York

Communicating effectively with women about breast cancer—whether about risk, diagnosis, prevention, or treatment—can be a challenge. This is both because the underlying issues are complex and because ongoing basic and clinical research continually yields new and/or updated information. These two issues are particularly pertinent when the subject is tamoxifen, since this most widely prescribed oncology drug remains under extensive and ongoing investigation.

Despite the need to integrate new developments into clinical practice, certain basic issues and concerns are common to all discussions between breast cancer patients and healthcare providers when the subject is tamoxifen. At the National Alliance of Breast Cancer Organizations (NABCO), Information Service professionals have noted that tamoxifen is the single most common subject of inquiries received from breast cancer survivors. They have also found, however, that a handful of issues remains unclear to some women, and that certain necessary facts about the use of tamoxifen can be inadvertently overlooked.

Successful communication between a physician to patient is defined as one in which the healthcare professional offers a thorough and thoughtful review of pertinent information; and where the patient understands the issues, feels that her questions have been answered, and leaves the session confident that her plan of action is the best one for her.

What follows is an inventory of issues that should be covered as part of successful patient communications about tamoxifen.

Why Use Tamoxifen?

The first and most important task of successful communication about tamoxifen is to explain the therapeutic rationale for use—whether it will be in the adjuvant setting, to control recurrent disease, or to act as a preventive in high-risk women. It may also be appropriate to discuss why the drug may *not* be an option, since many women with breast cancer may already be aware of tamoxifen and wonder why it is not being prescribed.

A complete discussion of tamoxifen should include:

- The histology of the patient's tumor, its hormone-receptor values, and other prognostic factors
- Results of studies on tamoxifen's benefits in this patient population, including quantitative assessments of reductions in risk recurrence and the risk of second breast cancers, or the probability of tamoxifen's ability to control recurring breast cancer
- How tamoxifen works
- How it will be administered, in what sequence, and for how long
- What systemic treatment alternatives to tamoxifen might also be considered, and their comparative benefits
- Additional benefits, still under study, that tamoxifen may confer in terms of cardiovascular health and osteoporosis, and how these benefits may vary in different patient groups (such as premenopausal women)
- Tamoxifen as a preventive for women at high risk of developing breast cancer.

Given the importance of accruing breast cancer patients to clinical trials, the provider should consider whether the patient is eligible for any trials using tamoxifen. If so, the provider should conduct a detailed review of the trial's design and objectives, and take the patient through each section of the informed consent form.

Side Effects

After explaining the benefits of the drug, the next subject to be covered is an explanation of its risks. All medical interventions carry risks as well as benefits, yet the woman with breast cancer requires a realistic picture of how she should expect to feel while on the drug, and what risks she will be assuming in exchange for tamoxifen's benefits in controlling her disease.

Any discussion of tamoxifen must include a review of its most frequent side effects (such as hot flashes or vaginal symptoms), the potential severity of such symptoms, and at what point symptoms should be reported. Providers should also, of course, suggest ways to manage these uncomfortable side effects, both through lifestyle modifications (such as exercise, fluid intake, or layered clothing) and the use of specific products (such as vaginal lubricants).

Medical professionals understand the distinction between "minor" side effects or toxicities and "major" toxicities that may be life-threatening. Nevertheless, it is important to be aware that each patient has her own reactions and thresholds for side effects. Some women, particularly premenopausal women, may find that tamoxifen-related hot flashes are extremely disruptive to their work and family lives, to the extent that the acute distress associated with these symptoms overshadows longer-term concerns about breast cancer. These patients need attention and interventions.

Answer straightforwardly, balancing reality and hope, and use humor when welcome and appropriate.

It is also often useful to review the following:
- How tamoxifen might interact with other planned or current treatments for breast cancer, or with other types of medications (including anticoagulants)
- What to do if a pill is skipped or if the patient cannot recall whether she has taken it
- How to obtain educational materials on the drug's benefits and side effects, including the manufacturer's package insert; any questions that arise as a result of reading the package insert should be raised with the medical team. [Many useful and often free resources are available to breast cancer patients for information and support (Table 1)]

Potentially Serious Risks

After reviewing potential side effects and management, the discussion should proceed to more serious risks. The risk of endometrial cancer in women who are taking tamoxifen is a subject that has received widespread media attention. It needs to be thoroughly discussed and understood (see Chapters 8 and 9). Many women are not aware that a number of commonly prescribed drugs, including some forms of estrogen replacement therapy (ERT), have also been associated with secondary cancer risk. Tamoxifen, however, is by no means alone in this regard. Though obvious, it can be useful to make clear that hysterectomized women (a frequently performed procedure in the US) have zero risk of endometrial cancer.

A discussion about the risks associated with tamoxifen treatment might also appropriately cover:
- The extent of endometrial and other cancer risks in women who have been diagnosed with breast cancer
- The extent to which tamoxifen's benefits in protecting against recurrent breast cancer or death from the disease vastly outweigh the small risk of endometrial cancer, which, when detected early, is curable
- Reports claiming that tamoxifen can cause other types of cancer, including liver cancer. The provider should explain that studies on this subject are

Table I

Organizations for Breast Cancer Patients and Professionals

- **The American Cancer Society** has voluntary programs concerned with breast cancer in its divisions and units nationwide. The ACS toll-free hotline, (800) ACS-2345, provides information on all forms of cancer, as well as referrals to the ACS-sponsored "Reach to Recovery" and "Look Good, Feel Better" programs. For more information, contact your local American Cancer Society office.

- **Cancer Care, Inc.,** based in New York City, is staffed by social work professionals offering support services, education and information, referrals and financial assistance. Cancer Care's toll-free counseling line provides assistance to cancer patients nationwide. Call (800) 813-HOPE.

- **The National Alliance of Breast Cancer Organizations (NABCO)** is the leading central information resource on breast cancer with a network of 375 breast cancer organizations. The quarterly NABCO News updates professionals and the public about developments in research, programs, and policy. The annual Breast Cancer Resource List compiles books, brochures, hotlines, and video resources useful to patients and professionals, as well as a list of more than 350 local breast cancer support groups nationwide. For more information, contact NABCO at 9 East 37th Street, 10th Floor, New York, NY 10016, (800) 719-9154.

- **The National Breast Cancer Coalition (NBCC)**, an advocacy organization, is the national voice seeking public policy change. The NBCC has had a major impact on research funding for breast cancer and on the practice of involving breast cancer survivors in decision making that affects their lives. The NBCC promotes increased breast cancer research, funding, legislation, and regulation that benefits breast cancer patients, survivors, and women at risk. For more information, contact the NBCC at 1707 L Street NW, Suite 1060, Washington, DC 20036, (202) 296-7477.

Table 1 *(Continued)*

- **The National Cancer Institute's Cancer Information Service** provides information and direction on all aspects of cancer through its regional network. Informational brochures are available without charge. Callers are referred to medical centers and clinical trial programs. Spanish speaking staff members are available. Call (800) 4-CANCER.

- **The National Coalition for Cancer Survivorship** is a national network of independent groups and individuals concerned with survivorship and sources of support for cancer patients and their families. NCCS is a clearinghouse for information and advocates for cancer survivors. 1010 Wayne Ave., 5th Floor, Silver Spring, MD 20910, (301) 650-8868. Website: www.cansearch.org. E-mail: info@cansearch.org

- **The Susan G. Komen Foundation** is a national volunteer organization seeking to eradicate breast cancer as a life-threatening disease, working through local chapters and *Race for the Cure* events in almost 100 cities. The Foundation is the largest private funder of breast cancer research in the US. The Komen Alliance is a comprehensive program for the research, education, diagnosis, and treatment of breast disease. Information on screening, BSE, treatment, and support is available by calling (800) I'M-AWARE or contacting The Susan G. Komen Foundation, Occidental Tower, 5005 LBJ Freeway, Suite 370, Dallas, TX 75244, (972) 855-1600.

- **Y-ME National Breast Cancer Organization** provides breast cancer information, support, and referrals through their national toll-free hotline, (800) 221-2141 (9:00 am to 5:00 pm CST, Monday through Friday, or 24 hours at (312) 986-8228). Trained volunteers, all of whom have had breast cancer, are matched by background and experience to callers whenever possible. Y-ME offers information on establishing local support programs, and has, in addition to their national headquarters in Chicago, 23 chapters nationwide. Y-ME has also started a hotline for men whose partners have had breast cancer. Call or write to Y-ME at 212 W. Van Buren Street, Chicago, IL 60607, 24-hour English hotline: (800) 221-2141; 24-hour Spanish hotline: (800) 986-9505.

ongoing, and that if indeed there is a risk, it is currently deemed not at all significant

- Information for premenopausal patients who might plan to become pregnant. Tamoxifen is not recommended for pregnant or lactating women.

Monitoring Women on Tamoxifen

A discussion about endometrial cancer risk provides a natural transition to a discussion of the optimal medical monitoring of women on tamoxifen. Outside the context of a clinical trial, women taking tamoxifen are, by definition, cancer survivors. As such, they should be reminded of the importance of a low-fat, high-fiber, balanced diet; maintaining lean body mass; and the avoidance of exposure to possible disease promoters or carcinogens, first and foremost of which is cigarette smoking.

Presumably, a program to monitor the patient's breast cancer—which would usually include routine clinical examinations and mammography—is in place, as well as other disease assessment procedures, such as bone scans or tumor marker assays. In addition to reinforcing compliance with this plan, the medical team should outline the following as part of the medical follow-up regimen for patients on tamoxifen:

- All women on tamoxifen should obtain regular gynecological examinations, at least annually.
- Patients should indicate to their gynecologists that they are taking tamoxifen. Although this seems to be an obvious point, we often hear about women, who, unaware of the current recommendation that breast cancer survivors not receive estrogen replacement therapy, avail themselves of topical estrogen preparations without consulting their oncology team.
- Unusual gynecological symptoms, such as bleeding, should be reported to the oncology team and should be immediately investigated by the gynecologist.
- A baseline ophthalmologic examination prior to beginning tamoxifen therapy. While this is a useful recommendation for any person, especially older patients, it is based on a recently reported association between tamoxifen and ocular symptoms.[1]

Many women wonder, "How will I know that the tamoxifen is working?" and "What will happen after I stop taking it?" The simple response is that it is presumed to be effective in the absence of recurrent or progressive disease, and its current recommended duration is up to 5 years. Many women correctly perceive, however, that in the adjuvant setting, medical science's current limited ability to accurately identify patients at highest risk for recurrent disease means that we are "overtreating" some women. The benefit/risk trade-off, understandably, can remain less than completely resolved in the minds of some patients. It might be useful to point out that communication about tamoxifen is ongoing and that any medical developments relevant to the patient's case will be promptly relayed to her. The patient, in turn, should be encouraged to bring questions about the drug to her medical team for satisfactory resolution.

Family Questions About Tamoxifen

The woman with breast cancer may raise questions about the potential merits of tamoxifen for her female relatives. First, it should be emphasized that tamoxifen is now available for the reduction of risk for breast cancer. However, her family members may want to learn more about the STAR trial, which is exploring both tamoxifen and raloxifene's ability to prevent breast cancer in high-risk women, and which, at this writing, is accruing participants. For more information about this trial, women should be referred to the National Cancer Institute's Cancer Information Service at (800) 4-CANCER.

Despite the fact that breast cancer continues to be many women's greatest health fear, an informed, more actively involved "new patient" is now emerging.

Second, physicians managing women with breast cancer need to be increasingly prepared to discuss the state of the art of investigating genetic susceptibility to breast cancer—a topic generating interest and excitement among both medical professionals and the public. Many women are not aware, for example, that fewer than 10% of breast cancer cases are currently thought to be the result of an inherited susceptibility. Moreover, although testing for BRCA-1 and BRCA-2 mutations is already available to qualified physicians and their eligible patients, such testing raises many complex ethical, medical, psychosocial, and legal questions. Furthermore, patients should be made aware that the clinical implications (and therefore, recommendations for action) of either a positive or negative test result—both for breast cancer survivors and women at risk—are still currently unclear and are the subject of continuing study.

Finally, the advantage of providing patients with written or videotaped materials about tamoxifen and breast cancer is that they can be shared with family members who are at best concerned and at worst fearful and confused about the prognosis of the woman close to them. An open and thorough discussion with information materials can go a long way toward correcting misperceptions. It can also offer family members a valuable background that can serve them well when they join the patient for office visits.

Facilitating Good Patient Communication

Whether the topic is tamoxifen or something else, following certain basic guidelines will contribute to the likelihood that the patient/medical professional communication will be a useful and positive one. Although many professionals (who routinely advocate for their breast cancer patients) naturally follow these guidelines, they are worth repeating:

• Conduct explanatory conversations in person, when the woman is dressed and in an office, rather than in an examining room setting.

• Encourage the patient to take notes, tape record these conversations, or bring in a family member or friend.

• Listen carefully to the patient's questions, as well as to other issues that might be implied or revealed.

• Answer straightforwardly, balancing reality and hope, and use humor when welcome and appropriate.

• If time is limited, the situation should be explained at the outset and the woman should be offered another time to continue the conversation (either in person or on the telephone), or to continue the discussion with another physician, nurse, or appropriate member of the medical team.

Caring professionals and breast cancer advocates have made tremendous progress in increasing public awareness of the facts about breast cancer and the need for women to take charge of their health. Continuing media coverage of breast cancer advocacy and scientific developments have contributed to the new approach to breast cancer being taken by an increasing number of women. Despite the fact that breast cancer continues to be many women's greatest health fear, an informed, more actively involved "new patient" is now emerging. This new breast cancer patient is prepared with background information about the disease and has opinions; requires treatment options; wants good communication, information, and the truth; is not passive, and may even hire and fire members of her medical team until she has it configured everything to her liking; knows the national public policy picture and often belongs to advocacy and information organizations; and expects medical professionals to be advocates for their patients and work for the cause.

For medical professionals, communicating well with an involved, informed patient has many benefits, which include an improved quality of life and ultimately, the potential for the patient's extended survival. ■

References

1. Nayfield SG, Gorin MB: Tamoxifen-associated eye disease: A review. *J Clin Oncol* 14:1018-1026, 1996.

This section of the book is dedicated to Amy Langer
in tribute to her great courage

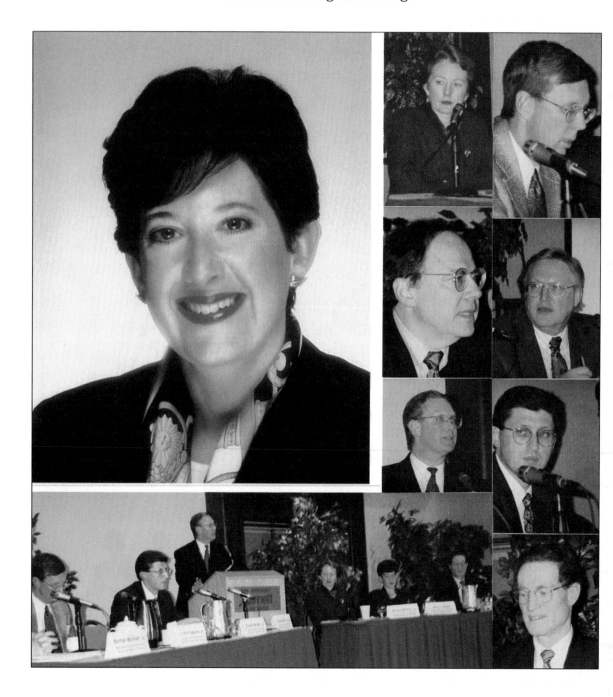

Chapter 14

Questions and Answers About Tamoxifen

V. Craig Jordan, PhD, DSc; Richard R. Barakat, MD;
I. Craig Henderson, MD; Amy S. Langer, MBA; Monica Morrow, MD;
C. Kent Osborne, MD; Joseph Ragaz, MD; and Norman Wolmark, MD

Jack Gentile, President, PRR, Inc.: "In addition to the journals, *ONCOLOGY* and *Managed Care & Cancer: The Journal of Cancer Economics,* PRR publishes two news magazines: *Oncology News International* for cancer specialists; *Primary Care & Cancer* for primary care physicians; and the new, *In Touch: The Good Health Guide to Cancer Prevention and Treatment,* a magazine dedicated to physicians, patients and their families. All of these publications offer their audiences an opportunity to write in and ask our panel of experts any questions they have relating to cancer.

"The most common questions we have received over the past couple of years from both our cancer specialty audience and the primary care physicians relate to the use of tamoxifen (Nolvadex) in breast cancer patients. The vast amount of reporting on tamoxifen in both professional publications and the popular media has inevitably led, however, to confusion and misinformation regarding the use of this drug. It is our hope that this roundtable discussion, which brings together seven breast cancer experts and a representative from a national breast cancer patient group, will offer a clearer picture of the role of tamoxifen in breast cancer and its proper use. Dr. V. Craig Jordan of Northwestern University will moderate the discussion."

Participants in the San Antonio Roundtable on Tamoxifen sponsored by PRR, Inc., publishers of *ONCOLOGY; Managed Care & Cancer: The Journal of Cancer Economics; Oncology News International; Primary Care & Cancer;* and *In Touch: The Good Health Guide to Cancer Prevention and Treatment.* From left to right, top (1)Amy Langer (large photo), Executive Director of the National Alliance of Breast Cancer Organizations (NABCO) (2) Monica Morrow, MD, of Northwestern University Medical School (3) C. Kent Osborne, MD, of the University of Texas Health Science Center, San Antonio (4) Norman Wolmark, MD, of the National Surgical Adjuvant Breast and Bowel Project (NSABP) and Allegheny University of the Health Sciences (5) I. Craig Henderson, MD, of the University of California, San Francisco (6) V. Craig Jordan, PhD, DSc, of Northwestern University Medical School (7) Richard Barakat, MD, of Memorial Sloan-Kettering Cancer Center (8) A view of the dais. Shown left to right: C. Kent Osborne, Richard Barakat, V. Craig Jordan, Monica Morrow, Amy Langer, and Joseph Ragaz, MD, of the University of British Columbia. Not shown are Norman Wolmark and I. Craig Henderson. (9) Joseph Ragaz.

Dr. V. Craig Jordan: "Over the past 25 years, we have seen dramatic developments in the use of tamoxifen. I think it's fair to say that it's the endocrine therapy of choice for selected patients with all stages of breast cancer and the first treatment to reduce the risk of breast cancer in well women. There has been a clearcut demonstration of its biological efficacy in the clinic, and obviously some troublesome side effects and concerns as well. The goal of this roundtable discussion is to put these side effects into perspective and to weigh the pros and cons of tamoxifen use from the patient's point of view. I have prepared a number of questions to ask the panel and will also take questions from the audience.

1. What are the major concerns about tamoxifen voiced by breast cancer patients, and how do you balance the possible side effects against the known benefits?

Dr. Jordan: "The first question involves the concerns about tamoxifen that physicians hear from their patients and that cancer survivors express within their patient organizations. Dr. Morrow, what has been your experience in this regard?"

Dr. Monica Morrow: "Five years ago, most patients' concerns were what I would consider the primary and appropriate concerns, namely, what will tamoxifen do to keep me from dying of breast cancer? More recently, secondary to adverse publicity surrounding the Breast Cancer Prevention Trial (BCPT) [in this trial, women at high risk for breast cancer were randomized to receive tamoxifen or placebo for 5 years] and the National Surgical Adjuvant Breast and Bowel Project (NSABP) studies, the main issue now among patients is side effects, primarily endometrial cancer, but also, to a much lesser extent, liver cancer, and, among premenopausal women, the misconception that tamoxifen will induce premature menopause.

"I put these concerns into perspective by stressing the risk-to-benefit ratio of tamoxifen use. The beneficial effects on survival of breast cancer patients who take tamoxifen far outweigh the possible adverse effects."

Ms. Amy S. Langer: "As knowledge of a drug's benefits increases over the years, so does knowledge of its side effects, and this is often what the media picks up. I think that some of the concerns about endometrial cancer raised by the media have been quite distorted. In fact, there have been very few cases of endometrial cancer reported in clinical trials of tamoxifen. It is incumbent on all of us to be sure that the facts about tamoxifen, including updated information from trials and the Oxford meta-analysis, are widely

Table I

Roundtable Participants

Moderator: **V. Craig Jordan, PhD, DSc**, Director, Lynn Sage Breast Cancer Research Program, Robert H. Lurie Comprehensive Cancer Center, Northwestern University Medical School

Richard R. Barakat, MD, Associate Attending Surgeon, Gynecology Service, Memorial Sloan-Kettering Cancer Center

I. Craig Henderson, MD, Adjunct Professor of Medicine, University of California, San Francisco

Amy S. Langer, Executive Director, National Alliance of Breast Cancer Organizations (NABCO)

Monica Morrow, MD, Director, Lynn Sage Breast Cancer Research Program, Robert H. Lurie Comprehensive Cancer Center, Northwestern University Medical School

C. Kent Osborne, MD, AB Alexander Distinguished Chair and Chief of Medical Oncology, The University of Texas Health Science Center, San Antonio

Joseph Ragaz, MD, Senior Medical Oncologist and Associate Professor, Vancouver Cancer Centre, British Columbia Cancer Agency, University of British Columbia

Norman Wolmark, MD, Chairman and Professor, Department of Human Oncology, Allegheny University of the Health Sciences, Pittsburgh; and Chairman of the National Surgical Adjuvant Breast and Bowel Project (NSABP)

---

disseminated, and that we try to convince the media of their crucial role in letting patients know the proven beneficial effects of tamoxifen use.

"When women taking tamoxifen call the National Association of Breast Cancer Organizations (NABCO) with concerns about endometrial cancer, we stress the importance of routine gynecologic surveillance. We also prefer to emphasize the positive data from the NSABP B-14 trial—that tamoxifen in node-negative breast cancer is clearly beneficial, compared with no tamoxifen, and that 5 years' duration is now the standard."

Dr. C. Kent Osborne: "I think that patient concerns about tamoxifen's side effects stem largely from misinformation that they have heard, not only from the media but also from physicians who may not understand the dual effects of antiestrogens like tamoxifen. These drugs have beneficial estrogen-agonist properties in some tissues and antagonist properties in the breast. Lacking this understanding, some patients and physicians may fear, incorrectly, that tamoxifen will have undesirable antiestrogen effects on cholesterol or bone density, or they may overestimate the risk of endometrial cancer. The net result of these misunderstandings is that women may stop taking the drug prematurely, in some cases, without telling their physician."

2. What do the clinical trials, specifically NSABP B-14, show about the question of endometrial cancer?

Dr. Jordan: I would like to specifically address the issue of increased risk of endometrial cancer risk because it seems to be the dominant negative side effect of tamoxifen. Dr. Wolmark, can you discuss the NSABP findings?"

Dr. Norman Wolmark: "The question of endometrial cancers should not be trivialized, and patients who take tamoxifen need to be apprised of the risk; but I also think that the risk needs to be placed in perspective. Tamoxifen is an extremely effective, relatively nontoxic drug in the treatment of breast cancer, particularly in the adjuvant setting. The NSABP protocol B-14—a randomized prospective trial—attempted to determine the benefit of tamoxifen in a specific subset of women: those with histologically negative nodes whose tumors were estrogen receptor-(ER) positive.

"Ten-year results now indicate that there is an unequivocal and significant prolongation of disease-free survival with tamoxifen (68%) vs placebo (57%). Overall, survival was also increased with tamoxifen use: from 75% for placebo to 78% for tamoxifen, a statistically significant increase. So basically, we have a prolongation in survival and a reduction in recurrence rate. This has to be weighed against the negative aspects, and the primary negative aspect is the occurrence of endometrial cancer.

"In the entire trial (1,400 women in each arm), there were 21 cases of endometrial cancer in patients randomized to receive tamoxifen. Certainly, that is more than would occur in the general, untreated, age-matched population; but to put it into perspective, it is certainly no more than would occur in women who are over age 50 and receiving unopposed estrogen replacement therapy.

"Overall, the benefits of tamoxifen in this population far outweigh the risks. And I think that, basically, women at large have been done a disservice by media reports of the risks of tamoxifen taken out of context of the benefits."

Dr. Jordan: "I would like to ask Dr. Ragaz how the endometrial cancer controversy is viewed in Canada?"

Dr. Joseph Ragaz: "Using data from the Canadian Registry, we estimated the late effects of tamoxifen on overall mortality. Calculations were done for each age cohort taking four principal conditions associated with tamoxifen effect: contralateral breast cancer, cardiac events, uterine cancer, and thromboembolic phenomena. Results have shown that, despite moderate excess of mortality from uterine cancer and thromboembolic events, there was a more substantial mortality reduction from contralateral breast cancer and cardiac events. The main conclusion of our work indicates that despite a dramatic rise in uterine cancer risk, mortality is only marginally affected, as only small absolute numbers will be affected. On the other hand, while only moderate relative risk (RR) reductions are seen for contralateral breast cancer and cardiac events, mortality will be reduced more significantly as large numbers across whole populations are affected.

The risk of endometrial cancer has to be emphasized, but it should not overshadow the potential benefit of tamoxifen in reducing overall mortality.

"On the other hand, while the increase in uterine cancer mortality is large, the absolute number of women affected is very small. In absolute terms, for each uterine cancer induced by tamoxifen, there would be a 5% to 10% reduction in breast cancer and cardiac mortality. So the risk of endometrial cancer is vastly overwhelmed by the benefits of tamoxifen when you look at its potential to improve late mortality.

"These data do not mean we should underestimate the importance of the risk of endometrial cancer. On the contrary, our knowledge of the increased risk should lead to improved screening, which may eventually lead to reductions in endometrial cancer mortality. So the risk of endometrial cancer has to be emphasized, but it should not overshadow the potential benefit of tamoxifen in reducing overall mortality."

3. Is endometrial cancer that occurs during tamoxifen therapy more aggressive?

Dr. Jordan: "I think one of the big issues with the endometrial cancer question really occurred in the early 1990s with the publication of an article based on the Yale-New Haven database suggesting that endometrial cancers in women who had taken tamoxifen were more aggressive. I would like to ask Dr. Barakat about his study of this issue at Memorial Sloan-Kettering Cancer Center, to be followed by some comments from Dr. Wolmark about the grade and stage of the endometrial cancers seen in the B-14 trial."

Dr. Richard R. Barakat: "When endometrial cancer does occur in women on tamoxifen, it is not more aggressive, as was suggested by the review of the

Yale-New Haven tumor registry. This report prompted us to review Memorial Sloan-Kettering's registry of breast cancer patients to specifically examine those who subsequently developed cancer of the uterus.

"We identified 27 patients who received tamoxifen and developed endometrial cancer after a breast cancer diagnosis. The results showed that 75% to 80% of the endometrial cancers in the tamoxifen group were low-grade, stage I, highly curable lesions—a distribution similar to that seen in the 50 breast cancer patients from the registry who had developed endometrial cancer but had not taken tamoxifen. This is also what you see in the general population—75% to 80% of endometrial cancers are confined to the uterus, stage I disease, usually with a low grade."

Dr. Wolmark: "Based on the NSABP experience, there is no evidence that the endometrial cancers found in women on tamoxifen are different from those that develop in patients who do not receive tamoxifen, with the majority of such lesions being low grade and confined. That's not to say there won't be deaths resulting from endometrial cancer that develops while taking tamoxifen, but we have not seen anything unique about endometrial cancers occuring in tamoxifen patients, relative to histology, distribution, or level of aggressiveness."

Dr. Jordan: "With my colleague at Northwestern, Dr. Vasileios Assikis, I recently published a review of international data that backs up both of the previous two speakers. Essentially, we found that the grade and stage of endometrial cancers associated with tamoxifen use are in exactly the same proportions as those seen in SEER data throughout the United States. So I think it is fair to say that all of the available evidence has been contrary to that single report of more aggressive endometrial cancers with tamoxifen use from the Yale-New Haven database."

4. Can anything be done to prevent the development of endometrial cancer during tamoxifen therapy or to diagnose it earlier?

Dr. Jordan: "Before we leave the endometrial cancer controversy, I would like to ask the panel to comment on any measures that can be taken to avoid the development of endometrial cancer in patients taking tamoxifen or to diagnose cases earlier. For example, the literature suggests that administration of a progestin can prevent hot flashes and postmenopausal symptoms. Is it possible, then, that progestins could be used to help prevent endometrial cancer in patients taking tamoxifen? I'll ask our gynecologist, Dr. Barakat, to respond."

Dr. Barakat: "As you know, there is really no proven medical screening for endometrial cancer, and there are many problems with the use of routine endometrial biopsies, ultrasonography, and vaginal sonography. In terms of progestins, we know they can be used to prevent the untoward effects of estrogen replacement therapy on the uterus, but whether we can give them safely with tamoxifen remains to be shown.

In terms of the overall quality of life of patients, we are probably on the verge of doing more harm than good by sending them for excessive endometrial screening.

"My understanding is that there is not a lot of concern about giving progestins to women with breast cancer, but there are preclinical data showing that it may have an adverse effect in terms of their breast cancer. Whether local progestin administration, for example, intrauterine progestin for a limited time, is beneficial remains to be proved. The biggest problem that I can see with giving women progestins comes from our medical oncology colleagues who really don't want us to use these agents, especially in high doses, in women with a history of breast cancer."

Dr. Osborne: "We really don't know how to monitor patients on tamoxifen for endometrial cancer and we certainly don't know how to prevent it. However, this is still being studied in the cooperative groups, and the Southwest Oncology Group (SWOG) is planning a trial to see whether progestins will reduce the incidence of endometrial cancer and whether screening with vaginal ultrasound, hysteroscopy, and biopsies will help to assess premalignant changes in the uterus. So hopefully in the next year or so, information will become available from these and other trials, and we'll have a better feel for how best to monitor these patients and—if endometrial cancer does occur—how to catch it.

"What bothers me most right now is that I think we've blown this whole thing out of proportion, and by performing endometrial screening, we are substantially increasing the cost of giving adjuvant tamoxifen with no evidence that the extra tests have any benefit. In terms of the overall quality of life of patients, we are probably on the verge of doing more harm than good by sending them for excessive endometrial testing."

Dr. Ragaz: "In British Columbia, our community oncologists do not universally accept that progestin use improves hot flashes and other side effects of tamoxifen. The prevalent opinion is that estrogen is beneficial. However, the issue of uterine cancer is forcing the issue of progestin use. We have proposed a randomized trial in breast cancer survivors of tamoxifen plus estrogen vs tamoxifen plus a progestin, and I know that the ECOG is also planning a randomized study of similar design. If this issue is to be addressed properly, it should be done within the context of randomized studies."

Ms. Langer: "As a nonphysician, I would just remind all of us that a very good way to avoid endometrial cancer is not to have an endometrium. In fact, in this country, more than one third of women who are at the age of increased breast cancer risk tend to be hysterectomized. So we should bear in mind that because of the natural patterns of medical care, a substantial proportion of women with breast cancer are not at risk of endometrial cancer because, like women of the same age in the general population, they may have already had a hysterectomy."

Dr. Morrow: "We don't really know what constitutes cost-effective screening for endometrial cancer, and, as has been suggested, this needs to be studied. One thing that everyone can agree on, however, is that women who are about to start tamoxifen should have a careful gynecologic examination to exclude preexisting endometrial cancer. In every report of tamoxifen-related endometrial cancer in the literature, there are many cases that occur within 2 to 6 months of starting the drug, and these are clearly not drug-induced cases. This is a group of patients who should be screened out prior to starting therapy."

5. Is there an increased risk of liver cancer from tamoxifen use?

Dr. Jordan: "Scientific observations from several years ago showed development of liver cancers in rats given large doses of tamoxifen. However, if these animal doses are translated into human doses, it would be the equivalent of a 14-year-old female taking 80 tamoxifen tablets daily until age 45 or 50. Dr. Wolmark, has increased liver toxicity been seen in any clinical trials?"

Dr. Wolmark: "Analysis of the cumulative data of the NSABP trials has shown no increased incidence of gastrointestinal cancers, including liver cancers, even with 10 years of tamoxifen use."

Dr. I. Craig Henderson: "The increased risks of liver cancer with tamoxifen use, if any, is so small that I tell my patients it is about what you would expect with the use of birth control pills."

Dr. Ragaz: "A 15-year review of the British Columbia tumor registry involving more than 27,000 breast cancer patients, most of whom had received tamoxifen, found 24 cases of gallbladder common duct cancer and 5 cases of liver disease—very similar to what we've seen in the population at large."

Ms. Langer: "I think those of us familiar with the data are reassured about liver cancer, but we do know that tamoxifen can induce some liver changes that are not easily interpretable by patients or their community physicians. Could someone comment on that?"

Dr. Osborne: "Liver function abnormalities occasionally show up in the blood tests that some of us obtain every 6 months following these patients, but in my experience, it is uncommon. I inform patients about the potential for some liver damage, but I have not seen a clinically important ramification of these liver abnormalities, and have never had to stop tamoxifen because of it. With almost any drug, there are going to be some patients who cannot tolerate it because of elevated liver function tests; but it is rare."

As a physician seeing tamoxifen patients for the past 20 years, I have never seen clinically significant eye changes associated with tamoxifen use.

Dr. Wolmark: "In the NSABP trials, we have not seen a difference in liver dysfunction between patients on tamoxifen and those on placebo."

6. Are there any concerns about tamoxifen's effects on the eyes?

Dr. Jordan: "I was surprised to learn that there are some concerns about possible adverse effects of tamoxifen use on the eyes. The package insert states that tamoxifen has the potential to cause cataracts and retinal problems. What information is there in the literature about eye problems, and do you feel that this is a concern for your patients? Dr. Osborne?"

Dr. Osborne: "This question has been addressed in the Breast Cancer Prevention Trial (see Chapter 16). We have not seen an increased incidence of cataracts that warrants major clinical concern. Those changes that have been noted are mainly ophthalmologic curiosities rather than any condition that would impair vision or lead to any kind of permanent dysfunction of the eye. So like other tamoxifen side effects, that too has been played out of proportion.

"Some early NCI trials of tamoxifen back in the early 1970s, in which patients received high doses for a long time period, did generate some eye changes, but only at the very high doses being given and only with prolonged treatment. Since then, there have been a few scattered studies suggesting that minor changes, corneal opacities, and so on, may occur. But in carefully done studies with careful ophthalmologic examination, these have not turned out to be significant. And certainly, as a physician seeing tamoxifen patients for the past 20 years, I have never seen clinically significant eye changes associated with tamoxifen use."

Dr. Morrow: "I agree. I think the concern came from uncontrolled, relatively anecdotal reports in older women who had aggressive screening. It was not surprising that some eye problems were found in these patients."

Dr. Henderson: "I think Dr. Osborne summarized it beautifully. The initial findings from the NCI were real, but the doses were very high, about 100 mg bid. I think all the other observations are really anecdotal and a remarkably small number when you consider the number of patient-years of follow-up we have on this drug—about 100 cases in 7 million women-years of experience."

Dr. Jordan: "Yes, they were really huge doses. And I think it was something like 100 anecdotal cases in about 7 million women-years of tamoxifen."

Dr. Ragaz: "We submitted about 80 of our long-term tamoxifen patients to regular ophthalmologic examination and found that up to 10% had mild keratopathy and gritty eyes (dry eyes). So our small, uncontrolled sample indicates that there may be some temporary, self-limiting keratopathy, but we did not see any lens problems."

7. What are the possible noncancer benefits of tamoxifen that you discuss with your patients, and is there evidence in the literature to support these discussions?

Dr. Jordan: "I would like to turn now to a question about other noncancer beneficial effects of tamoxifen and how they are integrated into the patient discussion. Dr. Morrow, could you comment?"

Dr. Morrow: "The risk-to-benefit ratio for the use of adjuvant tamoxifen therapy should be considered outside of the narrow confines of survival or death from metastatic breast cancer. For women with node-positive breast cancer, the overwhelming force of mortality is always the breast cancer, but in women with smaller, node-negative breast cancers, other causes of mortality—eg, cardiovascular disease, complications of osteoporosis, and other cancers—are a bigger issue.

"Data suggest that besides prevention of breast cancer recurrence, tamoxifen has additional benefits that might impact overall survival. Namely, it can lower cholesterol levels and reduce hospital admissions for cardiovascular disease, as demonstrated in the Stockholm trial; and, as shown in the Scottish studies, even in older women, tamoxifen may reduce mortality from cardiovascular disease.

"On the other hand, perhaps these findings are not absolute. The overview analysis of adjuvant tamoxifen from the Early Breast Cancer Trialists' Collaborative Group failed to demonstrate a reduction in nonbreast cancer mortality with use of tamoxifen."

Data suggest that besides prevention of breast cancer recurrence, tamoxifen has additional benefits that might impact overall survival.

Dr. Henderson: "I was a little disconcerted with the overview analysis results showing no reduction in nonbreast cancer mortality with tamoxifen use, and I remain unconvinced that the current analysis provides the final word on the subject. The contributions of various trials to the overview have not been analyzed. For example, this effect on nonbreast cancer mortality, which was rather striking at the last overview analysis, may be less so now because of the inclusion of many more trials with shorter follow-up.

"As Dr. Morrow said, I think that for breast cancer patients with a low risk of recurrence, these issues are very important in the decision to take tamoxifen."

Dr. Jordan: "Patients in many of the trials in the meta-analysis have not necessarily used tamoxifen for 5 years, whereas the data on hormone replacement therapy in postmenopausal women suggest that longer is better in regard to maintaining protection against cardiovascular disease."

Dr. Osborne: "I think we should certainly raise these issues with patients and tell them that there may be additional ancillary benefits of tamoxifen use, even though the long-term benefits are uncertain."

Dr. Wolmark: "The Breast Cancer Prevention Trial (BCPT), along with its primary end point of breast cancer prevention, has other specific end points designed to measure the benefit of tamoxifen relative to osteoporosis (prevention of fractures) and cardiovascular disease (reduction in cardiovascular deaths). There are women who do not have breast cancer but who are at high risk for developing the disease, either because they are over age 60, they have one or more first-degree blood relatives who have had breast cancer, or they have had lobular carcinoma in situ treated by lumpectomy alone."

8. What are the breast cancer benefits of tamoxifen besides increased survival?

Dr. Jordan: "There are other important cancer-related benefits associated with tamoxifen that we have not yet addressed, and I'll ask Dr. Wolmark to review these."

Dr. Wolmark: "Two other important benefits associated with tamoxifen beyond any survival benefits are the reduction in the incidence of contralateral breast cancer and the prevention of breast cancer recurrence in patients who have had lumpectomies.

"In all of the NSABP studies in which we've used tamoxifen as an adjunct of the treatment of breast cancer, we've noted that the incidence of breast cancer in the opposite breast has been reduced by 40% to 50%. It was this observation that provided the background and justification to start the Breast Cancer Prevention Trial.

"Use of tamoxifen in breast conservation patients who have received radiotherapy reduces the risk of recurrence by an additional 3% at 10 years. So the chances of women keeping that breast is significantly improved when tamoxifen or chemotherapy is added to the regimen. I think this is an important benefit of tamoxifen that is totally overlooked in most studies that assess the risk-to-benefit ratio."

Dr. Morrow: "Whether or not tamoxifen use improves survival in women who have had breast conservation, it adds to the quality of life of these patients, since those who chose breast preservation did so because they wanted to keep their breast."

9. What are the concerns of giving tamoxifen to the premenopausal patient?

Dr. Jordan: "I would now like to ask the panel about the use of tamoxifen in the premenopausal patient. Concerns have been raised about high circulating levels of estradiol that sometimes cause irregular menstrual cycles. What are your thoughts about the risks-to-benefits ratio of tamoxifen in premenopausal patients? Dr. Osborne?"

Dr. Osborne: "I would not be very concerned about the menstrual irregularities. They do occur in maybe 20% or so of patients, but this is not a major problem. A potential problem is that many patients on tamoxifen do get elevated estradiol levels—significantly elevated in some cases—and there is the concern that these high levels may make the tamoxifen less effective by competing with tamoxifen molecules for the estrogen receptors. There have been no adequate studies to address this potential problem, however. Tumors need to be biopsied to measure the amount of estrogen and the amount of tamoxifen in the tumor. These kinds of studies are needed to really pin this down. However, clinical results are newly released suggesting that tamoxifen is still effective in premenopausal women despite this rise in estrogen levels.

The important aspect of this issue is not the theoretical objections to using tamoxifen in premenopausal women, but the actual effects of its use in prolonging disease-free and overall survival.

"There are four randomized trials in metastatic breast cancer comparing tamoxifen with ovarian ablation. These are all small trials, but when you pool the information, the relative effectiveness of tamoxifen in premenopausal women is in the same ballpark as that of ovarian ablation. The recent meta-analysis also suggests that adjuvant tamoxifen in estrogen receptor-positive premenopausal patients who have not received chemotherapy does offer a disease-free and overall survival advantage. So I think that while there may be some concerns about this rising estrogen level in young women, it doesn't appear to be important as a cause of resistance to the drug."

Dr. Wolmark: "I think the important aspect of this issue is not the theoretical objections to using tamoxifen in premenopausal women, but the actual effects of its use in prolonging disease-free and overall survival. The NSABP protocol B-14 assessed tamoxifen in both pre- and postmenopausal women with node-negative, receptor-positive disease. The study showed absolutely no difference in the responsiveness to tamoxifen based on age. The premenopausal women had prolongation of disease-free and overall survival just as the postmenopausal women. So I think that the suggestion that premenopausal patients are tamoxifen resistant is not borne out by the data from randomized clinical trials.

"I think a lot of the concerns were based on the earlier trials from node-positive patients, from which people concluded that adding tamoxifen to chemotherapy in young premenopausal women was not as effective as adding tamoxifen to chemotherapy in patients over age 50. This still needs to be assessed today, but certainly from the node-negative trials, there is no suggestion that there is a relationship between patient age and tamoxifen benefit."

Dr. Jordan: "Dr. Morrow, you mentioned earlier that your younger patients were concerned about the possibility of tamoxifen-induced menopause. Do you want to elaborate on that?"

Dr. Morrow: "Certainly there is a percentage of women taking tamoxifen who will get menstrual irregularity, but I think it is important to remember that for the majority of premenopausal women, tamoxifen actually acts as a stimulant to ovulation. In fact, the agent had a brief life as a fertility drug. So premenopausal women who are on tamoxifen need to be cautioned that pregnancy is a possibility and that barrier contraception should be used."

Dr. Jordan: "Dr. Henderson, would you like to comment on the possibility of tamoxifen resistance in younger women?"

Dr. Henderson: "I think, clearly, the question of tamoxifen resistance in premenopausal patients with metastatic breast cancer is a moot point. You can tell whether a patient responds, and if she is responding, then therapy should be continued. In the adjuvant setting, however, it is a bit more complicated. I don't think there is any question that adjuvant tamoxifen imparts substantial benefits when used in premenopausal women. From the most recent overview, it would appear that the use of tamoxifen alone produces a benefit of the same magnitude as seen in postmenopausal women.

"The unanswered questions, however, revolve around two points. One, is tamoxifen really equivalent to chemotherapy in younger women? Indirect comparison suggests that it might be. Two, is it equivalent to oophorectomy? We've done several randomized trials in patients with metastatic breast cancer. None of them was completely reliable, since those physicians who believed ovarian ablation was preferable failed to submit their patients for tamoxifen therapy and vice versa. But the results did suggest a trend in favor of ovarian ablation.

"A third question, which may be of the greatest practical importance, is whether the optimal duration of adjuvant tamoxifen may be different in younger and older women. Indirect comparisons of duration seemed to show that for older women, there was clearly a difference between 2 years and 1 year of tamoxifen, but it was not so clear that there was a difference between say, 5 years and 2 or 3 years. Among younger women, however, there clearly was very little or no benefit seen with 1 year of tamoxifen, and it was really only when we began using tamoxifen for 5 years, particularly in the NSABP trials, that we established without question that there was a benefit in the younger women.

"So I think this is a question that remains open. I think that there is probably going to be an optimal duration of treatment with tamoxifen, and I think it may differ for younger and older women."

10. What can be said about the appropriate duration of tamoxifen?

Dr. Jordan: "That is a good point, and it leads to the next discussion: the issue of how long tamoxifen should be given. The National Cancer Institute has recommended that physicians limit tamoxifen use in the treatment of early breast cancer to 5 years in clinical practice. The NCI announcement came on the heels of the decision by the NSABP to stop clinical trial B-14 from comparing 5 and 10 years of tamoxifen use after surgery in women with node-negative, ER-positive breast cancer.

We would like to think that because node-positive patients have a slightly worse prognosis, giving more tamoxifen is better; but that may not be the case.

"In this trial, 1,172 women who had been on tamoxifen for 5 years and had not relapsed were randomized a second time to either 5 more years of tamoxifen, 20 mg/day, or placebo. After 4 years of follow-up, 92% of the placebo group was alive and free of disease, compared with 86% of the group scheduled to receive 10 years of tamoxifen.

"The NSABP study is really only the first piece of evidence suggesting the optimal duration for the pre- and postmenopausal, ER-positive, node-negative woman. And it looks like 5 years may be the right way to go; but the optimal duration might be different in node-positive women. Dr. Osborne, would you comment on this issue?"

Dr. Osborne: "Ideas on tamoxifen duration have changed over the last 10 years. Initially, it was felt that since tamoxifen seemed to be predominantly a cytostatic agent, it might be best to continue the drug for a longer period of time, maybe indefinitely. Now, additional data, both clinical and laboratory, are accumulating to suggest that we may have been wrong in our initial hypothesis. Molecular biology studies suggest that, in some cases, tamoxifen, an antiestrogen, can become a stimulatory agent in the breast. It raises the possibility that there may be an optimal duration for tamoxifen in the adjuvant situation—it may be shorter than we might have imagined before."

Dr. Jordan: "I would like to emphasize that the NSABP results should be provided as evidence for that particular group of patients only—ER-positive, node-negative women. I would like to see a more definitive comparison in different stages of the disease and in both pre- and postmenopausal women. Such efforts are currently underway (see Chapter 11); But, unfortunately, there cannot be a definitive answer given at this point in time for all stages of the disease."

Dr. Osborne: "We would like to think that because node-positive patients have a slightly worse prognosis, giving more tamoxifen is better; but that may not be the case. And I think outside of a clinical research trial, I wouldn't give the agent for more than 5 years, even in node-positive patients.

"The NSABP trial is not alone in showing that extending tamoxifen duration beyond 5 years adds no further benefit. There is a smaller trial from Scotland that showed similar results, and the Scottish trial included both node-negative and node-positive patients."

Dr. Morrow: "The duration question is not completely answered, and we have traditionally been relatively reluctant to stop tamoxifen in node-positive patients who are disease free. A study of long-term tamoxifen users is ongoing in the United Kingdom, but it might take 20 years to answer the question." (See Chapter 11.)

Dr. Wolmark: "The issue of 5 vs 10 years in node-positive patients remains a valid research question. However, we at the NSABP have stopped tamoxifen at 5 years for our node-positive breast cancer protocols, based on the data from the node-negative population. I think this is the best information we have, and this decision has to be made by individual patients together with their physicians."

Dr. Jordan: "In my opinion, the question of 5 vs 10 years is almost a null hypothesis. Nobody has really done a valid comparison to determine an optimal tamoxifen duration. You won't be able to detect any difference between 5 and 10 years with clinical trials as they are set up because they are not large enough. An average size clinical trial would show no difference, just as the NSABP trial showed no significant difference.

"My early concern with the NSABP study was that it would show a significant detrimental effect after 10 years, with a large increase in recurrent disease, but that has not turned out to be the case."

11. How do you manage the menopausal symptomatology associated with tamoxifen use?

Dr. Jordan: "I would now like to ask our panel how they manage the postmenopausal symptoms that may occur with tamoxifen use, such as hot flashes and vaginal dryness. Dr. Wolmark, what are your specific recommendations for patients who develop these symptoms while taking tamoxifen?"

Dr. Wolmark: "The treatment of hot flashes in women taking tamoxifen can be problematic because of the need to limit estrogen use. We've tried various interventions such as Bellergal-S [belladonna, phenobarbital, and ergotamine tartrate], the low–dose Catapres [clonidine] patch, and vitamin E. And although these treatments have all been successful on occasion, none can be recommended as a standard intervention.

"When hot flashes are severe enough to significantly interfere with a woman's quality of life, then more aggressive therapy should be considered, including intravaginal estrogen preparations and even systemic estrogens. I want to make it very clear that I am not recommending systemic estrogens as an adjunct to tamoxifen to deal with symptoms. Rather, its use should be restricted to select cases of women with severe acute symptoms."

Hot flashes are not all that common and may be attributed both to tamoxifen and to the fact that many postmenopausal women stop hormone replacement therapy once breast cancer is diagnosed.

Ms. Langer: "Younger women on tamoxifen may find it especially difficult to cope when thrust into menopausal symptoms. The thoughtful oncologist will often give brief estrogen interventions to alleviate severe acute symptoms. It may not be commonly known in the medical community that this practice is acceptable, especially among primary care physicians who may be following these patients long term."

Dr. Osborne: "Luckily, hot flashes are not all that common and may be attributed both to tamoxifen and to the fact that many postmenopausal women stop hormone replacement therapy once breast cancer has been diagnosed. Anecdotally, I have had success in a handful of patients using serotonin reuptake inhibitors such as venlafaxine (Effexor) at doses that are subtherapeutic for antidepressive activity."

Dr. Ragaz: "In my experience, women who increase their physical activity, through jogging or other regular exercise, often see a decrease in their hot flashes."

Dr. Jordan: "What about vaginal dryness? Dr. Osborne?"

Dr. Osborne: "Vaginal dryness is generally easily managed with use of vaginal creams. In a patient who is on tamoxifen, I have little fear of absorption of estrogen from the vagina. Short-term treatment of a few weeks is often effective, and you may not have to treat the patient again for months or even years."

Dr. Barakat: "Local applications of lubricating agents such as Replens or Astroglide gel may also help patients with vaginal dryness with sexual function."

Dr. Ragaz: "Some of our patients with vaginal dryness have reported benefits with use of over-the-counter lubricants containing primrose oil or jelly."

12. Should chemotherapy be added to tamoxifen or vice versa?

Dr. Jordan: "That concludes my own list of questions for the panel, and now I would like to put to them some questions that have been collected from the audience. The first concerns the use of adjuvant chemotherapy in patients taking tamoxifen and is addressed to Dr. Osborne."

Dr. Osborne: "I think there are still some uncertainties in this area, and there are ongoing clinical trials that should help better define where we stand. But if you look at individual trials of premenopausal women, or the meta-analysis, of women who are getting chemotherapy, there doesn't seem to be much of an additional advantage for adding tamoxifen. It may be because many of these patients are already getting another endocrine therapy in the form of chemically induced ovarian ablation.

"The key question in older women is not whether you should add tamoxifen to chemotherapy, because in this group of patients, tamoxifen is the standard agent. The question is whether you should add chemotherapy to tamoxifen. The majority of the studies don't show a survival advantage for the addition of chemotherapy to tamoxifen, although they do show a disease-free survival advantage. However, in the 3-arm NSABP trial, the arm containing doxorubicin/cyclophosphamide therapy did show a disease-free survival advantage in postmenopausal, ER-positive women getting tamoxifen.

"Although the NSABP trial needs to be confirmed, I think we must conclude from the available evidence that in postmenopausal women, there may be a slight advantage of adding a doxorubicin-containing regimen to tamoxifen; whereas in younger women, I'm not convinced of any advantage for the addition of tamoxifen to chemotherapy."

Dr. Ragaz: "The Oxford Overview analysis initially showed a slight benefit of tamoxifen added to chemotherapy in premenopausal patients, but in the latest review, this was not significant. I would caution, however, that in most of the studies in the overview, women had taken tamoxifen for only 2 years, and we now know that 5 years is more beneficial. So the overview may not fully answer the question. This question is presently being tested in the prospective Canadian NCI MA-12 study, which is randomizing ER-positive premenopausal patients on adjuvant chemotherapy. This study will address the survival impact of tamoxifen for 5 years against placebo after the completion of chemotherapy. Therefore, the answer to this question will soon become available."

Misconceptions within the patient population can lead to potentially serious consequences, such as stopping a drug that will provide survival benefits.

13. Should patients taking tamoxifen worry about the development of "fatty liver?"

Dr. Jordan: "A patient advocate from the Alamo Breast Cancer Foundation in San Antonio says that she has encountered several patients on tamoxifen who have developed "fatty livers," and knows of two women who have stopped taking tamoxifen because of this finding. She asks if any panel members have seen this in their patients, and is it a concern?"

Dr. Wolmark: "We have not seen that specific entity as a result of tamoxifen treatment in the NSABP trials. We are unaware of this common phenomenon of fatty replacement of the liver occurring as a result of therapy with tamoxifen."

Unknown physician from audience: "Fatty liver is a benign condition that is actually quite common if you look for it, particularly in women who are overweight or have mild diabetes. Breast cancer patients taking tamoxifen are closely monitored for possible metastases, including CT scans of the abdomen. In reading these scans, the radiologist may note a fatty liver. That's actually reassuring to the oncologist and the patient because it does not represent metastatic disease, and it's not a problem that progresses to chronic liver disease. It frequently goes away with time, weight loss, or diabetes control."

Dr. Jordan: "This illustrates how misconceptions within the patient population can lead to potentially serious consequences, such as stopping a drug that will provide survival benefits."

14. Does tamoxifen have a role in ductal carcinoma in situ (DCIS)?

Dr. Jordan: "The next question, from a medical oncologist at the Medical University of South Carolina, Charleston, asks whether the NSABP B-24 protocol will define the use of tamoxifen in noninvasive breast cancer. Dr. Wolmark?"

Dr. Wolmark: "The NSABP B-17 trial determined that in patients with noninvasive breast cancer (DCIS), lumpectomy with radiation provides better local ipsilateral control than lumpectomy alone. The B-24 protocol answers the question of whether adding tamoxifen to lumpectomy and radiation therapy in these patients will offer further improvement in local control.

"Unfortunately, we don't have the data from that trial yet. But if tamoxifen and radiotherapy in every other situation have been better than radiotherapy alone in controlling local ipsilateral recurrence, we're certainly hopeful that will be the case for DCIS, where one of the things we're trying to control is the subsequent occurrence of invasive cancer.

15. How long should a male breast cancer patient receive adjuvant tamoxifen?

Dr. Jordan: "Now we have a question from a male survivor of breast cancer who has been taking tamoxifen for 2½ years. He wants to know if the recommendation to stop tamoxifen after 5 years applies to male breast cancer patients as well. Dr. Osborne?"

Dr. Osborne: "Male breast cancer seems to behave, in many ways, just like the female counterpart. Since it is so uncommon, there are no large studies, as there are in female breast cancer, to address the question of duration. However, for a male breast cancer patient taking adjuvant tamoxifen after surgery who has never had disease recurrence, I would follow the same rules as female breast cancer. And my opinion is that outside of a clinical study, the drug should be stopped at 5 years. There are no data to suggest that longer than 5 years is better."

16. What happens if a patient stops taking tamoxifen on her own?

Dr. Jordan: "A member of the audience notes that physicians can't always control what their patients do; they can only advise. The question is: What happens if a patient stops taking tamoxifen on her own just to see if certain symptoms go away? Dr. Osborne, can you answer that?"

Dr. Osborne: "I'm sure that this is common, and I've had a number of patients tell me they have stopped the drug for a couple of weeks to see if it relieved symptoms. To really make an impact on the serum drug levels, however, you would have to stop taking tamoxifen for at least several weeks.

Health food store products are a bit of a black box because you don't know their exact components.

"We don't know what effect, if any, there would be on breast cancer survival if tamoxifen was stopped for a longer period of time, say 3 to 6 months. If the drug were restarted, perhaps the impact would be minimal, maybe not even measurable. After all, it's a small period of time relative to the 5 years that the woman may be taking tamoxifen. So I think if a patient came to me and said she had stopped for 3 months but then restarted, I would say she probably had nothing to worry about."

17. Is it safe for patients to use phytoestrogen products to treat menopausal symptoms associated with tamoxifen?

Dr. Jordan: "We have a question about how physicians should respond to patients on tamoxifen who want to try so-called natural estrogen products to relieve menopausal symptoms? Dr. Osborne, can you comment?"

Dr. Osborne: "Phytoestrogen products are being sold in health food stores as remedies for hot flashes; and although some of them may work, I have always been hesitant to suggest them to patients because of the uncertainty about what is in them. They could contain 'good estrogens' in the sense that they block the breast-cancer-promoting effects of the 'bad' natural estrogen produced by the body. Soy products, for example, contain estrogen, and it has been suggested that the high soy consumption in Asian countries has helped account for the lower incidence of breast cancer in Asian women. But these health food store products are a bit of a black box because you don't know their exact components."

Dr. Henderson: "Perhaps because I am from California, I have seen a number of patients on tamoxifen who have sought relief of hot flashes with phytoestrogen preparations. In general, I feel that these are probably neither safer nor more harmful than short courses of estrogen; but I try to make certain that patients who use them are fully informed."

18. Why do the effects of tamoxifen last so long?

Dr. Jordan: "Another audience member from the Alamo Breast Cancer Foundation wants to know why, if tamoxifen is cytostatic rather than cytotoxic, it continues to work after it is stopped. I would like to comment first, and then I'll turn the question over to Dr. Osborne.

"Tamoxifen may help control breast cancer in a variety of ways: Laboratory evidence suggests that, in addition to its cytostatic effects, tamoxifen also has a cytocidal effect, killing off breast cancer cells. It also appears to have a profound effect on angiogenesis, eradicating tumor cells by denying them a blood supply."

Dr. Osborne: "Just 1 year of tamoxifen therapy has been shown to reduce the risk of breast cancer recurrence 10 years later. So there seems to be some permanent effect. You don't have to kill the tumor cells to eradicate the tumor if you can stop tumor cell proliferation. Tumor cells continue to die off naturally, but the number of replacement cells is so large that the tumor grows bigger over time. If you can shut off that proliferation, which is what we think tamoxifen does, then you could eradicate all the tumor cells without directly killing any of them."

Dr. Jordan: "I think we have entered an age of uncertainty about how long to give tamoxifen. We have to trust the evidence emerging from clinical trials and reevaluate our previous model. However, it may be that the gains that we get in some patients with long-term tamoxifen use are offset by tamoxifen-stimulated growth in other patients. All patients are different, and this is why we must have huge clinical trials to answer the question."

Dr. Wolmark: "I would like to emphasize that just because we're recommending tamoxifen be stopped at 5 years, it doesn't mean that stopping tamoxifen will cause the tumor to start growing again. That's not what's happening. Whatever benefit is accumulated over that 5 years continues through 10 years of follow-up. What the NSABP study has shown is that adding 5 extra years of tamoxifen therapy does not increase the benefit and, also, that there's no rebound effect, no increased incidence of recurrence after tamoxifen is stopped."

Dr. Jordan: "That concludes our discussion. I would like to thank the entire panel for their excellent contributions, and I would also like to thank PRR, Inc. for putting on this event. Our hope was to be able to convey to a broader community the idea that the benefits of tamoxifen should be rationally weighed against the toxicities that have been seen. From the perspective of the benefits, I think the panel as a whole would agree that tamoxifen's benefits far outweigh any of the concerns that have been raised."

Chapter 15

Breast Cancer: Who and Why?

Monica Morrow, MD

Breast cancer is the most common cancer in American women and the second most common cause of cancer death. Current estimates indicate that the lifetime risk of developing breast cancer is 12.2%, or 1 in 8 women, and that the risk of breast cancer death is 3.6%, or 1 in 282.[1] The knowledge that breast cancer is a common disease, coupled with awareness on the part of both physicians and women of the factors that increase breast cancer risk, has caused concerns that breast cancer is an "epidemic," thereby leading many women to overestimate their level of risk.

Incidence

Everyone is familiar with the American Cancer Society statistic that 1 in 8 women will develop breast cancer. What many do not realize, however, is that this is a cumulative risk estimate, with half of a woman's risk occurring after the age of 65. As illustrated in Figure 1, age is a major breast cancer risk factor, with the majority of cancers occurring in women over age 55. The baseline risk for younger women, in the absence of other major risk factors, is quite low, and the chance of developing breast cancer between the ages of 35 and 55 is only 2.5% (Table 1).[2] It is also noteworthy that these figures represent the risk of *developing* breast cancer, not the risk of *dying* from breast cancer. The risk of dying of the disease is substantially lower—only 3.6% in a woman's lifetime.

If these statistics are true, how can we explain the large number of breast cancer cases being seen today, particularly in younger women? An examination of breast cancer incidence (number of cases per 100,000 women) from 1970 to 1993 reveals a small but real increase in the incidence of the disease (Figure 2). This increase is evident for all age groups, but certainly does not qualify as an epidemic. What has changed dramatically during that time period, however, is the number of younger women at risk. As illustrated in Figure 3, the aging of the post-World War II "baby boom" generation has resulted in an increase in the absolute number of women at risk for breast cancer and a corresponding increase in the absolute number of cases. Thus, in 1970, 5,120 cases of breast cancer in women under age 40 were reported to

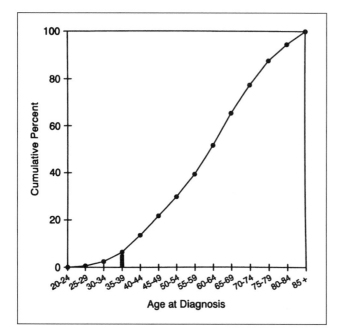

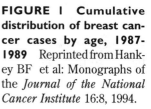

FIGURE 1 Cumulative distribution of breast cancer cases by age, 1987-1989 Reprinted from Hankey BF et al: Monographs of the *Journal of the National Cancer Institute* 16:8, 1994.

the Surveillance, Epidemiology, and End Results (SEER) program. This increased to 7,800 cases in 1980 and 10,050 cases in 1990, while the actual incidence of the disease remained fairly stable.[1]

Risk Factors

As with many other cancers, the etiology of breast cancer appears to be multifactorial. Both endogenous and exogenous factors are known to increase breast cancer risk. In addition to age, family history, reproductive history, and benign breast disease, endogenous factors also contribute to risk. Exposure to ionizing radiation is perhaps the most well-documented exogenous risk factor, but diet, alcohol, pesticides, and electromagnetic fields have all been suggested to increase breast cancer risk. While most people recognize the existence of risk factors, the magnitude of the increase in risk associated with these factors is often poorly understood, and knowledge of the interactions among risk factors is limited.

Family History

Family history is probably the most widely recognized breast cancer risk factor. It is now apparent that there are two very different levels of risk in women with family histories of breast cancer, one due to a genetically inherited predisposition to breast cancer, and the other associated with an increased familial incidence of breast cancer. At present, mutations in three genes, p53, BRCA-1, and BRCA-2, have been associated with a genetic predisposition to breast cancer. It is likely that additional genes will be identified in the future. Genetic breast cancer is uncommon, and is thought to account for only 5% to 10% of breast cancers in the US.[3,4] Familial characteristics suggestive of a genetic predisposition to breast cancer are listed in Table 2. The risk of genetic breast cancer associated with various combinations of these factors is shown in Table 3.

Since predisposing genes may be inherited from male or female relatives, and appear to be transmitted in an autosomal, dominant fashion,[4] a breast cancer risk assessment should include an evaluation of both maternal and paternal family histories. In an individual woman with breast cancer, the possibility that the disease resulted from a predisposing gene is related to the age at which disease developed. It is estimated that 12% of women diagnosed with breast cancer before the age of 30 carry such a gene, compared with 3% diagnosed between ages 40 and 49.

BRCA-1

Mutations of the BRCA-1 gene, located on chromosome 17q2l, are associated with a risk of both breast and ovarian cancer.[5] For women with these mutations, the risk of developing breast cancer before age 50 is estimated to be 50%, increasing to 85% by age 65. The risk of a second breast cancer is 65% by age 70.

Table 1

Probability of Developing and Dying of Breast Cancer

Age (Years)	Risk of Breast Cancer Development	Risk of Breast Cancer Death
Birth-110	10.2%	3.6%
65-110	6.53%	1.53%
20-40	0.49%	0.09%
35-55	2.53%	0.56%
50-70	4.67%	1.04%
65-85	5.48%	1.01%

Data from Seidman et al.[2]

The risk of ovarian cancer development is less well quantified and ranges from 20% to 50%. Mutations of BRCA-1 also appear to be associated with a 2-fold increase in the risk of prostate cancer and a small increase in the risk of colon cancer. Two specific mutations of BRCA-1 (185 delAG and 538 insC) were identified in 1% and 0.1% of Ashkenazi Jewish families. A specific mutation of BRCA-2 (6174 delT) has also been identified in 1.4% of this population.[6,7] These mutations may account for as many as 30% to 50% of breast cancer cases occurring in young Ashkenazi women; further studies, however, are needed to confirm this.

To date, more than 300 different mutations of the BRCA-1 gene have been identified. As more women are tested, more mutations will be identified. The level of cancer risk associated with each of these individual mutations is uncertain, since estimates of risks established to date were derived from the study of a relatively small number of families selected for their very high incidence of breast cancer.

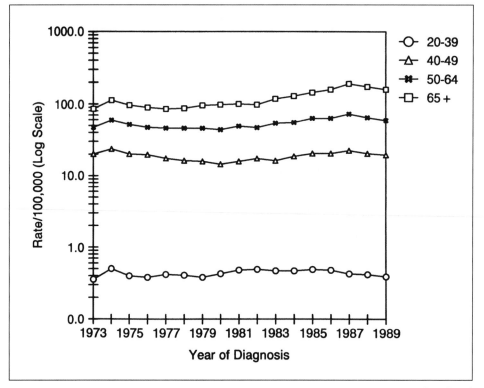

FIGURE 2 **Incidence rates for invasive breast cancer 1979-1989, by age** Reprinted from Hankey BF et al: Monographs of the *Journal of the National Cancer Institute* 16:8, 1994.

Table 2

Familial Characteristics Suggestive of a Genetic Predisposition to Breast Cancer

Multiple relatives (usually > 3) with breast cancer

History of breast and ovarian cancer

Early-onset breast cancer

Bilateral breast cancer

BRCA-2

Mutations of the BRCA-2 gene, located on chromosome 13, appear to carry the same level of breast cancer risk as mutations of BRCA-1.[8] With this genetic mutation, however, there may be a smaller increase in the risk of ovarian cancer. In addition, BRCA-2 mutations are associated with an increased risk of breast cancer in men.

In contrast to women with a genetic predisposition to breast cancer, women with an increased familial incidence of breast cancer have a much lower risk of the disease. The level of risk in familial breast cancer varies

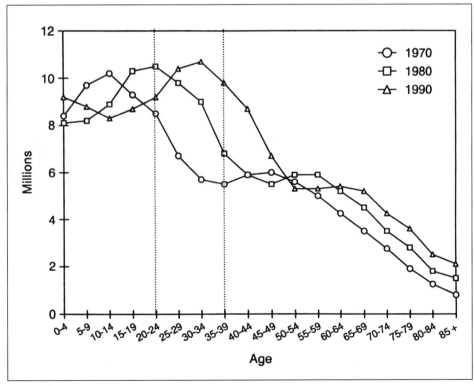

FIGURE 3 **Changes in the age distribution of the US female population by year**   Reprinted from Hankey BF et al: Monographs of the *Journal of the National Cancer Institute* 15:9, 1994.

Table 3

Estimated Probability of Breast Cancer Being Due to the BRCA-1 Gene

Criterion, Cancer, Age (y)	Probability Case Has a BRCA-1 Mutation
Single Affected	
Breast < 30	0.12
Breast < 40	0.06
Breast 40 - 49	0.03
Ovarian < 50	0.07
Sister Pairs	
Breast < 40, Breast < 40	0.37
Breast 40 - 49, Breast 40-49	0.20
Breast < 50, Ovarian < 50	0.61
Families	
Breast only ≥ 3 cases, diagnosed < 50	0.40
≥ 2 breast, ≥ 1 ovarian	0.82
≥ 2 breast, ≥ 2 ovarian	0.91

according to the degree of closeness with the affected relative and the age at which the relative developed the disease.[9,10] As illustrated in Table 4, the cumulative risk of breast cancer development in a woman with familial breast cancer rarely exceeds 30%.

The preceding discussion makes it clear that the ability to identify carriers of breast cancer predisposition genes is of great value when counseling women about their personal levels of breast cancer risk. Nevertheless, there are a number of issues surrounding the practice of genetic testing that must be considered.

First, genetic testing is a technique that is still in its infancy, and widespread standards for quality control have not yet been developed. In addition, false-positive and false-negative rates are unknown. Second, a positive test has the potential to produce severe anxiety, while a negative test may engender feelings of guilt, either of which can produce familial discord. In addition, genetic testing has the potential to reveal unsuspected information, such as the lack of a biologic relationship with a parent. A positive test also carries enormous implications for insurability, so confidentiality is a major issue.

Table 4

Breast Cancer Risk in Familial, Nonhereditary Cases

Affected Relative, Age	% Risk by Age 80
One first degree, < 50	13%-21%
One first degree, > 50	9%-11%
One second degree, < 50	10%-14%
Two second degree, < 50	21%-26%
Two first degree, < 50	35%-48%
Two first degree, > 50	11%-24%

Finally, a negative test does not necessarily eliminate the possibility of a genetic predisposition to breast cancer. For example, if a healthy woman with several affected relatives tests negative for a BRCA-1 mutation, it could mean that she does not carry the abnormal gene and is not at increased risk; or it could mean that BRCA-1 is not the gene responsible for breast cancer in her family. The information gained from testing will be greatly enhanced by testing a relative with breast cancer, as well as the non-affected woman who wants to know her genetic status.

The information presented above makes it clear that there are multiple uncertainties surrounding genetic testing. Many women do not consider prophylactic mastectomy an option regardless of their level of risk. Further, the effect of tamoxifen on breast cancer risk in women with mutations of a predisposition gene still remains uncertain (see Chapter 16). For these reasons, some women at risk for genetic breast cancer may opt not to be tested for predisposition genes. Genetic testing is not simply the ordering of a blood test. A counseling session prior to a decision to be tested should include a discussion of the problems and uncertainties associated with testing. In women who opt to be tested, a follow-up session to discuss the meaning of test results and to develop a surveillance strategy is a necessity.

Hormonal Factors

Breast cancer is clearly related to hormones, and numerous studies have linked breast cancer incidence to the age of menarche, menopause, and first pregnancy. The greatest risk is associated with a long period of uninterrupted menstrual cycles. There appears to be a 20% decrease in breast cancer risk for each year that menarche is delayed.[11] Other factors that delay the establishment of regular ovulatory cycles, such as physical activity, may also decrease risk.[12] Age at menopause also influences breast cancer risk, with women whose natural menopause occurs before age 45 having half the relative risk of breast cancer of women whose menopause occurs after age 55.[13] Oophorectomy results in similar risk reductions.

Table 5

Hormonal Risk Factors for Breast Cancer Development

Factor	Relative Risk
MENSTRUAL HISTORY	
Menarche < 12 yrs	1.3
Menopause > 55 yrs	1.5-2.0
Menopause < 45 yrs	0.77
PREGNANCY	
First live birth 25-29 yrs	1.5
First live birth after 30 yrs	1.9
First live birth after 35 yrs	2.0-3.0
Nulliparous	1.4-3.0

Parity and age at first birth have also been shown to influence risk. Nulliparous women are at greater risk than those who are parous, with a relative risk of about 1.4. The effect of term pregnancy on risk varies with age at first birth, with women whose first pregnancy occurs after age 30 having a 2- to 5-fold increase in risk compared with women whose first-term pregnancy is before age 18 or 19.[14,15] Abortion, whether spontaneous or induced, has no protective effect. Some studies have shown an increase in risk after incomplete pregnancy, while others show no effect.[16-18] The magnitude of increase in risk for hormonal risk factors is summarized in Table 5. Studies of the effect of lactation on breast cancer risk have had variable results, but some have suggested that lactation for prolonged periods of time may reduce breast cancer risk in premenopausal women, while having little effect on the risk of postmenopausal breast cancer.[19,20]

The effect of exogenous hormones, in the form of oral contraceptives and hormone replacement therapy, has been extensively studied; but clear evidence of a major influence on risk is lacking. Overall, there is no convincing evidence of an increased risk of breast cancer in women who have ever used oral contraceptives.[21-23] Studies of women with family histories of breast cancer or of benign breast disease have also failed to demonstrate an increased risk when oral contraceptives are used.

Studies of hormone replacement therapy have produced more variable results, but two meta-analyses suggest small but statistically significant increases in risk (relative risk 1.3 and 1.06) related to the duration of estrogen use.[24,25] For the majority of women, however, the benefits of hormone replacement therapy in reducing the risk of cardiovascular disease and osteoporosis outweigh the small increase in breast cancer risk.

Dietary Factors

The observation that national per capita fat consumption is correlated with breast cancer incidence and mortality suggests a possible relationship between diet and breast cancer risk. Nevertheless, epidemiologic studies of fat consumption and breast cancer risk have been inconclusive. In the largest prospective study of dietary fat, 89,538 nurses between the ages of 34 and 59 were studied. No relationship between the intake of total fat, saturated fat, cholesterol, or linoleic acid and breast cancer risk was found.[26] A review of 10 prospective studies (Figure 4) also failed to demonstrate a relationship between dietary fat (within the context of Western diets) and risk.[27] However, these studies do not exclude the possibility that a low dietary fat intake in childhood or extremely low-fat diets may alter risk.

Evidence supports a relationship between alcohol intake and breast cancer risk. A meta-analysis of 12 case control studies demonstrated a relative risk of 1.4 for each 24 grams of alcohol consumed per day (about 2 drinks),[28] data from prospective studies confirmed this risk.[29,30] It is unclear, however, whether it is drinking early in life or ongoing drinking that increases risk.

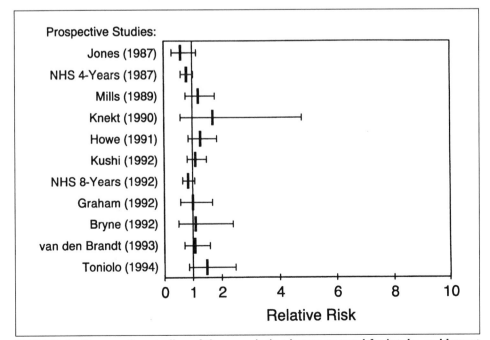

FIGURE 4   Prospective studies of the association between total fat intake and breast cancer   Vertical bars represent the relative risk for the highest category of fat intake. Reprinted from Hunter D, Willet W: *Dietary Factors in Diseases of the Breast,* p 203. Philadelphia, Lippincott-Raven, 1996. With permission.

Benign Breast Disease

Benign breast lesions are classified as nonproliferative, proliferative, or atypical. Nonproliferative lesions are not associated with increased breast cancer risk and accounted for 69% of 10,000 biopsies reported by DuPont and Page in 1985.[32] Proliferative disease is associated with a small increase in breast cancer risk (relative risk 1.5 to 2.0), while atypical hyperplasia carries the greatest risk of cancer development (relative risk 4 to 5).[31,32]

However, when strict diagnostic criteria are used, atypical hyperplasia is identified infrequently, and accounted for only

Table 6

Classification of Benign Breast Disease

Nonproliferative: No Increase in Risk

Adenosis	Fibrosis
Cysts—Micro or Macro	Mastitis
Duct ectasia	Metaplasia—squamous or apocrine
Fibroadenoma	Mild hyperplasia

Proliferative: 1.5- to 2.0-Fold Increase in Risk

Moderate or florid hyperplasia

Sclerosing adenosis

Papilloma with fibrovascular core

Atypia: 4.0- to 5.0-Fold Increase in Risk

Atypical hyperplasia—lobular or ductal

3.6% of the cases in the study by DuPont and Page. In this study, when atypical hyperplasia occurred in a woman with a family history of breast cancer, risk was substantially increased. The absolute risk of breast cancer development in women with a positive family history and atypical hyperplasia was 20% at 15 years, compared with 8% in women with atypical hyperplasia and a negative family history of breast cancer. Interestingly, no further increase in the risk of breast cancer was observed in women with proliferative disease who used estrogen after their breast biopsies.[33] These histologic diagnoses are classified under the headings of proliferative, nonproliferative, and atypical (listed in Table 6).

Another benign breast lesion that is clearly associated with an increased risk of breast cancer development is lobular carcinoma in situ (LCIS). In the past, LCIS was thought to be a malignant lesion, albeit one with a favorable prognosis. However, the finding that LCIS is associated with a risk of breast cancer development of approximately 1% per year, the observation that the risk of carcinoma is equal in both breasts, and the finding that neither the extent of LCIS in the breast nor its presence at a margin of resection influences the risk of subsequent cancer, have led LCIS to be regarded as a risk factor for breast cancer development—rather than an actual precursor of carcinoma.[34-39] The reported incidence and relative risk of carcinoma in patients with LCIS are summarized in Table 7.

Table 7

Risk of Invasive Carcinoma After LCIS

Author	Cases	% Invasive Cancer	Relative Risk
Haagensen et al [33]	287	18.0	6.9
Rosen et al [34]	99	34.5	9.0
Andersen [35]	47	26.4	12.0
Page et al [36]	44	23.0	9.0
Salvadori et al [37]	80	6.3	10.0
Ottesen et al [38]	69	11.6	11.0

Environmental Factors

Exposure to moderate- to high-dose ionizing radiation, either secondary to nuclear explosion or medical diagnostic and therapeutic procedures, increases breast cancer risk.[40-43] The level of risk is dependent on age at exposure, with a minimal increase in risk for exposure after age 40.[40-43] However, less than 1% of breast cancers are estimated to result from common radiologic diagnostic procedures such as chest x-rays or mammography.[44] In 1993, a markedly increased risk of breast cancer development was reported in women receiving mantle irradiation for the treatment of Hodgkin's disease before 15 years of age.[43] Other environmental factors, including exposure to electromagnetic fields, occupational exposures, and organochlorine pesticides, have been suggested to increase breast cancer risk,[45,46] but definitive data supporting these associations are still lacking.

Interactions Among Risk Factors

The majority of studies have focused on defining individual risk factors. This has created a lack of knowledge about interactions among the various known risk factors. In turn, this lack of knowledge has led to difficulties in the clinical identification of the "high-risk" woman.

Most women have a combination of factors that both increase risk and are protective, thereby complicating the assessment of an individual's level of risk. In addition, it is unclear whether the risk conferred by multiple risk factors is additive, multiplicative, or varies with the risk factor under study.

Interactions between a family history of breast cancer and other risk factors have been examined, often with conflicting results. As noted, Dupont

---

Table 8

History for Evaluation of Breast Cancer Risk

Patient Age

Reproductive History

Age of menarche

Parity, age at first birth

Age of menopause

Use of exogenous estrogen

Family History—Maternal and Paternal Relatives

Age at diagnosis, laterality of breast cancers

Presence of other cancer, especially ovarian

Number of unaffected relatives

Prior Biopsies

Number

Histologic diagnosis

Alcohol Intake

Exposure to Ionizing Radiation

---

and Page[31] observed that the combination of atypical hyperplasia and a family history of a first-degree relative with breast cancer increased the relative risk of breast cancer to 11 times that of the index population—compared to a relative risk of 4.4 for atypia alone. However, Rosen[35] found that the presence of a family history of breast carcinoma did not alter the level of risk after a diagnosis of LCIS—a lesion often considered part of a continuum with atypical hyperplasia.

An analysis of data from the Nurses' Health Study[47] found that in women with a mother or sister with breast cancer, known risk factors of age at menarche or menopause, parity, age at first birth, alcohol use, and the presence of benign breast disease did not further alter risk. Others [48,49] have reported that hormonal factors further modulated risk in women with a family history of breast cancer—although the effect varied with the factor under study.

Studies also occurred regarding the interaction between estrogen replacement therapy and other known breast cancer risk factors. Their results were variable, depending on the risk factor under study. In a meta-analysis of 16 published studies, Steinberg et al[50] found that the effect of estrogen replacement did not differ among parous and nulliparous women and those with or without benign breast disease. However, an enhanced risk was observed in women with a family history of breast cancer.

The analysis of the interaction among risk factors is further complicated by the fact that some factors may be important for the risk of premenopausal, but not postmenopausal cancer, and vice versa. Furthermore, these risks may not be constant over time. For example, a long duration of lactation appears to reduce premenopausal breast cancer risk; yet long lactation appears to have little impact on the risk of the more frequently encountered postmenopausal breast cancer.[51] In general, pregnancy reduces breast cancer risk; however, for a short period following pregnancy, risk is actually increased.[52]

Women with proliferative breast disease have a doubling of their relative risk of breast cancer; but 10 years after diagnosis, this risk returns to baseline. Similarly, the relative risk seen with a diagnosis of atypical hyperplasia is halved after a 10-year interval.[31]

A model to predict the risk of breast cancer development in women at a given age over a defined time interval was developed by Gail et al[54] using data from 4,496 matched pairs of cases and controls in the Breast Cancer Diagnosis and Demonstration Project. The model incorporated the risk factors of age at menarche, age at first live birth, number of first-degree relatives with breast cancer, and number of previous breast biopsies. The model was able to accurately predict risk in two validation studies of women undergoing annual mammographic screening.[55,56]

The model, however, overestimated breast cancer risk by 33% among women aged 60 and younger who did not undergo annual screening. There were several other limitations of the model, as well. Since only first-degree relatives were considered, it was not an appropriate model for women with extensive family histories of breast cancer, where risk may have been underestimated. In women with risk due to LCIS or atypical hyperplasia, the model underestimated risk, since the highest relative risk for breast biopsy was 2.0. Similarly, for the woman with nonproliferative disease, the model may have overestimated risk. In spite of these limitations, however, the model is still a clinically useful tool for identifying a woman's level of risk over a clinically relevant time period, after correction for competing causes of mortality.

From the preceding discussion, it can be appreciated that the problem of identification of the high-risk woman is far from solved. Many "risk factors" lack firm documentation of their clinical significance. Further, the interaction among risk factors and their variability over time is poorly understood.

The vast majority of data on risk comes from studies of white women. Little is known about the impact of ethnic diversity on the importance of these factors. In addition, there is no consensus regarding what level of increase in risk is necessary for a woman to be labeled high risk.

It is noteworthy that the majority of women with risk factors associated with the highest risk of breast cancer development will not develop breast carcinoma. Great caution must be exercised in labeling a woman as high risk, since such a label often results in increased anxiety for both the woman and

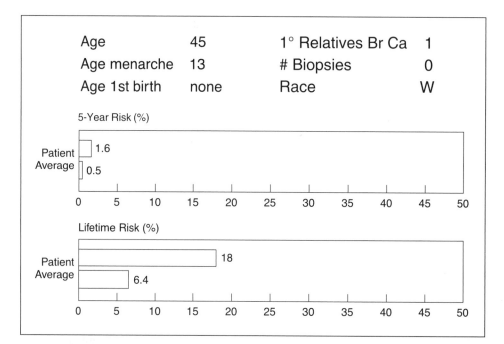

FIGURE 5 Risk assessment for breast cancer in a woman with 2 risk factors The woman illustrated here has a mother with breast cancer and has never had any children. The combination of these factors means that her 5-year risk of breast cancer development is 1.6%, compared to 0.5% in a woman with no risk factors. If she lives to age 70, her risk will be 18%, compared to 6.4% for the woman with no risk factors. This level of risk would not have qualified the woman to participate in the BCP Trial.

her physician, along with the potential for excessive numbers of mammograms and breast biopsies. It is also significant to note that approximately 50% of women who develop breast cancer have no risk factors beyond being an aging female.[53]

A risk evaluation begins with a careful history to evaluate the presence of known risk factors (Table 8) and a breast examination to exclude the presence of breast pathology and assess the difficulty of the examination. In women aged 40 and older, a mammogram should also be obtained. Since most women overestimate the risk of developing the disease, an attempt should be made to provide the patient with a quantitative estimate of her absolute risk of breast cancer over a defined time interval. The Gail model discussed above provides this information. These data were used in the NSABP P-1 prevention trial to estimate the risk level of participants. The risk levels calculated by this model are shown in Figures 5 and 6 for two sample patients.

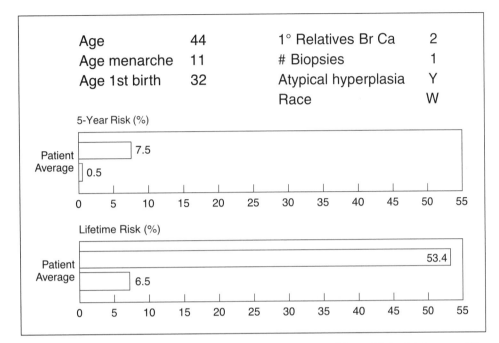

FIGURE 6 Risk assessment for breast cancer in a woman with multiple risk factors The
woman illustrated here had early menarche, late age at first birth, and has a mother and a sister
with breast cancer. In addition, she has had a breast biopsy showing atypical hyperplasia. This
combination of risk factors makes her 5-year risk of breast cancer development 7.5%, and her
lifetime risk, 53.4%.

At present, the options available to the high-risk woman are careful surveillance, prophylactic mastectomy, or tamoxifen.[57,58] The efficacy of careful
surveillance, which usually consists of a monthly breast self-examination, a
physician breast examination every 4 to 6 months, and an annual mammography, is still unknown. Prophylactic mastectomy, although clearly reducing
breast cancer risk, is not 100% protective. In this era of breast-conserving
treatment for carcinoma, prophylactic mastectomy is viewed by many as
excessively radical. There are no absolute indications for prophylactic mastectomy, since the acceptable degree of breast cancer risk will vary among
individuals. The long-term risk of breast cancer development in a population
of high-risk women undergoing prophylactic mastectomy is still uncertain.
The decision to use tamoxifen for risk reduction must be made after a careful
weighing of its risks and benefits, which are discussed in detail in the
following chapter.

For many high-risk women, though, tamoxifen is a welcome alternative to the "watch and wait" policy or prophylactic mastectomy.

Summary

Although a number of breast cancer risk factors have been identified, the mechanisms by which risk is increased remain uncertain, as are the interactions between factors that increase and decrease the risk of the disease. In addition, half of the women who develop breast cancer have no identifiable risk factors, indicating that strategies for the prevention and early detection of breast cancer must continue to be directed at the population of women as a whole in order to impact breast cancer morbidity and mortality. ∎

References

1. Miller BA, Feuer EJ, Hankey BF: The significance of the rising incidence of breast cancer in the United States, in DeVita VT, Hellman S, Rosenberg SA (eds): *Important Advances in Oncology 1994*, p. 193. Philadelphia, JB Lippincott, 1994.

2. Seidman H, Mushinski M, Gelb S: Probability of eventually developing or dying of breast cancer, United States. *CA Cancer J Clin* 35:36-56, 1985.

3. Claus E, Rich N, Thompson W: Genetic analysis of breast cancer in the Cancer and Steroid Hormone Study. *Am J Hum Genet* 48:232-242, 1991.

4. Weber B, Garber J: Familial breast cancer, in Harris J, Lippman M, Morrow M, Hellman S (eds.): p. 168. *Diseases of the Breast.* Philadelphia, Lippincott-Raven 1996.

5. Miki Y, Swensen J, Shattuck-Eidens D, et al: A strong candidate for the breast and ovarian cancer susceptibility gene BRCA-1. *Science* 266:66-71, 1994.

6. Strewing J, Abeliovich D, Peterz T, et al: The carrier frequency of the BRCA-1 185 delAG mutation is approximately 1 percent in Ashkenazi Jewish individuals. *Nat Genet* 11:198, 1995.

7. Neuhausan S, Gilewski T, Offit K, et al: Recurrent BRCA-2 6174 delT mutations in Ashkenazi Jewish women affected by breast cancer. *Nat Genet* 14:185,1996.

8. Wooster R, Neuhausen SL, Mangion J, et al: Localization of a breast cancer susceptibility gene, BRCA-2, to chromosome 13 q 12-13. *Science* 265:2088, 1994.

9. Hoskins KF, Stopfer JE, Calzone KA, et al: Assessment and counseling for women with a family history of breast cancer. A guide for clinicians. *JAMA* 273:577-585, 1995.

10. Claus EB, Risch NJ, Thompson WD: Autosomal dominant inheritance of early onset breast cancer. *Cancer* 73:643-651, 1994.

11. MacMahon B, Cole P, Brown J: Etiology of human breast cancer: A review. *J Natl Cancer Inst* 50:21-42, 1973.

12. Bernstein L, Ross R, Lobo R: The effects of moderate physical activity on menstrual cycle patterns in adolescence: Implications for breast cancer prevention. *Br J Cancer* 55:681-685, 1987.

13. Trichopoulos D, MacMahon B, Cole P: Menopause and breast cancer risk. *J Natl Cancer Inst* 48:605-613, 1972.

14. MacMahon B, Cole P, Lin T: Age at first birth and breast cancer risk. *Bull WHO* 43:209-221, 1970.

15. Trichopoulos D, Hsieh C, MacMahon B: Age at first birth and breast cancer risk. *Int J Cancer* 31:701-704, 1983.

16. Howe H, Senie R, Bzsuch H, et al: Early abortion and breast cancer risk in women under age 40. *Int J Epidemiol* 18:300-304, 1989.

17. Newcomb P, Storer B, Longnecker M, et al: Pregnancy termination in relation to risk of breast cancer. *JAMA* 275:283-287, 1996.

18. Adami H, Bergstrom R, Lund E, et al: Absence of association between reproductive variables and the risk of breast cancer in young women in Sweden and Norway. *Br J Cancer* 62:122-126, 1990.

19. Newcomb P, Storer B, Longnecker M, et al: Lactation and a reduced risk of premenopausal breast cancer. *N Engl J Med* 330:81-87, 1994.

20. Yuan J, Yu M, Ross R, et al: Risk factors for breast cancer in Chinese women in Shanghai. *Cancer Res* 48:1949, 1988.

21. Romieu L, Berlin J, Colditz G: Oral contraceptives and breast cancer: Review and meta-analysis. *Cancer* 66:2253, 1990.

22. Thomas D: Oral contraceptives and breast cancer: Review of the epidemiologic literature. *Contraception* 43:597-642, 1991.

23. Malone K, Daling J, Weiss N: Oral contraceptives in relation to breast cancer. *Epidemiol Rev* 15:80-97, 1993.

24. Silleros-Arena M, Delgado-Rodriguez M, Rodigues-Canteras R, et al: Menopausal hormone replacement therapy and breast cancer: A meta-analysis. *Obstet Gynecol* 79:286, 1992.

25. Steinberg K, Thacker S, Smith S, et al: A meta-analysis of the effect of estrogen replacement therapy on the risk of breast cancer. *JAMA.* 265:1985-1990, 1991.

26. Willett W, Stampfer M, Colditz G: Dietary fat and risk of breast cancer. *N Engl J Med* 316:22-28, 1987.

27. Hunter DJ, Willett WC: Dietary factors in the etiology and pathogenesis of breast cancer, in Harris JR, Lippman ME, Morrow M, Hellman S (eds): *Diseases of the Breast,* p. 201. Philadelphia, Lippincott-Raven, 1996.

28. Longnecker M, Berlin J, Orza M, et al: A meta-analysis of alcohol consumption in relation to breast cancer risk. *JAMA.* 260:652-656, 1988.

29. Gapstur S, Potter J, Sellers T, et al: Increased risk of breast cancer with alcohol consumption in postmenopausal women. *Am J Epidemiol* 136:1221-1231, 1992.

30. Friedenreich C, Howe G, Miller A, et al: A cohort study of alcohol consumption and risk of breast cancer. *Am J Epidemiol* 137:512-520, 1993.

31. Dupont W, Page D: Risk factors for breast cancer in women with proliferative breast disease. *N Engl J Med* 312:146-151, 1985.

32. Hutter R: Consensus meeting: Is fibrocystic disease of the breast precancerous? *Arch Pathol Lab Med* 110:171, 1986.

33. Dupont W, Page D, Rogers L, et al: Influence of exogenous estrogens, proliferative breast disease, and other variables on breast cancer risk. *Cancer* 63:948-957, 1989.

34. Haagensen CD, Bodian C, Haagensen DE. Lobular neoplasia (lobular carcinoma in situ), in *Breast carcinoma: Risk and Detection,* p 288. Philadelphia, WB Saunders, 1981.

35. Rosen PP, Lieberman PH, Braun DW Jr, et al: Lobular carcinoma in situ of the breast. *Am J Surg Path* 2:225-251, 1978.

36. Anderson JA: Lobular carcinoma in situ. A long-term follow-up in 52 cases. *Acta Path Microbiol Scan* 85:519-533, 1974.

37. Page DL, Kidd TE, Dupont WD, et al: Lobular neoplasia of the breast: Higher risk for subsequent invasive cancer predicted by more extensive disease. *Hum Pathol* 22:1232-1239, 1991.

38. Salvadori B, Bartoli C, Zurrida S, et al: Risk of invasive cancer in women with lobular carcinoma in situ of the breast. *Eur J Cancer* 27:35-37, 1991.

39. Ottensen GL, Graversen HP, Blichert-Tort M, et al: Lobular carcinoma in situ of the female breast: Short-term results of a prospective nationwide study. *Am J Surg Pathol* 17:14-21, 1993.

40. Tokunaga M, Land C, Yamamoto T, et al: Incidence of female breast cancer among atomic bomb survivors, Hiroshima and Nagasaki. *Radiat Res* 112:243-272, 1987.

41. Miller A, Howe G, Sherman G: Mortality from breast cancer after irradiation during fluoroscopic examinations in patients being treated for tuberculosis. *N Engl J Med* 321:1285-1289, 1989.

42. Hildreth N, Shore L, Dvorestsky P: The risk of breast cancer after irradiation of the thymus in infancy. *N Engl J Med* 321:1281-1284, 1989.

43. Hancock S, Tucker M, Hoppe R: Breast cancer after treatment of Hodgkin's disease. *J Natl Cancer Inst* 85:25-31, 1993.

44. Evans JS, Wennberg JE, McNeil BJ: The influence of diagnostic radiography on the incidence of breast cancer and leukemia. *N Engl J Med* 315:810-815, 1986.

45. Loomis D, Savitz D, Ananth C: Breast cancer mortality among female electrical workers in the United States. *J Natl Cancer Inst* 86:921-925, 1994.

46. Wolff M, Toniolo P, Lee E, et al: Blood levels of organochlorine residues and risk of breast cancer. *J Natl Cancer Inst* 85:648-652, 1993.

47. Colditz GA, Willett WC, Hunter DJ, et al : Family history, age, and risk of breast cancer: Prospective data from the Nurses' Health Study. *JAMA* 270:338-343, 1993.

48. Anderson DE, Badzioch MD: Combined effect of family history and reproductive factors on breast cancer risk. *Cancer* 63:349-353, 1989.

49. Brinton L, William R, Hoover R, et al: Breast cancer risk factors among screening program participants. *J Nat Cancer Inst* 62:37-44, 1979.

50. Steinberg KK, Thacker SB, Smith J, et al: A meta-analysis of the effect of estrogen replacement therapy on the risk of breast cancer. *JAMA* 265:1985-1990, 1991.

51. Newcomb PA, Storer BE, Longnecker MP, et al: Lactation and a reduced risk of premenopausal breast cancer. *N Engl J Med* 330:81-87, 1994.

52. Lambe M, Hsieh CC, Trichopoulos D, et al: Transient increase in the risk of breast cancer after giving birth. *N Engl J Med* 331:5-12, 1994.

53. Madigan M, Zeigler R, Benichon C, et al: Proportion of breast cancer cases in the United States explained by well established risk factors. *J Natl Cancer Inst* 87:1681-1685, 1995.

54. Gail M, Brinton L, Byar D, et al: Projecting individualized probabilities of developing breast cancer for white females who are being examined annually. *J Natl Cancer Inst* 81:1879-1886, 1989.

55. Bondy M, Lustbader E, Halabi S, et al: Validation of a breast cancer risk assessment model in women with a positive family history. *J Natl Cancer Inst* 86:620-625, 1994.

56. Spiegelman D, Colditz G, Hunter D, et al: Validation of the Gail et al model for predicting individual breast cancer risk. *J Natl Cancer Inst* 86:600-607, 1994.

57. Morrow M: Identification and management of the women at increased risk for breast cancer development. *Br Ca Res Treat* 31:53-60, 1994.

58. Bilimoria M, Morrow M: The woman at increased risk for breast cancer: Evaluation and management strategies. *CA Cancer J Clin* 45:263-278, 1995.

Chapter 16

Tamoxifen for Breast Cancer Prevention

V. Craig Jordan, PhD, DSc
Monica Morrow, MD

The Biological Basis for Prevention

There are currently (1999) 10 million women years of clinical experience with the use of tamoxifen in the treatment of all stages of breast cancer. The enormous clinical database, along with the low reported incidence of serious side effects, have acted as catalysts to support the testing of tamoxifen as a preventive in well women at high risk for breast cancer. In October, 1998, the US Food and Drug Administration approved tamoxifen for reducing the incidence of breast cancer in women at high risk for developing the disease.

As long ago as 1936, Lacassagne[1] predicted that a therapeutic intervention could be developed that would "prevent or antagonize the congestion of oestrone in the breast." Unfortunately, no therapeutic agent had been available, and all his predictions had been based upon the known effect of early oophorectomy on the development of mammary cancer in high-incidence strains of mice. Clearly, even Lacassagne could see that indiscriminate oophorectomy of young women was an inappropriate intervention! However, it should be remembered that during the past 3 decades, a burst of literature on the prevention of rodent mammary cancer has supported the clinical use of tamoxifen to prevent breast cancer.

Beginning in 1973, animal studies with tamoxifen were undertaken for two reasons: first, to establish the efficacy of tamoxifen in well-described models of carcinogenesis, and secondly, to discover whether tamoxifen would always be an inhibitor, or whether the drug would exacerbate tumorigenesis. Two animal model systems were used extensively: the carcinogen-induced rat mammary carcinoma model and the mouse mammary tumor virus (MMTV) infected strains of mice. In studies, the mammary carcinogens dimethylbenzanthracene- (DMBA)[2] and N-nitrosomethylurea- (NMU),[3] induced tumors in young female rats. The timing of the carcinogenic insult was very important because as the animals aged, they became resistant to mammary carcinogens. Tumorigenesis did not occur in oophorectomized animals and the sooner oophorectomy was performed after the carcinogenic insult, the more effective the prevention of tumor development.[4]

The administration of tamoxifen to carcinogen-treated rats prevented the initiation of carcinogenesis—animals remained tumor free.[5,6] The short-term administration of tamoxifen at different times after the carcinogenic insult was effective in reducing the number of tumors. Nevertheless, most animals developed at least one tumor after therapy was stopped.

In contrast, continuous tamoxifen therapy that was started 1 month after the administration of carcinogens almost completely inhibited the appearance of mammary tumors (see Chapter 2, Figure 7). Under these circumstances, tamoxifen prevented promotion and suppressed the appearance of "occult" disease. In fact, when treatment was stopped prematurely (eg, a 3- to 4-month duration of therapy), the microfoci of transformed cells grew into palpable tumors. Since the timing of initiation in human breast cancer is unknown, and since, unlike the laboratory model, not all women will develop tumors, tamoxifen was given to target populations to suppress and reverse the promotional effects of estrogen during carcinogenesis.

Until recently, there was a paucity of information about the efficacy of tamoxifen to inhibit mouse mammary tumorigenesis. In part, this was due to the observation that tamoxifen was estrogenic in short-term tests in oophorectomized and immature mice. However, the finding that long-term tamoxifen therapy rendered the oophorectomized mouse vagina and athymic mouse uterus refractory to estrogenic stimuli prompted a reconsideration of the value of tamoxifen as a preventive in mouse mammary tumor models. High-incidence strains of mice that developed mammary tumors were infected with mouse mammary tumor virus (MMTV) (see Appendix 1), which was transferred to their offspring in the mothers' milk. Tumorigenesis appeared to be ovarian dependent, as the highest incidence of tumors appeared in females. Furthermore, tumorigenesis could be delayed or prevented, depending on the animal's age at oophorectomy. Steroid hormones activated the proviral MMTV, which, in turn, initiated an increase in growth factors from the viral integration site Int. 2 in the mouse mammary DNA. Promotion of the initiated cells with steroid hormones and prolactin then completed tumorigenesis.

It was also clear in the mouse model, *unlike the human*, that early pregnancy promoted the early appearance of mammary tumors. Long-term tamoxifen therapy, after an early pregnancy to promote tumorigenesis, was equivalent to oophorectomy performed at 4 months, in reducing tumorigenesis by 50% at 14 months of age. Tamoxifen was actually superior to oophorectomy because oophorectomized animals continued to develop tumors, whereas animals previously treated with tamoxifen did not develop any more tumors,[7] even after therapy was stopped.

These initial observations were followed by another study of tumorigenesis in virgin mice. According to this study design, mice developed mammary tumors during their second year of life. Again, long-term tamoxifen therapy started at 3 months of age was superior to oophorectomy at 3 months. Fifty percent of the oophorectomized animals developed tumors by the third year of life, whereas 90% of the tamoxifen-treated mice remained tumor free.[8] The general conclusions of this study are illustrated in Figure 1.

In mice, long-term tamoxifen therapy started at 3 months of age was superior to oophorectomy at 3 months.

Overall, results of the mouse model studies are particularly interesting because they have changed our view of the interspecies pharmacology of tamoxifen: Within a few weeks, the pharmacology of tamoxifen changes from being an estrogen in the uterus and tamoxifen then becomes an antiestrogen. Clearly, an understanding of this process may have important implications for the long-term use of tamoxifen as an adjuvant therapy and a preventive for breast cancer.

Prevention: From the Laboratory to the Clinical Trial

Twenty-five years ago, tamoxifen was shown to prevent the induction[5,6] and promotion[9] of carcinogen-induced mammary cancer in rats. Similarly, tamoxifen was also shown to prevent the development of mammary cancer induced by ionizing radiation in rats.[10] These laboratory observations, coupled with the emerging preliminary clinical observation that adjuvant tamoxifen could prevent contralateral breast cancer in women,[11] provided a rationale for Dr. Trevor Powles, who in 1986, established the Vangard study at the Royal Marsden Hospital in England to test whether tamoxifen could prevent breast cancer in high-risk women.[12]

This chapter will explore the progress that has been achieved in the last decade to answer the question: "Does tamoxifen have worth in the prevention of breast cancer in select high-risk women?" The first results of three international trials that address this question—the Royal Marsden study, the NSABP/NCI study, and the Italian study—have been reported.

Royal Marsden Study

Powles and coworkers recruited 2,484 women aged 30 to 70 to a placebo-controlled trial using 20 mg of tamoxifen daily for up to 8 years. Women were

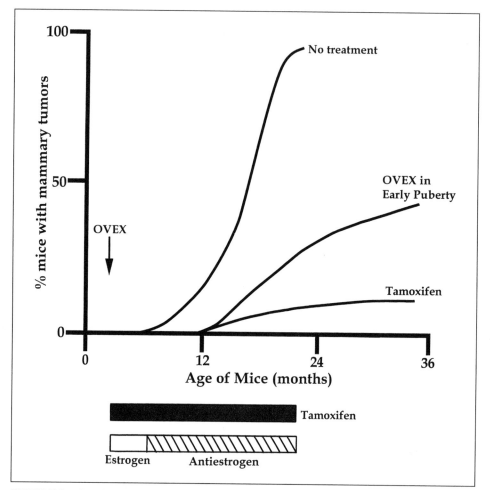

FIGURE I   Ovariectomy vs tamoxifen in the mouse model   We compared the effectiveness of ovariectomy (ovex) with long-term tamoxifen treatment in preventing mouse mammary cancer. Virgin mice from inbred high-incidence strains were infected with MMTV and developed mammary tumors spontaneously in the second year of life. The effect of early ovariectomy was to reduce the number of mice that developed tumors. Long-term tamoxifen treatment, however, was even more effective. The bar beneath the black band in the figure denoting the duration of tamoxifen therapy describes the pharmacology of tamoxifen therapy in the mouse uterus. The drug was initially able to stimulate an increase in uterine weight (an estrogen-like effect); but with continuous therapy, uterine weight decreased and tamoxifen acted as an antiestrogen.

eligible if their risk of breast cancer was increased due to family history. Each participant had at least one first-degree relative with breast cancer under age 50; or a first-degree relative affected at any age, plus an additional affected first- or second-degree relative; or a first-degree relative with bilateral breast cancer. Women with a history of benign breast biopsy and an affected first-degree relative of any age were also eligible. Women with a history of venous thrombosis, any previous malignancy, or an estimated life expectancy of fewer than 10 years were excluded.[13, 14] A total of 2,494 women consented to participate in the study, and 23 were excluded from final analysis due to the presence of preexisting ductal carcinoma in situ (DCIS) or invasive breast carcinoma.[14] The trial was undertaken to evaluate the problems of accrual, acute symptomatic toxicity, compliance, and safety as a basis for subsequent large national, multicenter trials designed to test whether tamoxifen can prevent breast cancer.

The Marsden group has made an extensive study of gynecological complications associated with tamoxifen use in healthy women.

However, the trial has also been analyzed for breast cancer incidence.[14]

Acute symptomatic toxicity was low for participants on tamoxifen or placebo, and compliance remained correspondingly high: 77% of women on tamoxifen and 82% of women on placebo remained on medication at 5 years, as predicted. There was a significant increase in hot flashes (34% vs 20%)—mostly in premenopausal women ($P < 0.005$); vaginal discharge (16% vs 4%; $P < 0.005$); and menstrual irregularities (14% vs 9%; $P < 0.005$), respectively. At the most recent follow-up, 320 women had discontinued tamoxifen and 176 had discontinued placebo prior to the study's completion ($P < 0.005$).

Until their report in 1994,[13] the Marsden group observed no thromboembolic episodes; a detailed analysis of other coagulation parameters in a sequential subset of women also found no significant changes in Protein S, Protein C, or cross-linked fibrinogen degradation products. At 70 months, no significant difference in the incidence of deep vein thrombosis or pulmonary embolism was observed between groups. A significant fall in total plasma cholesterol occurred within 3 months and was sustained over 5 years of treatment.[15-17] The decrease affected low-density lipoprotein, with no change in apolipoproteins A and B or high-density lipoprotein cholesterol.

In contrast, tamoxifen exerted antiestrogenic or estrogenic effects on bone density, depending on menopausal status. In premenopausal women, early findings demonstrated a small but significant ($P < 0.05$) loss of bone in both the lumbar spine and hip at 3 years.[17] It will be most important to evaluate the results at 5 and 8 years of therapy, as current indications suggest bone stabilization rather than continued loss. In contrast, postmenopausal women had increased bone mineral density in the spine ($P < 0.005$) and hip ($P < 0.001$) compared to nontreated women.

Finally, the Marsden group has made an extensive study of gynecological complications associated with tamoxifen treatment in healthy women. Since ovarian and uterine assessment by transvaginal ultrasound became available some time after the trial's start, many subjects did not have a baseline evaluation. Ovarian screening demonstrated a significantly increased risk ($P < 0.005$) of detecting benign ovarian cysts in premenopausal women who had received tamoxifen for more than 3 months compared to controls. There were no changes in ovarian appearance in postmenopausal women.[13] A careful examination of the uterus with transvaginal ultrasonography using color Doppler imaging in women taking tamoxifen showed that the organ was usually larger; moreover, women with histological abnormalities had significantly thicker endometria.[18] Of particular interest in this regard was the recent observation that 20 mg of tamoxifen daily exerted a time-dependent proliferation of the endometrium in premenopausal and early postmenopausal women. This effect appeared to be mediated by the stromal component, since no cases of cancer or even epithelial hyperplasia were observed among the tamoxifen-treated group in the Italian study with 33 women.[19]

Although the Vangard study has provided invaluable information about the biological effects of tamoxifen in healthy women, the trial was not designed to answer the question of whether tamoxifen prevents breast cancer. In spite of this, an analysis of breast cancer incidence was reported at a median follow-up of 70 months, when 42% of the participants had completed therapy or withdrawn.[14] During the study, 336 women on tamoxifen and 305 on placebo received hormone-replacement therapy. No difference in the incidence of breast cancer was observed between the groups. There were 34 carcinomas in the tamoxifen group and 36 in the placebo group—a relative risk of 1.06. Of the 70 cancers, only 8 were ductal carcinoma in situ. An analysis of the subset of women on hormone-replacement therapy did not demonstrate an interaction with tamoxifen treatment.

NSABP/NCI Study

This study opened in the United States and Canada in May of 1992 with an accrual goal of 16,000 women to be recruited at 100 North American sites. It closed after accruing 13,338 in 1997 due to the high-risk status of the participants. The study design is illustrated in Figure 2. Those eligible for entry included any woman over the age of 60, or women between the ages of 35 and 59 whose 5-year risk of developing breast cancer, as predicted by the Gail model,[20] was equal to that of a 60-year-old woman. Additionally, any woman over age 35 with a diagnosis of lobular carcinoma in situ (LCIS) treated by biopsy alone was eligible for entry to the study. In the absence of LCIS, the risk factors necessary to enter the study varied with age, such that

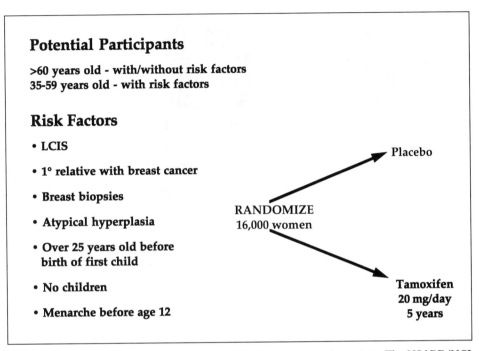

Potential Participants

>60 years old - with/without risk factors
35-59 years old - with risk factors

Risk Factors

• **LCIS**

• **1° relative with breast cancer**

• **Breast biopsies**

• **Atypical hyperplasia**

• **Over 25 years old before birth of first child**

• **No children**

• **Menarche before age 12**

RANDOMIZE
16,000 women

Placebo

Tamoxifen 20 mg/day 5 years

FIGURE 2 Study design of the NSABP/NCI chemoprevention trial The NSABP/NCI chemoprevention trial tested the worth of tamoxifen to reduce the risk of breast cancer in high-risk women. After recruitment of 11,000 women, the risk factors for the study population were so high that an accrual goal of only 13,000 women needed to be met. This was accomplished by summer, 1997.

a 35-year-old woman must have had a relative risk (RR) of 5.07, whereas the required RR for a 45-year-old woman was 1.79. Routine endometrial biopsies to evaluate the incidence of endometrial carcinoma in both arms of the study were also performed.

The breast cancer risk of women enrolled in the study was extremely high, with no age group having an RR of less than 4—including the over-60's group. Recruitment was also balanced, with about one-third younger than 50 years, one-third between 50 and 60 years, and one-third older than 60 years. Secondary end points of the study included the effect of tamoxifen on the incidence of fractures and cardiovascular deaths. Most importantly, the study plans to provide the first information about the role of genetic markers in the etiology of breast cancer. It will also establish whether tamoxifen has a role to play in the treatment of women who are found to carry somatic mutations in the BRCA-1 gene. (Laboratory results are not yet available.)

The first results of the NSABP study were reported in September, 1998, after a mean follow-up of 47.7 months. There were a total of 368 invasive and

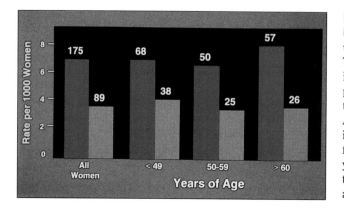

FIGURE 3   Incidence of invasive carcinoma in the tamoxifen prevention trial There were 175 cases of invasive carcinoma in the placebo group and 89 in the tamoxifen group ($P<0.0001$). A reduction in risk was seen in all age groups, ranging from 44% in women 49 or younger to 51% for women in their 50s, and 55% in women aged 60 and older.

noninvasive breast cancers in the participants; 124 in the tamoxifen group and 224 in the placebo group. A 49% reduction in the risk of invasive breast cancer was seen in the tamoxifen group (Figure 3), and a 50% reduction in the risk of noninvasive breast cancer was observed (Figure 4). A subset analysis of women at risk due to a diagnosis of LCIS demonstrated a 56% reduction in this group (Figure 5). The most dramatic reduction was seen in women at risk due to atypical hyperplasia, where risk was reduced by 86% (Figure 6).

The benefits of tamoxifen were observed in all age groups, with a relative risk of breast cancer ranging from 0.45 in women aged 60 and older to 0.49 for those in the 50- through 59-year age group, and 0.56 for women aged 49 and younger (Figure 3). A benefit for tamoxifen was also observed for women with all levels of breast cancer risk within the study, indicating that the benefits of tamoxifen are not confined to a particular lower risk or higher risk subset (Figure 7). Benefits were observed in women at risk on the basis of family history and those whose risk was due to other factors (Figure 8).

As expected, the effect of tamoxifen occurred on the incidence of estrogen receptor (ER)-positive tumors, which were reduced by 69% per year. The rate of ER-negative tumors in the tamoxifen group (1.46 per 1,000 women) did not significantly differ from the placebo group (1.20 per 1,000 women) (Figure 9). Tamoxifen reduced the rate of invasive cancers of all sizes, but the greatest difference between the groups was the incidence of tumors 2.0 cm or less (Figure 10). Tamoxifen also reduced the incidence of both node-positive and node-negative breast cancer (Figure 11). The beneficial effects of tamoxifen were observed for each year of follow-up in the study. After year 1, the risk was reduced by 33%, and in year 5, by 69% (Figure 12).

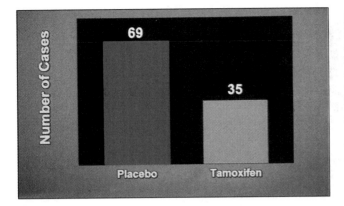

FIGURE 4 Incidence of DCIS in the tamoxifen prevention trial There was a relative risk of DCIS of 0.50 (95% CI 0.33-0.77) in tamoxifen-treated patients. The average annual rate of noninvasive breast cancer per 1,000 women was 1.35 in the tamoxifen group and 2.68 in the placebo group.

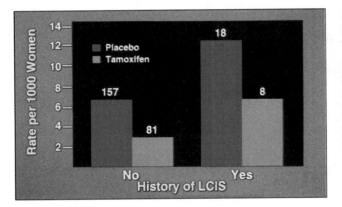

FIGURE 5 Incidence of breast cancer in women with LCIS in the tamoxifen prevention trial Tamoxifen reduced the relative risk of breast cancer in women with LCIS to 0.44 (95% CI 0.16-1.06). In women without LCIS, the relative risk was 0.51 (95% CI 0.39-0.68).

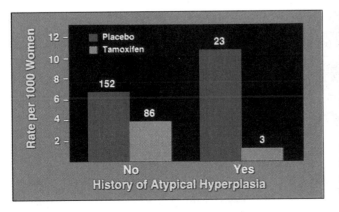

FIGURE 6 Incidence of breast cancer in women with atypical hyperplasia in the tamoxifen prevention trial Tamoxifen reduced the relative risk of breast cancer in women with atypical hyperplasia to 0.14 (95% CI 0.03-0.47). In women without atypical hyperplasia, the corresponding relative risk was 0.56 (95% CI 0.42-0.73).

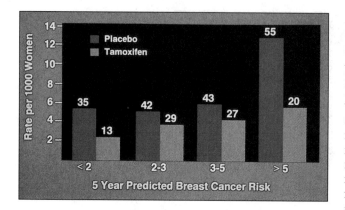

FIGURE 7 Effect of risk status on breast cancer prevention with tamoxifen A reduction in breast cancer incidence was seen at all levels of risk within the prevention trial. For women with a 5-year risk of ≤ 2%, the relative risk was 0.37. When risk was 2% to 3%, the relative risk was 0.68; and when the risk was 3% to 5%, the relative risk was 0.66. For women with a 5-year risk of 5% or greater, the relative risk was 0.34.

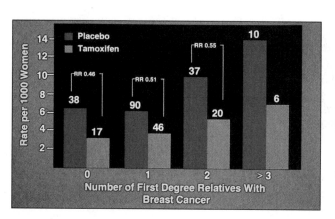

FIGURE 8 Effect of family history on breast cancer prevention with tamoxifen The benefit of tamoxifen was equal in women with no first-degree relatives with breast cancer, a single, affected first-degree relative, two affected first-degree relatives, or three or more affected first-degree relatives.

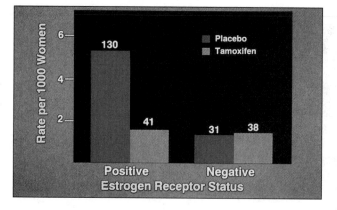

FIGURE 9 Effect of receptor status on breast cancer prevention with tamoxifen The annual rate of ER-positive breast cancer in the tamoxifen group was 1.58 per 1,000 women, compared to 5.02 per 1,000 women in the placebo group—a 69% reduction. There was no difference in the incidence of ER-negative tumors in the tamoxifen and placebo groups.

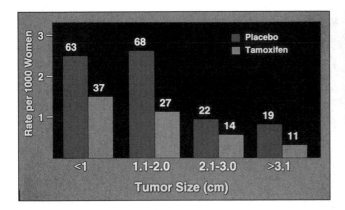

FIGURE 10 Tumor size in the tamoxifen prevention trial Tamoxifen reduced the incidence of both small and large breast cancers; but the greatest differences were seen in the incidence of tumors 2.0 cm or less.

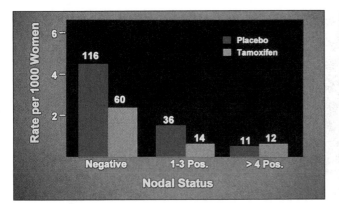

FIGURE 11 Nodal status in the tamoxifen prevention trial The rate of node-negative breast cancer in the placebo arm was 4.48 per 1,000 women compared to 2.31 per 1,000 in the tamoxifen arm. The rate of cancers with 1 to 3 positive nodes was also reduced; 1.39 per 1,000 in the placebo group and 0.54 per 1,000 in the tamoxifen group.

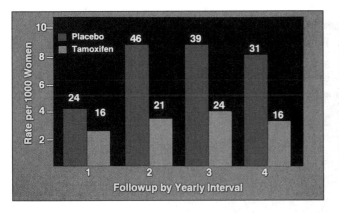

FIGURE 12 Breast cancer incidence by follow-up interval in the tamoxifen prevention trial A reduction in breast cancer incidence was seen in tamoxifen-treated women in each year of follow-up in the trial. The rates of reduction in years 1 through 6 were 33%, 55%, 39%, 49%, 69%, and 55%.

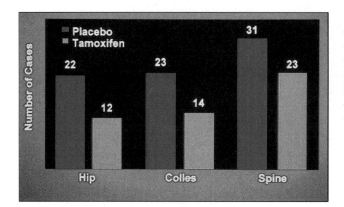

FIGURE 13 Fractures in the tamoxifen prevention trial A 45% reduction in hip fractures, a 39% reduction in Colles fractures, and a 26% reduction in spinal fractures were observed in tamoxifen-treated women.

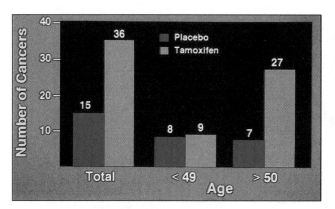

FIGURE 14 Endometrial carcinoma in the tamoxifen prevention trial Tamoxifen increased the relative risk of endometrial carcinoma to 2.53. In women aged 50 and older, tamoxifen increased the relative risk to 4.01 (95% CI 1.70-10.90).

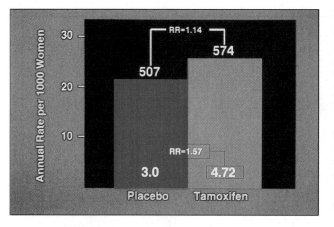

FIGURE 15 Cataracts in the tamoxifen prevention trial The occurrence of cataracts in the placebo group was 21.72 per 1,000 and 24.82 per 1,000 in the tamoxifen group. The relative risk of 1.14 was marginally significant (95% CI 1.01-1.29). The rates of cataract surgery were 3.0 and 4.72 per 1,000 women in the placebo and tamoxifen groups, respectively.

Tamoxifen also reduced the incidence of osteoporotic fractures of the hip, spine, and radius by 19% (Figure 13). However, the difference approached, but did not reach, statistical significance. This reduction was greatest in women aged 50 and older at study entry. No difference in the risk of myocardial infarction, angina, coronary artery bypass grafting, or angioplasty was noted between groups.

This study confirmed the association between tamoxifen and endometrial carcinoma. The relative risk of endometrial cancer in the tamoxifen group was 2.5. The increased risk was seen in women aged 50 and older, whose relative risk was 4.01 (Figure 14). All endometrial cancers in the tamoxifen group were grade 1 and none of the women on tamoxifen died of endometrial cancer. There was 1 endometrial cancer death in the placebo group. Although there is no doubt that tamoxifen increases the risk of endometrial cancer, it is important to recognize that this increase translates to an incidence of 2.3 women per 1,000 per year who develop endometrial carcinoma.

More women in the tamoxifen group developed deep vein thrombosis (DVT) than in the placebo group. Again, this excess risk was confined to women aged 50 and older. The relative risk of DVT in the older age group was 1.71. (95% CI 0.85 to 3.58). An increase in pulmonary emboli was also seen in the older women taking tamoxifen, with a relative risk of approximately 3. Three deaths from pulmonary emboli occurred in the tamoxifen arm, but all were in women with significant comorbidities. An increased incidence of stroke (RR 1.75) was also seen in the tamoxifen group, but this did not reach statistical significance.

An assessment of the incidence of cataract formation was made using patient self-report. A small increase in cataracts was noted in the tamoxifen group—a rate of 24.8 women per 1,000 compared to 21.7 in the placebo group (Figure 15). There was also an increased risk of cataract surgery in the women on tamoxifen. These differences were marginally, statistically significant, and observed in the older patients in the study. These findings emphasize the need to assess the patient's overall health status before making a decision to use tamoxifen for breast cancer risk reduction.

An assessment of quality of life showed no difference in depression scores between groups. Hot flashes were noted in 81% of the women on tamoxifen compared to 69% of the placebo group, and the tamoxifen-associated hot flashes appeared to be of greater severity than those in the placebo group. Moderately bothersome or severe vaginal discharge was reported by 29% of the women in tamoxifen group and 13% in the placebo group. No differences in the occurrence of irregular menses, nausea, fluid retention, skin changes, or weight gain or loss were reported.

Italian Study

The third tamoxifen prevention study, performed in Italy, began in October, 1992, and randomized 5,408 women aged 35 to 70 to 20 mg of tamoxifen daily for 5 years.[22] Women were required to have had a hysterectomy for a nonneoplastic condition to obviate concerns about an increased risk of endometrial carcinoma. There was no requirement that participants be at risk for breast cancer development, and in fact, those who underwent premenopausal oophorectomy with hysterectomy actually had a slightly reduced risk of breast cancer development. Women with endometriosis, cardiac disease, and deep venous thrombosis were excluded from the study. Although 5,408 women were randomized into this study, 1,422 withdrew and only 149 completed 5 years of treatment.

The incidence of breast cancer did not differ between groups, with 19 cases in the tamoxifen group and 22 in the placebo group. Tumor characteristics, including size, grade, lymph node status, and receptor status, also did not differ between groups.

The incidence of thrombophlebitis was increased in the tamoxifen group. A total of 64 events were reported, 38 in the tamoxifen group and 18 in the placebo group ($P = 0.0053$). However, 42 of these were superficial phlebitis.

No differences in the incidence of cerebrovascular ischemic events were observed.

Conclusions

Based on a single trial with a positive result and two with negative results, it may seem, at first glance, that the role of tamoxifen in breast cancer prevention remains unresolved.

However, critical differences exist between these three studies (see highlighted properties in Table 1).

The negative finding in the Italian study[22] is readily explained by the relatively low risk of breast cancer development in the study population, the high dropout rate, and the small number of participants who completed 5 years of treatment.

In fact, the Italian study shows a trend towards significance among women who took tamoxifen for more than 1 year, suggesting that with further follow-up, the results of this study may become more positive. At present, the only conclusion that can be drawn from this study is that tamoxifen's possible benefits are likely to be small in women with an average or decreased risk of breast cancer.

The Royal Marsden study was initially described as a pilot study to examine toxicity and compliance,[12] which would serve as a feasibility

Table I

A Comparison of Patient Characteristics in the
Tamoxifen Prevention Trials

Characteristic	NSABP	Royal Marsden	Italian
Sample Size	13,388	2,471	5,408
Women years of follow-up	46,858	12,355	5,408
Participants < age 50	40%	62%	36%
1° relative with breast cancer	55%	55%	18%
> 2 1° relatives with breast cancer	13%	17%	2.5%
Use of HRT	0%	42%	8%
Breast Cancer Incidence/1,000:			
Placebo	6.7	5.5	2.3
Tamoxifen	3.4	4.7	2.1

assessment for a larger trial to determine if tamoxifen prevents breast cancer. In spite of being designed as a pilot study, the trial is now said to have a 90% power to detect a 50% reduction in breast cancer incidence, yet shows no effect.[14] The authors suggest that the positive results of the NSABP trial at 3.5 years of follow-up are most likely due to the treatment of clinically occult carcinoma, rather than the prevention of new breast cancers. Their negative trial with a follow-up of 6 years reflects the absence of prevention.

However, of the 368 total cancers in the NSABP study,[21] 104 (28%) were DCIS, compared to 11% of the 70 cancers in the Royal Marsden study. The higher percentage of DCIS in the NSABP trial indicates that the detection of subclinical cancers occurred, and that any treated occult cancer was not truly amenable to detection by currently available means. Whether occult carcinoma was treated or true prevention occurred, a significantly greater number of women were spared surgery, irradiation, and chemotherapy. The data from the overview analysis do not support the contention that these cancers will become clinically evident when tamoxifen is stopped, since the reduction in contralateral breast cancer persists through 10 years even though tamoxifen treatment was stopped at 5 years.[23]

Overall, the results of the NSABP trial,[21] with its large study population, clearly support the benefit of tamoxifen for breast cancer prevention in high-risk women. These findings are consistent with laboratory observations and with the contralateral breast cancer risk reduction seen with tamoxifen therapy. Based on this, the use of tamoxifen should be seen as a welcome alternative to clinical follow-up or prophylactic mastectomy in the management of the high-risk woman. ■

References

1. Lacassagne A: Hormonal pathogenesis of adenocarcinoma of the breast. *Am J Cancer* 27:217-225, 1936.

2. Huggins SC, Grand LC, Brillantes FP: Mammary cancer induced by a single feeding of polynuclear hydrocarbons and their suppression. *Nature* 189:204-207, 1962.

3. Gullino PM, Pettigrew HN, Grantham FH: N-Nitrosomethylurea as mammary gland carcinogen in rats. *J Natl Cancer Inst* 54:401-414, 1975.

4. Dao TL: The role of ovarian hormones in initiating the induction of mammary cancer in rats by polynuclear hydrocarbons. *Cancer Res* 22:973-981, 1962.

5. Jordan VC: Antitumour activity of the antioestrogen ICI 46,474 (tamoxifen) in the dimethylbenzanthracene (DMBA)-induced rat mammary carcinoma model. *J Steroid Biochem* 5:354, 1974.

6. Jordan VC: Effect of tamoxifen (ICI 46,474) on initiation and growth of DMBA-induced rat mammary carcinomata. *Eur J Cancer* 12:419-425, 1976.

7. Jordan VC, Lababidi MK, Mirecki DM: The antiestrogenic and antitumor properties of prolonged tamoxifen therapy in C3H/OUJ mice. *Eur J Cancer* 26:718-721, 1990.

8. Jordan VC, Lababidi MK, Langan Fahey S: Suppression of mouse mammary tumorigenesis by long-term tamoxifen therapy. *J Natl Cancer Inst* 83:492-496, 1991.

9. Jordan VC, Allen KE, Dix CJ: Pharmacology of tamoxifen in laboratory animals. *Cancer Treat Rep* 64:745-759, 1980.

10. Welsch CW, Goodrich-Smith M, Brown CK, et al: Effect of an estrogen antagonist (tamoxifen) on the initiation and progression of gamma radiation-induced mammary tumors in female Sprague-Dawley rats. *Eur J Cancer* 17:1255-1258, 1981.

11. Cuzick J, Baum M: Tamoxifen and contralateral breast cancer. *Lancet* 2:282, 1985.

12. Powles TJ, Hardy JR, Ashley SE, et al: A pilot trial to evaluate the acute toxicity and feasibility of tamoxifen for prevention of breast cancer. *Br J Cancer* 60:126-133, 1989.

13. Powles TJ, Jones AL, Ashley SE, et al: The Royal Marsden Hospital pilot tamoxifen chemoprevention trial. *Breast Cancer Res Treat* 31:73-82, 1994.

14. Powles T, Eeles R, Ashley S, et al: Interim analysis of the incidence of breast cancer in the Royal Marsden hospital tamoxifen randomized chemoprevention trial. *Lancet* 362:98-101, 1998.

15. Jones AL, Powles TJ, Treleaven J, et al: Haemostatic changes and thromboembolic risk during tamoxifen therapy in normal women. *Br J Cancer* 66:744-747, 1992.

16. Powles TJ, Tillyer CP, Jones AL, et al: Prevention of breast cancer with tamoxifen: An update on the Royal Marsden pilot program. *Eur J Cancer* 26:680-684, 1990.

17. Powles TJ, Hickish T, Kanis JA, et al: Effect of tamoxifen on bone mineral density measured by dual-energy X-ray absorptionetry in healthy premenopausal and postmenopausal women. *J Clin Oncol* 14:78-84, 1996.

18. Kedar RP, Bourne TH, Powles TJ, et al: Effects of tamoxifen on uterus and ovaries of postmenopausal women in a randomized breast cancer prevention trial. *Lancet* 343:1318-1321, 1994.

19. Decensi A, Fontant V, Bruno S, et al: Effect of tamoxifen on endometrial proliferation. *J Clin Oncol* 14:434-440, 1996.

20. Gail MH, Brinton LA, Byar DP, et al: Projecting individualized probabilities of developing breast cancer for white females who are being examined annually. *J Natl Cancer Inst* 81:1879-1186, 1989.

21. Fisher B, Constantin JP, Wickerham DL, et al: Tamoxifen for prevention of breast cancer: Report of the National Surgical Adjuvant Breast and Bowel Project P-1 Study. *J Natl Cancer Inst* 90:1371-1388, 1998.

22. Veronesi U, Maisonneuve P, Costa A, et al: Prevention of breast cancer with tamoxifen: Preliminary findings from the Italian randomised trial among hysterectomised women. *Lancet* 362:93-97, 1998.

23. Early Breast Cancer Trialists' Collaborative Group: Tamoxifen for early breast cancer: An overview of the randomised trials. *Lancet* 351:1451-1467, 1998.

Chapter 17
The STAR Trial

V. Craig Jordan, PhD, DSc

In 1987, tamoxifen and raloxifene were shown to preserve bone density in ovariectomized rats and to prevent estrogen-induced increases in uterine weight.[1] We also showed that both tamoxifen and raloxifene prevented rat mammary carcinogenesis.[2] We had discovered the target site selectivity of antiestrogens: They are estrogen-like at some sites, eg, bone, but inhibitors of estrogen action at other sites, eg, the breast and the uterus. We reasoned that it would be possible to use tamoxifen or other compounds[1,3] to prevent osteoporosis in postmenopausal women, but at the same time, prevent breast cancer in broad groups of women without risk factors other than age. Others[4,5] confirmed the laboratory results with tamoxifen, and we have since effectively translated the concepts to the clinic:

Tamoxifen maintains bone density in the lumbar spine,[6] neck of the femur,[7] and radius,[8] but not by the same magnitude as would be expected from hormone replacement therapy (HRT). Lumbar spine data obtained from a double-blind, placebo-controlled trial of 140 postmenopausal women are shown in Figure 1. The increase in bone density was only about 1%. Be that as it may, tamoxifen reduced hip fracture, measured as a secondary end point in the National Surgical Adjuvant Breast and Bowel Project (NSABP) prevention trial P-1, by 50% (see Chapter 16). These results are proof that targeted antiestrogen to prevent breast cancer might afford additional physiologic support for the patient.

Despite these positive data, tamoxifen is not FDA approved for the treatment and prevention of osteoporosis. Drug development over the past 30 years has focused on breast cancer treatment and prevention and the elucidation of potential toxicities. Today, tamoxifen is listed by the World Health Organization (WHO) as an essential drug for the treatment of breast cancer. It is also the first FDA approved drug to reduce cancer incidence in well women at elevated risk for breast cancer. However, our concept of a multifunctional drug[3] has acted as a catalyst for the development of other drugs for different uses.

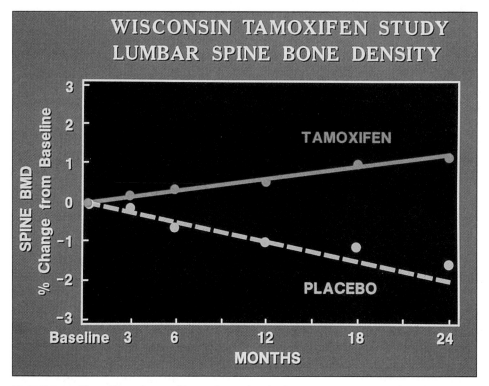

FIGURE I   The effect of tamoxifen on bone density in 140 postmenopausal, node-negative breast cancer patients randomized to receive tamoxifen or placebo for 2 years. Bone mineral density (BMD) was determined by Dr. R. Mazess using dual-photon absorptiometry. Adapted from Love RR et al.[6]

A New Approach to Prevention

In 1990, we proposed a new direction for drug development at the Eighth Cain Memorial Award Lecture:[3]

We have obtained valuable clinical information about this group of drugs that can be applied in other disease states. Research does not travel in straight lines, and observations in one field of science often become major discoveries in another. Important clues have been garnered about the effects of tamoxifen on bone and lipids; it is possible that derivatives could find targeted applications to retard osteoporosis or atherosclerosis. The ubiquitous application of novel compounds to prevent diseases associated with the progressive changes after menopause may, as a side effect, significantly retard the development of breast cancer. The target population would be postmenopausal women in general, thereby avoiding the requirement to select a high-risk group to prevent breast cancer.

We proposed the development of the ideal antiestrogen that would be targeted to produce specific actions at different sites in a woman's body. The

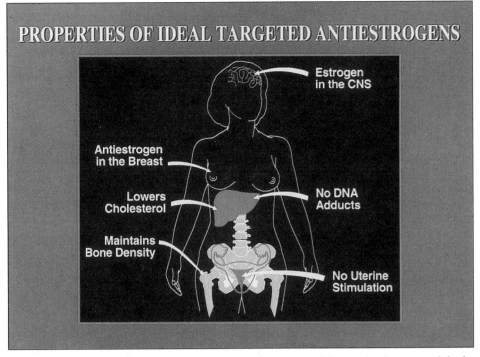

PROPERTIES OF IDEAL TARGETED ANTIESTROGENS

Estrogen in the CNS

Antiestrogen in the Breast

Lowers Cholesterol

No DNA Adducts

Maintains Bone Density

No Uterine Stimulation

FIGURE 2   The ideal antiestrogen produces specific actions at different sites in a woman's body.

properties of this ideal agent, or designer estrogen,[9] are summarized in Figure 2. Such an agent would have all the benefits of estrogen for the postmenopausal woman, but with the added advantage of preventing breast and endometrial cancer.[10,11] Today, this concept has become known as selective estrogen receptor modulation, and the agents are known as SERMs.

Tamoxifen is the first drug in this class and the pioneer that made SERM research a reality. Raloxifene is next in line to be clinically tested.

What Is Raloxifene?

Raloxifene, originally called keoxifene, was first reported by scientists at Eli Lilly, Indianapolis, to be an antiestrogen with a high affinity for the estrogen receptor (ER). Much like its earlier analogue, LY117018, however, raloxifene has mild estrogen-like properties in the uterus.[12] In fact, at very high doses, LY117018 can block the antiuterotropic effects of a variety of steroidal and nonsteroidal compounds in the rat.[13] The drug has antitumor effects in the rat, but is less potent than tamoxifen.[2,14] Although the original direction for raloxifene's clinical development was breast cancer therapy, Eli Lilly chose to abandon this approach towards the end of the

1980s. However, the discovery that raloxifene might prevent osteoporosis,[1] prevent breast cancer,[2] and at the same time, have minor estrogen-like effects in the uterus, laid the foundation for subsequent confirmation of bone data in animals.[15] These discoveries also led to the completion of clinical trials that demonstrated maintenance of bone density in postmenopausal women at risk for osteoporosis.[16]

Raloxifene is currently FDA approved for the prevention of osteoporosis. Raloxifene, 60 mg daily, produces a 1% to 2% increase in postmenopausal bone density—an increase equivalent to that noted with tamoxifen (Figure 1). Raloxifene also reduces fractures by about 30% to 40%. In addition, raloxifene is also approved to prevent osteoporosis in Europe and in more than a dozen other countries.

As part of a safety profile for any estrogen-like drug for the prevention of osteoporosis, raloxifene had to be evaluated for breast safety. To this end, Eli Lilly organized an independent oncology advisory committee to adjudicate all breast cancers diagnosed in the randomized, placebo-controlled trials for the prevention of osteoporosis. The committee (Table 1) was assembled to provide expertise in diagnosis, breast cancer prevention, and breast oncology. Committee members met every 6 months to review pathology, mammograms, and patient records to determine whether disease was preexisting at the time of entry to the trial and whether the cancer was invasive or

---

Table 1

The raloxifene oncology advisory committee*

Alberto Costa, MD – European Institute for Oncology, Milan (breast surgeon, co-PI Italian tamoxifen prevention trial)

V. Craig Jordan, PhD, DSc – Northwestern University Medical School, Chicago (committee chairperson)

Marc E. Lippman, MD – Georgetown University Medical School, Washington, DC (Director, Lombardi Comprehensive Cancer Center)

Monica Morrow, MD - Northwestern University Medical School, Chicago (breast surgeon, Director, Lynn Sage Breast Cancer Program)

Larry Norton, MD – Memorial Sloan-Kettering Cancer Center, New York (Head, Division of Oncology)

Trevor J. Powles, FRCP, PhD – Royal Marsden Hospital, London (Medical Oncologist, PI Royal Marsden, Tamoxifen Prevention Study)

---

* responsible for the evaluation and adjudication of breast cancer cases in the 10,533 patients participating in randomized, placebo-controlled trials to prevent osteoporosis

noninvasive. All patients who developed breast cancer in all trials were adjudicated blind, and the results were then collated and analyzed by Biostatistician Steven Eckert of Eli Lilly.

Breast cancer incidence was a secondary end point for toxicologic monitoring in the randomized trials of osteoporosis. Nevertheless, the pharmacology of raloxifene and the animal data predicted that the drug was likely to reduce, rather than increase, breast cancer incidence. As a result, the oncology advisory committee saw the process of adjudication and cancer monitoring as a hypothesis-driven experiment to confirm the pharmacology of the drug group.

Henceforth, raloxifene, a drug used to prevent osteoporosis, became a Trojan horse for the prevention of breast cancer[1,3] in low-risk women. It reduced the incidence of breast cancer in the 10,355-woman analysis in placebo-controlled trials by about 50%. A total of 58 invasive and noninvasive breast cancers were noted during the 33-month median evaluation period. There was a decrease in estrogen receptor positive disease in the raloxifene group. However, there was no change in negative disease.[17] These encouraging preliminary data, as well as the clinical data on osteoporosis, formed the basis for the next breast cancer prevention trial, the P-2 Study of Tamoxifen And Raloxifene (STAR).

The STAR Trial

The STAR trial is a phase III, double-blind trial that will assign eligible postmenopausal women to either daily tamoxifen (20 mg orally) or raloxifene (60 mg orally) therapy for 5 years. Trial participants will also complete a minimum of 2 additional years of follow-up after therapy is stopped.

The STAR trial's primary aim is to determine whether long-term therapy is effective in preventing the occurrence of invasive breast cancer in postmenopausal women who are identified as being at high risk for the disease. The comparison is to be made to the established drug, tamoxifen. Its secondary aim is to establish the net effect of raloxifene therapy, ie, cardiovascular data, fracture data, and general toxicities.

The P-2 trial is summarized in Figure 3.

Who is eligible?

Three groups of women are eligible:

1) Postmenopausal women over the age of 60, regardless of their risk level for developing breast cancer

2) Postmenopausal women with a diagnosis of lobular carcinoma in situ (LCIS)

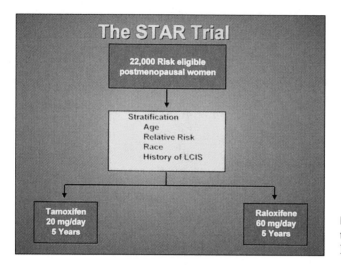

FIGURE 3 The design of the Study of Tamoxifen and Raloxifene (STAR) trial.

3) Postmenopausal women between the ages of 35 and 59 who possess risk factors that place them at high risk for developing breast cancer. Risk determination is based on a computerized calculation using the modified Gail model previously utilized in the P-1 trial. This group of women must have a combination of risk factors that increases the risk of developing breast cancer.

These risk factors (see Chapter 15) are based on:
- Age
- Number of first-degree relatives (mother, daughters, and sisters) who have been diagnosed with breast cancer
- Whether a woman had any children and her age at first delivery
- The number of times a woman has had breast lumps biopsied, especially if the tissue were shown to have atypical hyperplasia
- The woman's age at her first menstrual period

There will also be a list of pre-entry requirements that need to be completed by the study participants prior to randomization:
- Complete medical history, including an individual assessment of breast cancer, cardiovascular, and osteoporosis risk factors
- Signed consent form
- Detailed family history of breast cancer and cardiovascular disease, demographic information, and a review of existing symptoms
- Clinical breast examination
- Gynecologic examination (including a bimanual pelvic exam and Pap

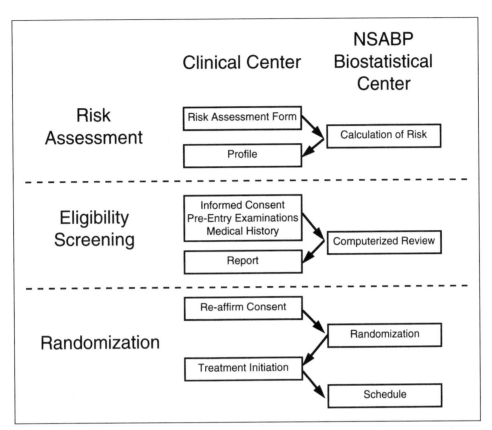

FIGURE 4 The proposed enrollment process for the NSABP Protocol P-2 STAR trial

test; and an invitation to give the potential participant a screening endometrial biopsy or transvaginal ultrasound)

• Bilateral mammography within the last 365 days
• CBC, differential, and serum chemistries, including liver and renal function studies
• Blood collection for the serum and lymphocyte bank
• Submission of tumor blocks for participants with a prior history of lobular carcinoma in situ or atypical hyperplasia

The entry process, illustrated in Figure 4, will occur at official recruitment sites in Canada and the United States. Follow-up visits to monitor health and collect study data will be explained at the recruitment sites.

Since tamoxifen is now approved as the standard of care for the reduction in the incidence of breast cancer in women at risk, the study will also seek to address questions about the new drug, raloxifene.

Only with the STAR trial can an effective risk/benefit profile be established for raloxifene as a breast cancer preventive. It is also important to note that premenopausal women will not be recruited. Unlike tamoxifen, there has been no extensive clinical experience with raloxifene in premenopausal women. An evaluation of the safety of raloxifene in premenopausal women is planned before alterations in the entry criteria for the STAR protocol can be made.

Important Scientific Questions

The official aims stated above will be answered by the results of the P-2 trial within 5 years. There are, however, other scientific questions that I believe are important new concepts for prevention, especially with drugs that have multiple applications and FDA approvals.

The overall questions can be summarized as follows:

What will be the optimal duration of SERM therapy as a breast cancer preventive?

With tamoxifen, we know some answers. Five years of treatment reduces new (contralateral) breast cancers by 47% (see Chapter 5); and this is the approximate figure for reduction in primary breast cancer in high-risk women (see Chapter 16). Preliminary data demonstrate that longer therapy does not increase or decrease the effectiveness of tamoxifen to reduce the risk of new breast cancers.[18] However, the numbers are too small for real certainty.

A remarkable clinical finding with tamoxifen is that a 5-year "pulse" somehow alters the breast, so that 5 years after treatment cessation, the development of breast cancer is still prevented in the contralateral breast.[19] This is also true for tamoxifen in animals. A critical duration and dose prevent the development of mammary tumors by changing the environment of the mammary tissue.[20] In other words, the number of tumors observed after tamoxifen therapy never catches up to those observed in the controls. Thus, tamoxifen, given as a limited pulse, can produce optimal protection long after the drug has been stopped. Although we have tested 5 years of treatment in clinical trials, it may be that a longer pulse might eventually prove to produce a lifetime of protection.

The concept of the duration of the pulse to alter the breast is extremely important since the competing forces of prevention and drug resistance may come into play with an indefinite drug schedule. At present, it is unclear which pharmacological property of tamoxifen is responsible for changing the breast—It may not solely be antiestrogenicity.

What do we know about the safety of SERM therapy?

As of 1999, there are no long-term antitumor data with raloxifene or any SERM other than tamoxifen. Even though both are antiestrogens in the breast, the physical pharmacologies of tamoxifen and raloxifene are different; raloxifene is designed to be a long-term therapy to prevent osteoporosis. It will be critical to observe whether the long-term follow-up of the P-2 trial affords the same protection of the breast as tamoxifen. Looked at another way, it is significant that tamoxifen (in limited use) might provide a lifetime of protection for women at risk for breast cancer, whereas raloxifene (with continuous use) might not. Additionally, if raloxifene is taken for decades to prevent osteoporosis, at what point will an increased incidence of raloxifene-resistant breast cancer catch up? Alternatively, will true breast cancer prevention occur with extended use, and will the rate drop below the current target of 50% risk reduction?

Regrettably, the answer to the posed scientific questions will require another 3 decades of clinical testing. It has already taken 2 decades of human testing to prove the scientific principles described in the laboratory via large populations treated with tamoxifen. The same will prove true with SERMs for the prevention of multiple diseases in women.

Conclusion

The successful demonstration that tamoxifen can reduce the incidence of primary breast cancer, and the October, 1998 FDA approval for its broad clinical use in high-risk women now provide a new dimension of healthcare opportunities for women. This landmark mandates that other drugs be compared to this standard of care so that they are safe and effective for their proposed applications. The side-by-side evaluation of raloxifene and tamoxifen will establish the risks and benefits of both agents within the next 5 years. It is fair to state that through its reinvention from a contraceptive to a breast cancer treatment, tamoxifen has now become the leader of a new era of preventive therapeutics.[21] ∎

References

1. Jordan VC, Phelps E, Lindgren UJ: Effects of antiestrogens on bone in castrated and intact female rats. *Breast Cancer Res Treat* 10:31-35, 1987.

2. Gottardis MM, Jordan VC: The antitumor actions of keoxifene (raloxifene) and tamoxifen in the N-nitrosomethylivea induced rat mammary carcinoma model. *Cancer Res* 47:4020-4024, 1987.

3. Lerner LJ, Jordan VC: Development of antiestrogens and their use in breast cancer: Eighth Cain Memorial Award Lecture. *Cancer Res* 50:4177-4189, 1990.

4. Turner RT, Wakley GK, Hannon KS, et al: Tamoxifen prevents the skeletal effects of ovarian hormone deficiency in rats. *J Bone Miner Res* 2:449-456, 1987.

5. Turner RT, Wakley GK, Hannon KS, et al: Tamoxifen inhibits osteoclast-mediated resorption of trabecular bone in ovarian hormone-deficient rats. *Endocrinol* 122:1146-1150, 1988.

6. Love RR, Mazess RB, Barden HS, et al: Effect of tamoxifen on bone-mineral density in postmenopausal women with breast cancer. *N Engl J Med* 326:852-856, 1992.

7. Ward RL, Morgen G, Dalley D, et al: Tamoxifen reduces bone turnover and prevents lumbar spine and proximal femoral bone loss in early postmenopausal women. *Bone Min* 22:187-194, 1993.

8. Kristensen B, Ejlerrsen B, Dalgaard P, et al: Tamoxifen and bone metabolism in postmenopausal low-risk breast cancer patients: A randomized study. *J Clin Oncol* 12:992-997, 1994.

9. Jordan VC: Designer estrogens. *Scientific Am* 279:60-67, 1998.

10. Tonetti DA, Jordan VC: Targeted antiestrogens to treat and prevent disease in women. *Mol Med Today* 2:218-223, 1996.

11. Jordan VC: After the menopause: Tamoxifen and other new prevention maintenance therapies. *J Women's Health* 6:257-259, 1997.

12. Black LJ, Jones CD, Falcone JF: Antagonism of estrogen action with a new benzothiophene-derived antiestrogen. *Life Sci* 32:1031-1036, 1983.

13. Jordan VC, Gosden B: Inhibition of the uterotrophic activity of estrogens and antiestrogens by the short-acting antiestrogen LY117018. *Endocrinol* 113:463-468, 1983.

14. Clemens JA, Bennet DR, Black LJ, et al: Effects of a new antiestrogen keoxifene (LY156758) on growth of carcinogen-induced mammary tumors and on LH and prolactin levels. *Life Sci* 32:2869-2878, 1983.

15. Black LJ, Sato M, Rowley ER, et al: Raloxifene (LY139481 HCL) prevents bone loss and reduces serum cholesterol without causing uterine hypertrophy in ovariec-tomized rats. *J Clin Invest* 93:63-69, 1994.

16. Delmas PD, Bjarnason NH, Mitlak BH, et al: Effects of raloxifene on bone-mineral density, serum cholesterol concentrations and uterine endometrium in postmenopausal women. *N Engl J Med* 337:1641-1647, 1997.

17. Jordan VC, Glusman JE, Eckert S, et al: Incident primary breast cancer is reduced by raloxifene: Integrated data from multicenter, double-blind, randomized trials in 12,000 postmenopausal woman. *Proc Am Soc Clin Oncol* 17:466 (Abstract), 1998.

18. Fisher B, Dignam J, Bryant J, et al: Five versus more than five years of tamoxifen therapy for breast cancer patients with negative lymph nodes and estrogen receptor-positive tumors. *J Natl Cancer Inst* 88:1529-1542, 1996.

19. Early Breast Cancer Trialists' Collaborative Group: Tamoxifen for early breast cancer: An overview of the randomized trials. *Lancet* 351:1451-1467, 1998.

20. Jordan VC, Allen KE: Evaluation of the antitumor activity of the nonsteroidal antiestrogen monohydroxytamoxifen in the DMBA-induced rat mammary carcinoma model. *Eur J Cancer* 16:239-251, 1980.

21. Jordan VC: Tamoxifen: The herald of a new era of preventive therapeutics. *J Natl Cancer Inst* 89:747-749, 1997.

Chapter 18

Y-ME Hotline: The 20 Most Frequently Asked Questions About Tamoxifen

V. Craig Jordan, PhD, DSc
Monica Morrow, MD

Y-ME is a national breast cancer organization headquartered in Chicago that serves hundreds of thousands of American women who have been diagnosed with breast cancer. Y-ME operates a hotline staffed 24 hours a day to respond to questions concerning breast cancer diagnosis, treatment, and recovery. It provides educational meetings and support groups throughout the country, including educational workshops for the lay public, special programs for teenage girls, and a wig and prothesis bank. Y-ME publishes a bimonthly newsletter as well as pamphlets targeting special audiences, such as single women or male partners of breast cancer patients. Many of Y-ME's services are also available in Spanish. Y-ME promotes the psychosocial needs of people with breast cancer and encourages women to be active participants in their medical care.

The 20 most frequently asked questions about tamoxifen on the Y-ME hotline follow:

1. How do I deal with hot flashes?

For some, but not all women, hot flashes and menopausal symptoms are extremely troublesome. In general, younger women are more likely to experience symptoms than women in their late 50s and 60s. However, it must be stressed that based on controlled clinical trials, the increase in symptoms is modest compared to symptoms noted in patients taking placebo.

Although there are many natural or drug remedies, it is clear that there is no simple solution for everyone. Regrettably, no scientific evidence supports over-the-counter remedies. However, some women can benefit from some available agents. Women should consult their physician if symptoms become severe; at that point, the benefits of tamoxifen should be weighed against the difficulties of the symptoms. Clonidine has been found to be effective if used at night to reduce hot flashes and night sweats. However, if you are using tamoxifen as a preventive, it may not be critical to take tamoxifen at this time in your life. In this case, waiting a year, then retrying with a 5-year course may be one solution. This is not recommended if you have had a previous diagnosis of breast cancer. Some physicians may recommend the use of progestins. These are safe in the short term in combination with tamoxifen, but we do not know whether they will, years later, destroy the value of tamoxifen in the breast. Certainly, it is known from animal studies that this is true, ie, the effects of tamoxifen as an anticancer agent can be reversed by progesterone. Progestins should not be used long term with tamoxifen, as we do not have any evidence from clinical trials that this approach is safe.

2. I didn't take tamoxifen when I was diagnosed with breast cancer. Will I benefit now?

This is a very important issue, but there are no clinical trial data to provide an absolute answer of yes. However, your physician could consider several facts in coming to a joint decision about the appropriateness of delayed tamoxifen treatment. If the original diagnosis was estrogen receptor- (ER) positive, the first line of therapy will be tamoxifen should a recurrence ever occur. We know that earlier treatment provides survival advantages, so it's possible that the delayed treatment would provide health benefits.

Additionally, it is known that a woman with one breast cancer is at elevated risk for a second breast cancer in the contralateral breast. Tamoxifen has been shown to reduce the incidence of second primary breast cancer, regardless of whether the original tumor was ER positive or negative. Additionally, tamoxifen is proven to reduce the risk of primary breast cancer and ductal carcinoma in situ (DCIS) in clinical trials, so there is every reason to suppose it would be effective in the remaining breast tissue of either breast. Finally, women with a diagnosis of breast cancer are generally asked to avoid hormone replacement therapy (HRT). Tamoxifen will not increase coronary heart disease or weaken bones. Indeed, tamoxifen can even aid the breast cancer survivor by decreasing fractures.

3. I took tamoxifen for only 2 years. Will I benefit if I restart it and take it for another 3 years?

From the overview of all randomized clinical trials conducted worldwide during the past 2 decades, we know that 5 years of adjuvant tamoxifen treatment is superior to 2 years in both disease-free and overall survival of breast cancer patients. Additionally, we know that 5 years of tamoxifen is superior to 2 years of tamoxifen in controlling contralateral breast cancer. A physician should consider these issues when asked the question of restarting tamoxifen after a period off the drug. However, there are no clinical data to support the advantages of "pulsing" (ie, tamoxifen with 2 years as an adjuvant, followed by no drug for several years, followed by 3 more years of tamoxifen). What is known, however, is that the patient will receive tamoxifen treatment upon recurrence if the original diagnosis was ER positive.

There are few concerns that a physician should have when considering treatment for a total of 5 years with tamoxifen. Therefore, the clinical decision to treat a patient with tamoxifen as a "delayed adjuvant" must take into account the patient's history and type of disease. The clinician must then make a decision based on the known risks that are acceptable for the use of tamoxifen in well women who are at elevated risk for breast cancer.

4. What factors would put me at high risk for breast cancer?

Most women overestimate their risk of breast cancer. Although we can name many breast cancer risk factors, the majority of these factors only slightly increases a woman's risk of developing the disease. The more common risk factors, such as early onset of menses (before age 12), having no children or having a first child after 30, late menopause, or the use of hormone replacement therapy only slightly increase risk. The presence of one of these risk factors would not be enough, in and of itself, to classify a woman as high risk.

Single factors that would put a woman at high risk are uncommon. The presence of a genetic mutation in the BRCA-1 or BRCA-2 genes increases breast cancer risk over a woman's lifetime to 50% to 80%. In the absence of a genetic mutation, the risk seen with a family history of breast cancer is much lower. The precise level of risk will vary with the number of affected relatives and the age of the woman at risk. For example, a 35-year-old woman whose mother had breast cancer at age 60 has only approximately a 5% risk of developing breast cancer over the next 20 years. The benign breast condition called lobular carcinoma in situ (LCIS) increases risk to approximately 1% per year. Although this may not sound like a particularly high level of risk, it is many times higher than the risk in a woman without LCIS. The other benign breast condition that increases risk is called atypical hyperplasia. Women with atypical hyperplasia have about an 8% to 10% risk of cancer development over 10 years. However, the combination of atypical hyperplasia and a mother or sister with breast cancer increases the 10-year risk of breast cancer development to 20%. In the absence of these risk factors, a woman's level of risk can only be determined by considering her age and the balance of factors, which conversely protect and increase breast cancer risk.

Computer programs are available which will calculate a woman's risk of breast cancer development for the next 5 years until age 90. This type of information is often useful in determining the appropriate risk management strategy.

5. I am 35 and have been advised to take tamoxifen for 5 years. How long will tamoxifen take to work and how long will the benefits last?

Experience with tamoxifen as a treatment for breast cancer shows that the antitumor effects occur within 2 months. However, for the most benefit, tamoxifen, should be taken for 5 years. This conclusion is based on an enormous number of clinical trials from around the world. Five years is better than either 1 or 2 year(s) of treatment. However, we know not only about treatment, but also about breast cancer prevention from the preexisting clinical trials.

Five years of tamoxifen reduces the incidence of primary (new) breast cancers in the contralateral breast by 50%. However, the effects of tamoxifen continue to protect the breast even after the drug is stopped. Strong data from the Overview Analysis in Oxford suggest that tamoxifen continues to reduce the incidence of new breast cancer by 50% for 5 years after the drug is stopped. Preliminary evidence also suggests that tamoxifen keeps working for 10 years after a woman stops taking it. The fact that the medical community does not know the duration of the positive effects of tamoxifen is not because it stops working, but because further decades of monitoring are necessary to document the long-term benefits of tamoxifen.

6. I am postmenopausal. Is my risk of side effects higher from tamoxifen than a premenopausal woman and why?

Postmenopausal women have a higher number of serious side effects compared to premenopausal women. Postmenopausal women have double the risk of endometrial cancer when they take tamoxifen. This should, however, be placed into perspective. One thousand 60-year-old postmenopausal women will have a diagnosis of one good grade, early-stage endometrial cancer per year. If those women are all using tamoxifen, then this number becomes 2 endometrial cancers per year per 1,000 women. Additionally, postmenopausal women taking tamoxifen have an increase in blood clots at the same rate as hormone replacement therapy or raloxifene. The risks are all the same, but again, the rate is very small. Serious blood clots can occur, but these are associated with other diseases a patient might have. Your physician can judge the risks before starting tamoxifen.

On the other hand, premenopausal women develop endometrial cancer at an extremely low rate, and tamoxifen does not increase the incidence of endometrial cancer in premenopausal women. Additionally, premenopausal women do not have an increased risk of blood clots while taking tamoxifen. Premenopausal women suffer fewer serious side effects because they continue to menstruate, thereby cleaning out the womb of cancer cells. They also get fewer blood clots because they are generally healthier and more active than older women.

7. I am a postmenopausal woman at high risk for breast cancer. Why is my risk for side effects with tamoxifen higher than a premenopausal woman's?

It is known that endometrial cancer occurs more frequently in well women who are postmenopausal than in premenopausal women. This is because 1) cancers are associated with advancing age, and 2) cancer cells are shed by the monthly cycle in premenopausal women.

Studies from autopsy data have shown that the numbers of endometrial cancers in a woman's uterus are 4 times the clinically detected rate based on symptoms (ie, spotting or bleeding) that are followed up by a gynecologist. On average, 60-year-old women have a diagnosis of one endometrial cancer per 1,000 women per year. They are usually very early stage disease and can be cured by hysterectomy. Women who take tamoxifen have an increased incidence of 2 endometrial cancers per 1,000 women. We would expect to find this increase based on the known number of endometrial cancers already in the womb. Tamoxifen has a slight estrogen-like effect that may increase endometrial tumor growth and allow early detection. Tamoxifen is, however, not as powerful as estrogen in stimulating tumor growth.

Blood clots may also occur with advancing years, a lack of exercise, long periods of bed rest, and other comorbidities like cancer and diabetes. Hormone replacement therapy, raloxifene, and tamoxifen all increase blood clots to the same extent in postmenopausal women. However, in all cases, this is a very small incidence. Clearly, a woman would need to be informed that the risk of blood clots with hormone replacement therapy and raloxifene used to prevent osteoporosis is the same as the risk of clots with the use of tamoxifen to prevent breast cancer.

8. If I think I am high risk for breast cancer and wanted to consider tamoxifen, what questions would I ask my doctor?

Women seeing a physician for risk assessment should ask for a numeric estimate of their short-term risk of breast cancer development (usually 5 years), as well as their lifetime risk. They should determine what risk factors are present. Early evidence suggests that tamoxifen may be particularly beneficial in reducing risk in women at risk on the basis of benign breast diseases, lobular carcinoma in situ, and atypical hyperplasia. Women considering tamoxifen for risk reduction should question the amount that their level of risk would be reduced by tamoxifen. If postmenopausal, they should ask about other beneficial effects of the drug, such as protection against osteoporosis and reduction in blood cholesterol. Premenopausal women should ask whether they can take the drug while they are trying to become pregnant and about the need for barrier contraception while on tamoxifen. Women should also ask about the side effects of tamoxifen, their potential severity, and the likelihood of these side effects occurring based on their age and health status. Women should inquire about the length of tamoxifen therapy, and whether breast cancer protection ends when the drug is stopped. It is also appropriate to ask about other strategies for the management of high-risk women, such as close clinical follow-up or prophylactic mastectomy, what each entails, and how effective they might be.

9. In layman's language, what makes healthy, premenopausal women high risk and in potential need of tamoxifen therapy as a preventive for breast cancer?

Since breast cancer is an age-related disease, premenopausal women have a relatively low baseline risk of developing the disease. To be considered high risk, premenopausal women must usually have several breast cancer risk factors. The younger a woman is, the more risk factors she needs to be considered high risk. Mutation in a gene that predisposes to breast cancer, such as BRCA-1 or BRCA-2, increases risk, regardless of a woman's age. For most premenopausal women, a single relative with breast cancer, even if a mother or sister, is not a high enough level of risk to warrant tamoxifen treatment. Women who have not had children or who have had their first child after age 30 have a small increase in risk. Again, these alone are not indications for tamoxifen. Most benign breast conditions do not increase risk, nor do "lumpy" breasts on clinical examination. Benign breast conditions that do increase risk are atypical hyperplasia and lobular carcinoma in situ. These problems are seen in fewer than 5% of premenopausal women who have breast biopsies. In the NSABP Breast Cancer Prevention trial, a 5-year risk of breast cancer development equal to that of a 60-year-old woman was needed to be eligible to enter the study. This level of risk is a useful benchmark for premenopausal women who are concerned about whether or not they need tamoxifen treatment.

10. I am a healthy, premenopausal, high-risk woman who is taking tamoxifen. How long will I need to stay on it to prevent breast cancer?

There is enormous clinical experience with the use of tamoxifen. Over the past 20 years, the duration of tamoxifen treatment has extended from 1 to 5 years. It is now clear that 5 years of tamoxifen is superior to shorter durations (1 or 2 years) to prevent primary breast cancer in the contralateral (opposite) breast in women with previous breast cancer. Overall, 5 years is the recommended therapy.

11. How long do I have to take tamoxifen?

Tamoxifen is the single most effective agent for the adjuvant treatment of breast cancer in postmenopausal women.

This is a matter between you and your doctor. The standard duration of tamoxifen treatment in all US clinical studies is 5 years. Nevertheless, many patients have taken tamoxifen for more than 5 years, and clinical trials are now testing the value of indefinite tamoxifen treatment.

Nonetheless, the National Cancer Institute has issued a Physicians' Alert stating that, for node-negative patients, 10 years of tamoxifen provides no greater benefit than 5 years. However, these results were based on the recurrences of breast cancer in only one clinical trial; many in the clinical trial community believe that more information is needed. In fact, clinical trials conducted in England are now addressing the issue of duration of tamoxifen therapy by recruiting 20,000 women who have stopped tamoxifen at various times to determine the risks and benefits in large patient populations.

12. What are the side effects of tamoxifen therapy? Are they temporary or permanent?

There are a variety of minor side effects associated with tamoxifen that should be discussed with your doctor. A comparison of side effects in placebo-controlled trials is illustrated in Table 1. The most common concern is postmenopausal symptoms. A minority of patients may suffer severe symptoms, but these will diminish with time. Some side effects, such as hot flashes, occur more frequently in younger women. Less than 5% of women stop tamoxifen because of side effects. Postmenopausal women should be aware that there is also a modest increase in the detection of endometrial cancer in women taking tamoxifen. In general, 1 postmenopausal woman in 1,000 will develop endometrial cancer each year. In postmenopausal women taking tamoxifen, the rate is 2 women who may have endometrial cancer diagnosed per 1,000 per year. Any signs of vaginal spotting or bleeding should be reported to your doctor and followed up with a gynecologic examination [see Chapters 8 and 9].

Table I

Percentage of Women Who Reported an Adverse Side Effect in the NSABP-14 5-Year Tamoxifen Trial (20 mg Daily) Vs Placebo

Both pre- and postmenopausal women participated in the study. These are the only side effects noted by the nearly 3,000 women involved in the trial. It should be recognized that all side effects were not experienced by all women.

Adverse Effect	Nolvadex (n = 1424)	Placebo (n = 1420)
Hot flashes	63.9%	47.6%
Weight gain (> 5%)	38.1%	40.1%
Fluid retention	32.4%	29.7%
Vaginal discharge	29.6%	15.2%
Nausea	25.7%	23.9%
Irregular menses	24.6%	18.8%
Weight loss (> 5%)	22.6%	18.0%
Skin changes	18.7%	15.3%
Increased blood urea nitrogen (BUN)	18.1%	20.2%
Diarrhea	11.2%	14.0%
Increased serum glutamic-oxaloacetic transaminase (SGOT)	4.8%	2.8%
Increased alkaline phosphatase	3.0%	4.6%
Vomiting	2.1%	1.7%
Increased bilirubin	1.8%	1.2%
Increased creatinine	1.7%	1.0%
Thrombocytopenia*	1.5%	1.2%
Leukopenia**	0.4%	1.1%
Thrombotic events Deep vein thrombosis	0.8%	0.3%
Pulmonary embolism	0.4%	0.1%
Superficial phlebitis	0.3%	0.0%

*Defined as a platelet count of < 100,000/mm³

**Defined as a white blood cell count of < 3,000/mm³

13. How does tamoxifen work?

Tamoxifen has target site-specific actions. The drug acts as an antiestrogen to block breast cancer growth, but it also has an estrogenic effect to help maintain bone density and to decrease circulating cholesterol. Prolonged (5 years or more) use of tamoxifen is associated with a decrease in myocardial infarction (heart attacks). The way tamoxifen works as an antibreast cancer drug depends principally on its ability to block the growth effects of estrogen in the breast cancer. A majority of breast cancers contain estrogen receptors (locks) that bind estrogen (keys) in a woman's body. The estrogen fits the estrogen receptor (ER) in the tumor cell and turns on all of the reactions necessary to instruct the cell to divide. As a result, the tumor grows relentlessly with estrogen as the fuel. Tamoxifen binds to the estrogen receptor and blocks the ability of estrogen by stopping estrogen binding. It blocks the estrogen receptor—blocks the lock—as long as the drug is taken. In turn, tamoxifen cannot switch on the proper mechanism to instruct the tumor to grow, so the cells die and the tumor shrinks.

Another way to understand the different effects that tamoxifen can produce around a woman's body is to view it as a programmed elevator key: The estrogen makes the elevator stop at all the floors, while the tamoxifen key only allows stops at some floors. Estrogen stimulates all sites around a woman's body *including* the breast cancer; but tamoxifen stimulates all the sites *except* the breast cancer.

14. What happens if I don't take, or stop taking, tamoxifen?

Forgetting to take the medication once in a while is not a cause for concern. Although 20 mg daily (one 20 mg tablet or two 10 mg tablets) is recommended, there is usually sufficient tamoxifen in the blood to protect you if tablets are forgotten.

Tamoxifen works as an anticancer agent if the drug is present to suppress the tumor. Without the drug, estrogen can reactivate the growth mechanism.

15. How should I monitor myself for side effects and problems?

The most important method is simply to report any major changes in your normal activities to your physician or healthcare professional. Tamoxifen is remarkably free from serious side effects, but it is often tempting to blame tamoxifen for problems normally associated with menopause or aging.

The side effects of tamoxifen are listed in Table 1. It is unlikely that an individual will experience all or even most of these side effects. This list includes symptoms from thousands of different women over many years. The single most important concern is the early detection of endometrial cancer (see Chapters 8 and 9). If you experience any vaginal spotting or bleeding after menopause, you should tell your physician, who will then order a full gynecological examination.

16. How effective is tamoxifen?

Tamoxifen is the single most effective agent for the adjuvant treatment of breast cancer in postmenopausal women. Each woman will respond differently, depending upon the type and stage of breast cancer. However, the Overview Analysis of clinical trials convincingly demonstrates a survival advantage for women taking tamoxifen. On average, this can translate to a year or two more of life for women taking tamoxifen compared with women not taking tamoxifen. Tamoxifen is the only therapy that reduces the incidence of breast cancer in the opposite breast and also reduces the risk of local recurrence of breast cancer in the affected breast in women treated with lumpectomy and radiotherapy.

17. Where can I get tamoxifen at a reasonable price?

The price of tamoxifen has remained remarkably stable for the past 10 years. It is controlled in the United States through patent protection. Moreover, Zeneca Pharmaceuticals believes that no woman who needs Nolvadex be denied the drug because of her economic circumstances. Truly needy women can apply through their physicians to Zeneca's assistance program. Between 1978 and 1996, Zeneca provided more than $114 million worth of tamoxifen to needy patients.

18. Should I take tamoxifen if I'm ER negative or premenopausal?

Tamoxifen is more effective in some circumstances than in others. Although tamoxifen works most effectively in patients with estrogen receptor-rich disease, estrogen receptor-poor patients can also benefit. The point where the tumor is described as estrogen receptor positive or negative varies from place to place. For example, most laboratories have used a value of 10 femtomoles/mg protein as their cut-off point; values greater than 10 are considered estrogen receptor positive; and those less than 10 are considered negative. In San Antonio, however, the cut-off point is 3 femtomoles/mg protein. New techniques of immunocytochemistry do not have a quantitative scale at all. Therefore, it is best to consider patients as estrogen receptor rich or poor.

Tamoxifen is equally effective at reducing the risk of contralateral breast cancer whether or not the first tumor was ER rich or ER poor.

Clinical trials with node-positive breast cancer patients over age 50 have noted that estrogen receptor-poor patients have a survival advantage after taking tamoxifen. Although most physicians would follow the consensus guidelines that only node-positive patients with receptor-rich tumors should be given tamoxifen, the FDA-approved indications do not rule out tamoxifen for receptor-poor patients with node-positive disease.

Although tamoxifen works most effectively in patients with estrogen receptor-positive disease, estrogen receptor-poor patients can also benefit.

The above situation contrasts with node-negative disease and premenopausal patients. Tamoxifen is FDA approved for the adjuvant treatment of pre- and postmenopausal, node-negative patients with estrogen receptor-rich primary tumors. Tamoxifen is also approved for the treatment of patients who are premenopausal with stage IV (advanced), estrogen receptor-positive breast cancer.

19. Can I get pregnant while on tamoxifen?

Tamoxifen should not be given to a woman who is known to be pregnant because of possible birth defects and harm to the fetus. Women who are of reproductive age *must* use barrier contraception to prevent pregnancy. Premenopausal women who take tamoxifen are at risk for pregnancy. Women who may wish to conceive after a diagnosis of breast cancer should consult their physician because tamoxifen should not be prescribed. If a woman chooses to become pregnant after a course of tamoxifen, the drug should be stopped for up to 6 months before pregnancy is considered.

20. How is tamoxifen different than chemotherapy?

Tamoxifen is generally classified as an antiestrogen rather than a chemotherapy. In general, cytotoxic chemotherapy attacks all dividing cells in a woman's body—not just the cancer cells. As a result, chemotherapy is associated with a high level of toxic side effects. In contrast, tamoxifen does not have dangerous effects on normal cells, but it does stop the growth of tumors. It causes death in the tumor cells, but does not injure other tissues. Side effects of tamoxifen are very low compared with any of the cytotoxic chemotherapies. ■

For additional information about Y-ME, please write to:
Y-ME
National Breast Care Organizations
212 W. Van Buren, 4th Floor
Chicago, IL 60607-3908

24-hour National hotline: 1-800-221-2141
24-hour Spanish-language hotline: 1-800-986-9505

Fax: 312-294-8597

Appendix 1

Translational Research: Applying Laboratory Discoveries to Patient Care

V. Craig Jordan, PhD, DSc

The precise biological events that occur in the breast to cause cancer are currently unknown. However, research over the past 50 years has provided remarkable insight into the working of the normal cell and this, in turn, has acted as a framework to understand the process of carcinogenesis. If we can understand the normal cell, then perhaps we can detect differences in a cancer cell and attempt to correct the change.

The course of human disease has been documented by the medical profession throughout this century. Cancer of the breast has the ability to spread through the body, and based on the principle of "seed and soil," the "seed," or metastases, from the primary tumor in the breast, travels throughout the body in the blood and lymphatic systems to lodge in distant organs of preference (Figure 1). The metastasis finds the correct "soil" to nurture growth. To survive, chemical signals are transmitted from the metastases that encourage the growth of new blood vessels towards the growing metastasis. This process is called angiogenesis. The blood vessels supply nutrients and oxygen to the dividing metastasis that enable the tumor to continue growth at the expense of the host. Ultimately, the spread and unregulated growth of metastases throughout the body will overwhelm the host.

Clinical research has allowed physicians to determine the degree of spread from the breast by examining the axillary lymph nodes for the microscopic presence of tumor. Patients are then classified as good prognosis (node negative for tumor) or poor prognosis (many lymph nodes containing tumor) (Figure 2).

Twenty years ago, patients were treated with breast surgery alone in the belief that, because some patients would be cured, the wise strategy was to wait for a recurrence in those who were not cured, and treat these latter patients on recurrence or progression. Now, adjuvant treatment with chemotherapy or tamoxifen is used after primary surgery to prevent recurrence by

BREAST CANCER DISTANT METASTASES

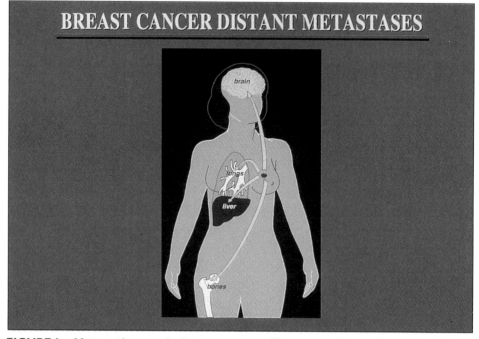

FIGURE 1   **Metastatic spread of breast cancer**   The tumor cells travel through the blood and lymphatic system to lodge in organs of preference throughout the body, if not treated. The diagram illustrates some, but not all, of the sites of potential metastatic spread. The metastases then continue to grow at the expense of the host in their new environment.

destroying unseen micrometastases around the body. This is the current strategy that is used to provide the best survival opportunity. The objective of all therapy with medicines is to destroy the metastases without harming the host; however, this is a difficult balance. Toxicities occur when chemotherapy attacks both normal and cancer cells. However, the enormous success of tamoxifen, with its low incidence of side effects and targeted mode of action, has changed the strategy for treatment.

The current goal of research is to target vulnerable growth pathways in the tumor and to develop nontoxic treatments. The clinical description of human disease has been complemented by efforts in the research laboratory to understand, under controlled conditions, the causes of mammary cancer in animals. Several principles have emerged that have ultimately provided an insight into the control and prevention of human disease. However, research does not travel in straight lines and the results and accomplishments in a laboratory model do not always provide solutions. Rather, in many instances, research only provides clues as to where to look for more information about human disease.

The description of the process of mammary carcinogenesis in laboratory animals has revealed targets to treat and to prevent breast cancer. For most of this century, it has been known that strains of mice can be bred that have a high incidence or a low incidence of mammary cancer. In the 1930s, a virus, called Bittners Milk Factor, was found to be transferred to the offspring in the mother's milk. This principle is unique to the mouse, and the virus, called mouse mammary tumor virus (MMTV), is *not* generally believed to be involved in human disease. However, the virus has taught the research community a lot about carcinogenesis in the mouse. The gene has been thoroughly investigated and is now a research tool in molecular biology. Applications of this knowledge have been enormous and the success has opened the door for the discovery of "oncogenes" (ie, cancer-causing genes).

In 1962, Nobel laureate Professor Charles Huggins showed how a single dose of a polycyclic hydrocarbon derived from tar could produce mammary cancer in susceptible strains of rats. Throughout all of this century, chemicals had been linked to cancer, but the sensitivity and ease with which the tumors were produced in rats was the key. Mammary carcinogenesis was completely dependent on the age of the animals and the hormonal state; ie,

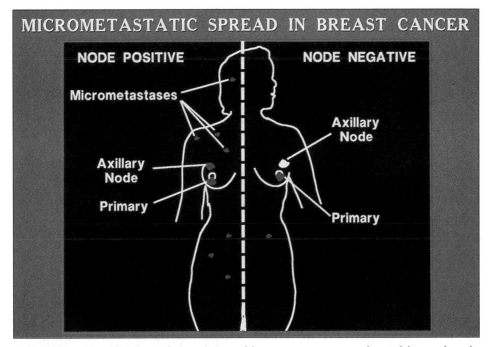

FIGURE 2 Classification of the stages of breast cancer as node positive and node negative The presence of microscopic tumor in the axillary lymph nodes is a marker of the spread of micrometastases throughout a patient's body.

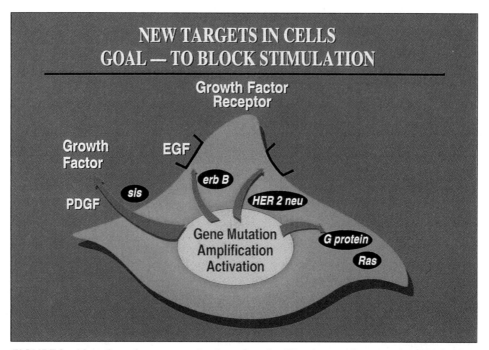

FIGURE 3   Mutation of oncogenes in the normal cell leads to an increase in stimulatory-growth pathways   The diagram shows only a few examples of the many dozens of reported changes. Growth factors, like platelet derived growth factor (PDGF), can be increased, and this activated oncogene product is called *sis*. Estrogen receptor-negative breast cancers have increased surface receptors that respond to epidermal growth factor (EGF). This is a normal stimulatory growth factor that is produced in many anatomic sites in the body; but the receptor also responds to the oncogenic stimulatory growth factor, called transforming growth factor alpha (TGFα). The breast cancer cells produce an excess of the stimulatory growth factor that encourages growth through the EGF receptor known as *erb* B. A similar cell surface receptor called *HER-2/neu* is an oncogene product found in about 20% to 30% of poor prognosis breast cancers. Currently, attempts to target therapy to attack the *HER-2/neu* target have met with some success in the laboratory; there are encouraging clinical data to suggest that the oncogene is a marker for sensitivity to chemotherapy. The G proteins are signal transduction pathways that relay messages from the exterior to the interior of the cell. They operate as on/ off switches. About 10% of breast cancers have a mutation at an oncogene product called *ras* that is stuck in the "on" position. Additionally, we know that the chemical carcinogens that produce mammary tumors in rats specifically mutate the *ras* gene.

the presence or absence of the sex steroids, estrogen and progesterone. However, some strains of rats were completely resistant to the chemical carcinogen. This again highlights the difference between laboratory animals and women. The animals were inbred to be vulnerable to the carcinogenic insult, and it is now clear that the same process cannot readily happen in women. The human is outbred and not inbred, so, in general, we are not vulnerable to carcinogens and we survive through sophisticated repair mechanisms in our cells. Nevertheless, some principles have translated from the laboratory to the clinic.

It is known from atom bomb survivors at Hiroshima and from adolescents who received radiation treatments for Hodgkin's disease, that there is an increased susceptibility in young girls for radiation to initiate breast cancer. A significant radiation insult to young girls increases the risk for breast cancer in later life. This is also true for the young laboratory rat of the correct strain—whether the carcinogenic insult is radiation or chemical. There is only a narrow window of time when the mammary gland is vulnerable to the initiation of cancer. However, in the laboratory, it was found that female sex hormones are essential. Cancer does not occur if the animal has no ovaries. We also know that restricting the influence of the ovaries can have a profound

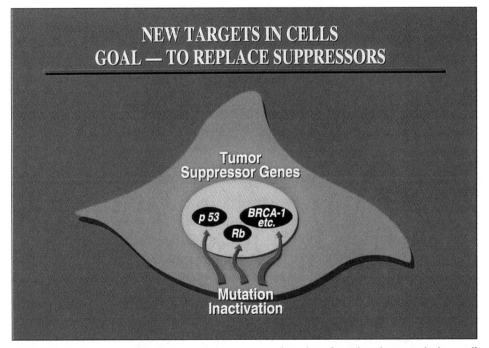

FIGURE 4 Tumor suppressor genes are proteins that function by restricting cell replication A mutation, or small change in the protein, will change its shape and it will not be able to perform its function as a cellular brake. The Rb or retinoblastoma protein was discovered to be responsible for the genetically transmitted cancer of the eye, called retinoblastoma. Susceptible individuals are at genetic risk of having their low compliment of Rb destroyed by mutation of the tumor-suppressor gene DNA. This destruction of the brake causes cancers in the affected individuals. The protein, p53, is mutated in all different sorts of cancers and the unmutated protein appears to be a tumor-suppressor gene. The breast cancer susceptibility gene BRCA-1 is mutated in high-risk individuals with a genetic family history of breast cancer. (See Appendix 3.)

effect on the development of breast cancer in humans. Men have less than 1% of the incidence of breast cancer compared with women. Women who have an oophorectomy for medical reasons in their mid 30s generally have half the incidence of breast cancer in later life, compared with women who have a natural menopause at 50. Therefore, it is believed that estrogen is intimately involved in the development and the growth of breast cancer.

But does estrogen cause breast cancer?

Laboratory studies have dissected the process of carcinogenesis into two stages: initiation and promotion. Initiation involves a genotoxic insult that alters the pattern of DNA—the blueprint for future generations of cells. The DNA can be altered by genotoxic chemicals or radiation, but in general, the cell can quickly repair the damage before the imprint, or mistake, is made permanent in future generations of cells through rapid replication.

What controls the replication of cells and growth in general?

Normal cells maintain their boundaries through a carefully regulated conversation with their neighbors. This is accomplished by a balance of negative and positive chemical messengers, called growth factors, that locally affect the cells. A stimulatory-growth factor will instruct cells to divide when an injury needs to be repaired, and an inhibitory growth factor will prevent the cells from growing further once tissue repairs are complete. Those chemicals that act as accelerators or brakes on the same cell where they are made are called autocrine growth factors; but if they affect an adjacent cell, they are called paracrine growth factors.

The process of carcinogenesis is initiated by mutations of proto-oncogenes that lie buried and quiescent within the blueprint of our DNA. A proto-oncogene is converted to a growth-stimulating oncogene by either increasing the production of a mutant growth factor or its cell surface receptor (Figure 3). The cells' own growth mechanisms are dysregulated and begin responding to the hyperstimulation of growth messages.

However, an increase in accelerator growth signals is only one side of the story. Cells have regulator proteins within the nucleus that stop dysregulated growth. These are called tumor suppressor genes. The tumor suppressor gene can also be mutated so that the stop signal for replication in the cell is no longer recognized (Figure 4).

It is, therefore, clear that a very complex sequence of events must occur—and not be corrected by cellular repair mechanisms—before cancer is initiated. The mistake must be consolidated at an early stage to allow the cancer any hope of progressing to invasive disease. This event is, therefore, rarely successful. However, if initiation *is* successful, estrogen provides the fuel to drive the damaged cells through replication before the repair of mutations is

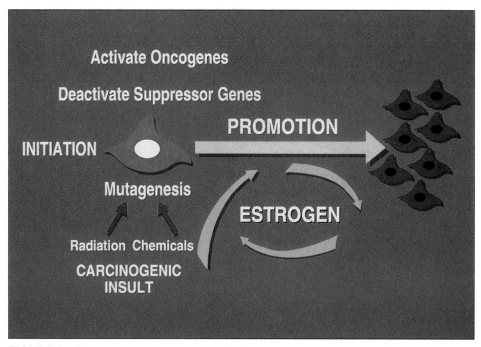

FIGURE 5 The mutation of oncogenes, or tumor suppressor genes, by initiators of carcinogenesis acts to disrupt the integrity of the DNA The damage is consolidated by rapid cycles of cell replication so that the mistakes do not get repaired. Estrogen acts to promote and consolidate the carcinogenic insult that ultimately results in tumor formation.

complete. The mistakes to the DNA blueprint are copied faithfully in future generations to form a cancer cell. Estrogen allows the microfoci of deranged cancer cells to expand, and they may even amplify their estrogen-receptor (ER) population to maintain the growth response. Other tumor cell populations may develop new growth pathways by mutations of other growth regulator genes. The ER will then become vestigial and redundant.

Cancer is characterized by genetic instability. The possibility of the mutant cell surviving at the expense of its female host can be unlimited. The diagrams illustrated in Figure 5 show the activation of oncogenes, the destruction of tumor-suppressor genes by mutagens (chemicals or radiation), and finally, the process of carcinogenesis being promoted to completion by estrogen. The malignant cell can then initiate disease progression by metastasizing in other parts of the body.

The knowledge of carcinogenesis has now promoted a focused evaluation of new therapeutic strategies to either prevent or at least localize breast cancer. Diligent laboratory research has made these opportunities possible. Some of the strategies are illustrated in Figure 6.

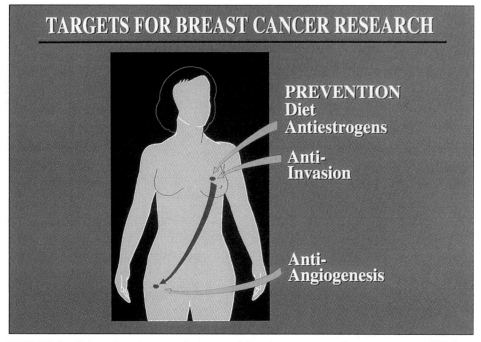

FIGURE 6 Strategies that are being evaluated to prevent breast cancer Lifetime nutritional factors may be important to prevent breast cancer, but tamoxifen is being tested in clinical trials in the United States, Britain, and Italy to block the promoting effects of estrogen. Additionally, drugs that prevent tumor invasion could prevent spreading. However, when malignant cells *do* spread to distant sites, an antiangiogenic drug might prevent the formation of blood vessels and starve the metastasis. Without nutrients from the host, the tumor will die.

There is currently intense interest in developing a nutritional strategy to prevent cancer. The epidemiologic data point to a varying incidence of different cancers in different countries. Might it be the environment, or perhaps diet?

A whole host of dietary factors may be involved, and laboratory research has identified several protective factors like antioxidants, phytoestrogens, and various fish oils that can alter carcinogenesis in animals. Similarly, a high-fat diet has been implicated in increased cancer risk. However, it is not easy to alter the lifestyle of the nation from conception to the grave to prove the role of nutrition in the development of cancer. Indeed, it is well known that it is very difficult for our society to control food consumption in general.

Antiestrogens, on the other hand, can be used in the context of clinical trials to answer a straightforward question: "Does 5 years of tamoxifen therapy prevent breast cancer in a woman at high risk?" That question has been successfully addressed through a nationwide clinical trial comparing tamoxifen treatment with placebo. Biases are avoided by coding the treatments and observing the results only after years of data collection of the positive and negative effects of treatment. Without clinical trials, the question of the safety and worth of tamoxifen as a preventive could not be answered. The alternative was the judgment of an individual physician to recommend treatment based on his or her prejudice or anecdotal experience. This was the method of medicine up to the 1960s, and to all extents, it should be prevented so that our communities remain protected.

The exciting possibility of prevention was tested in the tamoxifen trial. The question, "Can an *antiestrogen* prevent breast cancer with a minimum number of side effects?" has been answered. Already, a spectrum of new antiestrogens and approaches to this research question are being positioned by the pharmaceutical industry so, by the turn of the century, numerous new antiestrogens will be benefiting from the information obtained with tamoxifen today. Raloxifene (Evista) is a result of that research knowledge.

Translational research from the 1987 discovery that raloxifene and tamoxifen preserved bone density resulted in the use of raloxifene to prevent osteoporosis. But the fact that raloxifene could prevent breast cancer simultaneously is currently being tested in the STAR trial (study of tamoxifen and raloxifene). (See Chapter 17.)

Two other major research questions focus on the concept of restricting the spread of cancer when it occurs. New drugs are being developed that prevent malignant cells from destroying normal tissue around them. This process of destruction allows the micrometastasis to enter the blood and lymphatics in the breast and spread throughout the body. The chemicals secreted by the tumor cells—called proteases and collagenases—invade the surrounding tissue in front of the malignant cell like a snowblower invading into deep snow to create a path to the road. The drug target, for example, would be the snow blower, which could be stopped by a fallen branch jammed in the blades. Clearly, these drugs could be used as preventives in high-risk women. If a tumor occurred in the breast, it would not spread throughout the body and could be detected and completely cured by surgery.

The final point of attack is when the micrometastasis has found a suitable "soil" and needs to grow through unlimited access to nutrients from the host. If a strategy can be devised to stop angiogenesis—the process of obtaining a blood supply—then the micrometastasis will starve to death.

Conclusions

Overall, ideas developed in the laboratory are being rapidly translated into practical weapons to treat and prevent breast cancer. Only through continued research will our ability to control breast cancer be assured. It is essential to train and support a new generation of physicians interested in laboratory science and scientists interested in the control of breast cancer. People make discoveries and people advocate new ideas to change the approach to a cure for breast cancer. The support of young investigators in centers of research excellence with a proven record of successful accomplishment is the best investment for the future of scientific discovery. ■

Appendix 2

How Does Tamoxifen Work?

V. Craig Jordan, PhD, DSc

There is no simple answer to the complex issue of the molecular events that not only cause tamoxifen to act as a targeted antitumor agent in the breast, but which also cause additional positive effects around a woman's body (Figure 1). A possible explanation must be divided into three different aspects: (1) the local antitumor actions of tamoxifen in breast cancer cells, (2) the peripheral antitumor actions of tamoxifen, and (3) the physiological actions of tamoxifen.

Local Antitumor Actions of Tamoxifen in Breast Cancer Cells

In the 20 years since Dr. Marc E. Lippman first showed that tamoxifen inhibits the growth of estrogen receptor- (ER) positive breast cancer cells in culture, this model has been used extensively to dissect the molecular components of estrogen and antiestrogen actions. The molecular mechanism by which estrogen can control replication is illustrated in Figures 2a and 2b. A cascade of events in the cell is triggered by estrogen from the circulation which diffuses into the cell to bind to an estrogen receptor in the nucleus. The receptor complex becomes activated by changing its shape; two complexes are then believed to work in concert to activate estrogen-responsive genes composed of DNA. The genes are then decoded by the transcription complex to make messenger RNA that makes a new protein in the cell cytoplasm. This process is called translation. Simply stated, the release of a trigger mechanism has the effect of making multiple new proteins that all have separate functions and, once orchestrated correctly, will convince the machinery of the cell to replicate itself through the duplication of DNA (the blueprint of the cell).

Some of the critical genes for replication are currently elusive, although the application of knowledge derived from the laboratory during the past decade has revolutionized our understanding of the molecular biology of cell replication. The key, though, is the trigger mechanism. If this can be blocked or immobilized, the cell will not divide on command.

Tamoxifen is a nonsteroidal antiestrogen that binds to the estrogen receptor, but cannot produce the correct folding in the protein to switch on the

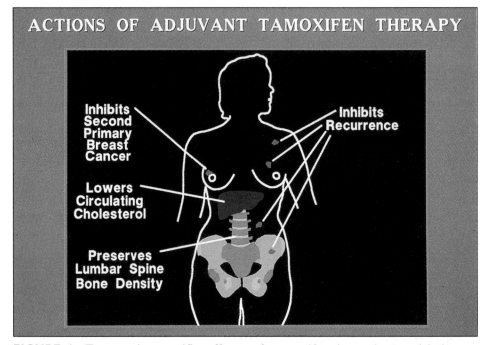

FIGURE I   Target site-specific effects of tamoxifen in patients with breast cancer   Tamoxifen is proven to increase survival by preventing disease recurrence. It is the only therapy that reduces the incidence of contralateral breast cancer. These effects can be considered antiestrogenic actions of tamoxifen. In contrast, tamoxifen maintains bone density and lowers circulating cholesterol in postmenopausal patients. These important physiologic effects may help prevent osteoporosis and coronary heart disease in postmenopausal women at high risk for these diseases.

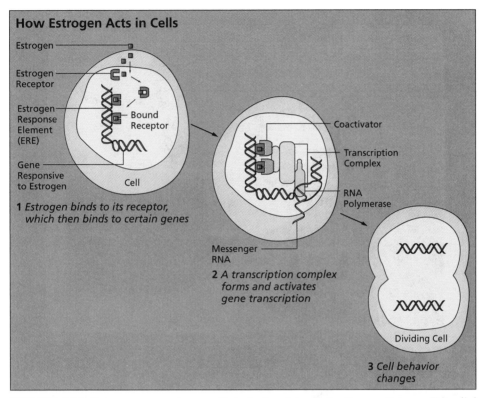

How Estrogen Acts in Cells

Estrogen

Estrogen Receptor

Estrogen Response Element (ERE)

Bound Receptor

Gene Responsive to Estrogen

Cell

1 *Estrogen binds to its receptor, which then binds to certain genes*

Coactivator

Transcription Complex

RNA Polymerase

Messenger RNA

2 *A transcription complex forms and activates gene transcription*

Dividing Cell

3 *Cell behavior changes*

FIGURE 2(a) Estrogen receptor-mediated signal transduction pathway   Estradiol diffuses through the cellular membranes to the nucleus where it binds to the ER. The receptor complex undergoes a conformational change and locks the steroid into the protein structure like the closing of the jaws of a crocodile. The receptor complex dimerizes and interacts with the estrogen response element (ERE), located near the target gene. These events cause the recruitment of other proteins called coactivators that form a transcription complex that opens up the DNA, allowing RNA polymerase to bind and transcribe messenger RNA. In the case of breast cancer, these events act as a trigger to cause the cells to replicate.

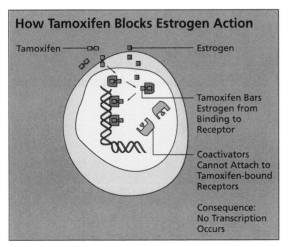

How Tamoxifen Blocks Estrogen Action

Tamoxifen

Estrogen

Tamoxifen Bars Estrogen from Binding to Receptor

Coactivators Cannot Attach to Tamoxifen-bound Receptors

Consequence: No Transcription Occurs

FIGURE 2(b) Tamoxifen binds to the ER receptor, but stops the conformational changes that lock the molecule into the protein. Instead, tamoxifen acts to wedge into the receptor, and the side chain acts like a stick in the jaws of a crocodile. As a result, coactivators cannot bind to the receptor complex and critical genes are not transcribed. These events prevent cell division.

Adapted from Jordan VC: *Scientific Am* 279:60-67, 1998.

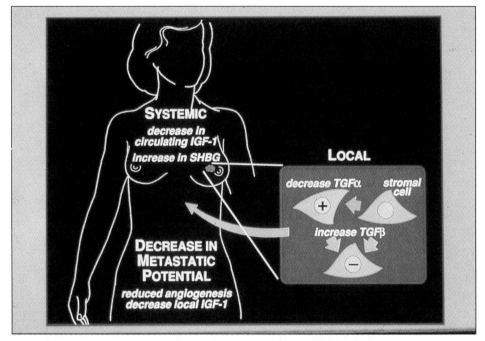

FIGURE 3   Overall effects of tamoxifen as an antitumor agent.   The effects of tamoxifen in a breast tumor [inset] are to decrease the secretion of stimulatory growth factors, such as transforming growth factor alpha (TGFα), and to increase the secretion of an inhibitory growth factor, such as transforming growth factor beta (TGFβ). TGFβ is known to inhibit the growth of estrogen receptor-negative cells, and it is believed that this is how tamoxifen can be effective in the patient with an estrogen receptor-poor tumor. TGFβ functions as a paracrine growth factor, controlling the growth of an adjacent cell. Similarly, tamoxifen is thought to increase TGFβ production in the stromal cells in the tumor. The stromal cells act as a skeleton or support for the cancer cells in the tumor. Although these local antitumor effects may be essential, tamoxifen can also decrease the local and circulating levels of a stimulatory growth factor called insulin-like growth factor-1 (IGF-1). This growth factor stimulates the growth of both ER-positive and ER-negative tumors. Tamoxifen lowers the available level of circulating estrogen in a postmenopausal woman's body by increasing the level of sex hormones binding globulin (SHBG), a blood transport protein that binds estrogenic steroids. If the steroids remain bound in the blood, they cannot diffuse into the estrogen receptor-positive tumor. Finally, tamoxifen may contribute to survival by decreasing tumor invasion and preventing the metastases from developing new blood vessels, ie, angiogenesis.

optimal sequence of events that efficiently makes specific replication proteins. The cells cannot sustain cycles of replication and will remain quiescent for as long as tamoxifen is present, blocking the receptors. The tamoxifen receptor complex will either initiate the death of the cells in the tumor or stop new cell replication. A breast tumor may decrease in size because most cells start to die as a result of tamoxifen therapy. Tumors go into remission because the cells necessary for the growth of the tumor cannot be replaced.

Usually, tumors are composed of mixtures of both estrogen receptor-positive and estrogen receptor-negative cells (Figure 3). This "community" of cells helps and supports each other through the growth factor secretion so that some resistant cells can survive at the expense of their neighbors. Conversely, inhibitory growth factors secreted from estrogen receptor-positive tumor cells in response to tamoxifen therapy can potentially control the growth of adjacent estrogen receptor-negative cells. This stasis (inactivity) of growth for a mixed cell population could account for responses that were clinically observed in a few patients with "estrogen receptor-poor" tumors.

The Peripheral Antitumor Actions of Tamoxifen

There are three potential points of attack that could be responsible for the survival advantages seen in patients treated with adjuvant tamoxifen therapy (Figure 3). Tamoxifen could reduce metastatic spread by

- Reducing the production of estrogen-regulated proteases that are required to maintain invasion.
- Reducing the circulating level and local production of stimulatory growth factors (for example, insulin-like growth factor [IGF]1) that might be essential to maintain the growth response of early micrometastases.
- Reducing the angiogenic potential of micrometastases.

Each of these concepts has been noted in laboratory studies, but it is unclear whether they contribute singly or together to the effectiveness of tamoxifen.

It should be pointed out, however, that the associated antitumor actions all support the overall direct antitumor effects of tamoxifen on metastasis.

Physiological Actions of Tamoxifen

The actions of tamoxifen in the postmenopausal woman are a paradox. The ability to inhibit breast cancer growth is classified as an antiestrogenic action, whereas the action of tamoxifen on the level of circulating cholesterol and bone could be viewed as estrogenic. However, close examination of the actual effects shows that the changes produced by tamoxifen cannot be explained in these simple terms. Tamoxifen produces a selective estrogenic effect on

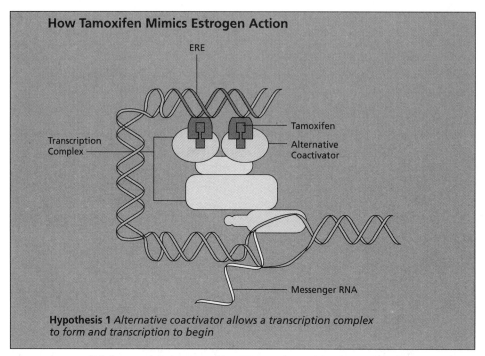

FIGURE 4(a)   It is known that the tamoxifen ER complex can bind to EREs. It is possible that complexes can recruit novel coactivators located specifically in a target site where tamoxifen produces estrogen-like effects. It is theorized that the distribution of coactivators governs estrogenic or antiestrogenic activity at different sites around the body.

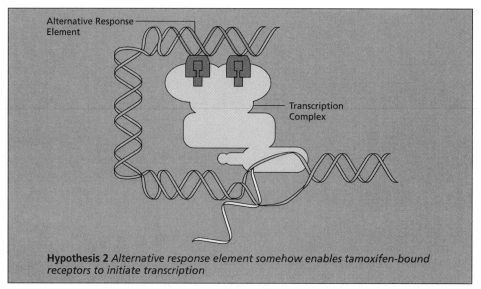

FIGURE 4(b)   It is possible that the altered tamoxifen ER complex binds preferentially to an alternative response element in the promoter region of a target gene. The novel DNA-binding sites could act as an initiation site to recruit a transcription complex. The theory predicts that novel DNA binding sites are located specifically at target sites around the body. These are believed to control estrogenic responses to tamoxifen.

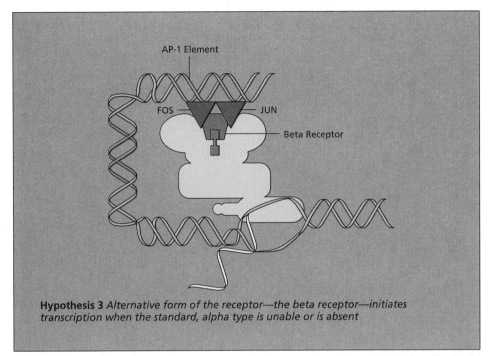

Hypothesis 3 *Alternative form of the receptor—the beta receptor—initiates transcription when the standard, alpha type is unable or is absent*

FIGURE 4(c) A second estrogen receptor called ER beta has recently been described. The classical estrogen receptor is now referred to as ER alpha. The two estrogen receptors appear to be differentially distributed throughout the body so ER beta could play a role in drug action. It is known that the new receptor has a different ligand binding site from ER alpha. One theory is that tamoxifen binds to ER beta, but the complex now has a protein-protein interaction with the fos and jun complex called AP-1. This interaction results in a stimulatory response that could activate an estrogen-responsive gene with an "antiestrogen" such as tamoxifen.

Adapted from Jordan VC: *Scientific Am* 279:60-67, 1998.

postmenopausal bone. Similarly, the effect on cholesterol is to lower low-density lipoprotein cholesterol, but unlike estrogen, tamoxifen does not increase high-density lipoprotein cholesterol.

The most unusual effects are observed in the postmenopausal uterus, where tamoxifen produces estrogen-like symptoms in some women, but a complete antiestrogenic effect in others. There is a selective effect in the uterine cells of the majority of women. Stromal tissue of the endometrium is increased, whereas the epithelium does not undergo hyperplasia. The reason for the target site-specific effects of tamoxifen around a woman's body is unknown. Current research is investigating the possibility that genes are selectively activated by the tamoxifen-estrogen-receptor complex, or that groups of helper proteins that facilitate gene activation may only be found at some sites recognized as estrogen target tissues (see Figures 4a, 4b, and 4c). This is an area of intense scientific research that could provide vital information to develop new target site-selective antiestrogens in the future. ■

Appendix 3

Breast Cancer Susceptibility Gene BRCA-1

V. Craig Jordan, PhD, DSc

The past decade has witnessed a successful collaboration between epidemiology and molecular biology. Familial breast and ovarian cancer clusters have been documented that account for 10% to 15% of the annual incidence of breast cancer in the US. The gene responsible for susceptibility to this form of cancer is referred to as BRCA-1. This gene is mutated at different places in the germline. In hereditary breast and ovarian cancers, the growth of a tumor results from the loss of a normal allele.

The fact that there are many potential sites of mutation makes the job of determining the precise sequence of the entire BRCA-1 gene in a woman time consuming and expensive. Nevertheless, absolute confirmation that an individual is carrying the mutated BRCA-1 gene dramatically alters the person's risk for breast and ovarian cancers compared to that of the general population This relationship is illustrated in Figure 1 and Figure 2.

Women with a BRCA-1 mutation have an 80% cumulative risk of developing breast cancer by the age of 70. In contrast, women without this mutation have only an 8% cumulative risk of developing breast cancer. Women with a BRCA-1 mutation also have a 44% cumulative risk of developing ovarian cancer compared with a 0.6% risk in women without the mutation.

A woman who has had one breast cancer has an increased risk of developing a second breast cancer in the other (contralateral) breast. Identification of a BRCA-1 gene mutation in a woman with breast cancer is associated with a nearly 50% risk of contralateral breast cancer by age 50 (Figure 3); in contrast, breast cancer survivors without BRCA-1 mutations have only a 7% to 10% risk of contralateral breast cancer.

Although the precise function of the BRCA-1 gene is unknown (Figure 4), exciting clues to its properties make research on the protein extremely important. The gene encodes 1863 amino acid RING-finger protein (220-kD), which has led some to suggest that the protein functions as a tumor suppressor in the nucleus of the cell by blocking excessive gene activation. However, other research suggests that BRCA-1 is a secreted protein that belongs to the granin family. During pregnancy, the messenger RNA for BRCA-1 increases

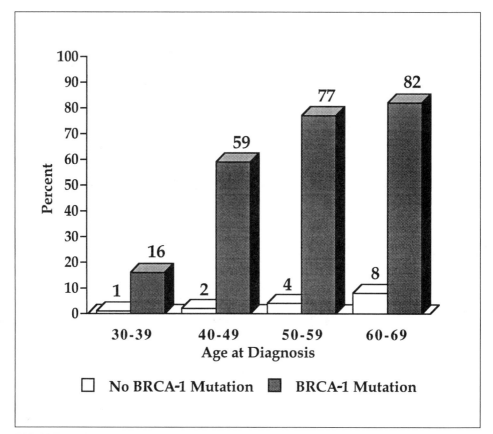

FIGURE I Cumulative Risk of Developing Breast Cancer by Age Group Women are divided according to presence or absence of a mutation in the BRCA-1 gene. Modified from Easton DF, Bishop DT, Ford D, et al: Genetic lineage analysis in familial breast cancer and ovarian cancer: Results from 214 families. *Am J Human Genetics* 52:678-701, 1993 (with permission).

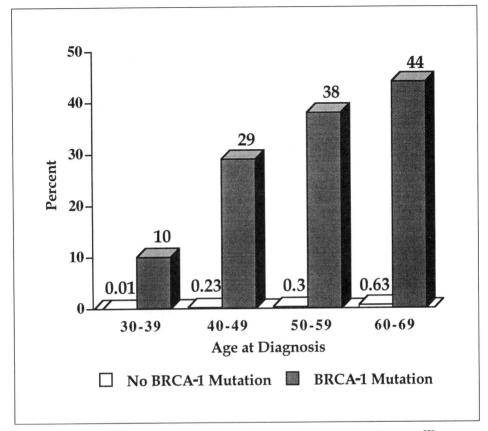

FIGURE 2   Cumulative Risk of Developing Ovarian Cancer by Age Groups   Women are divided according to the presence or absence of a mutation in the BRCA-1 gene. Modified from Easton DR, Bishop DT, Ford D, et al: Genetic lineage analysis in familial breast cancer and ovarian cancer: Results from 214 families *Am J Human Genetics* 52:678-701, 1993 (with permission).

in breast epithelial cells; there are reports that the human and mouse protein is expressed in response to estrogen. By all indications, it appears that the protein is an inhibitory growth regulator, or brake, that is capable of preventing growth. Clearly, if this protein is mutated or damaged, the inhibitory function cannot be carried out and growth will become relentless. Most inherited BRCA-1 mutations produce truncated proteins that vary from 5% to 99% of the full-length protein. Whereas point mutations in BRCA-1 of sporadic tumors are very rare, complete somatic deletion of one allele of BRCA-1 occurs in approximately 50% of sporadic breast cancers. Further clinical risk factors are considered in Chapter 15.

There is currently no information about the therapeutic role of tamoxifen in women who test positive for BRCA-1 mutations. Information about the

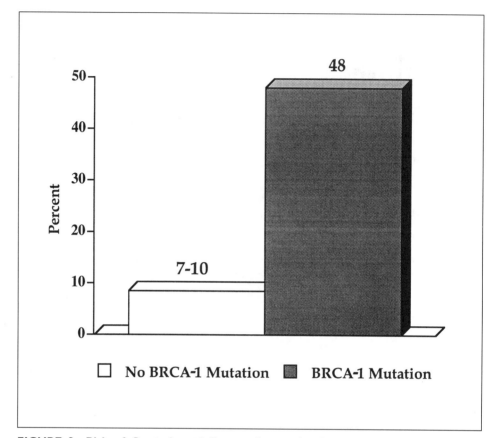

FIGURE 3   Risk of Contralateral Breast Cancer by Age 50 in BRCA-1 Mutation Cancers   Data from Ford D, Easton DF, Bishop DT, et al: Risk of cancer in BRCA-1 mutation cancers. *Lancet* 343:692-695, 1994 (with permission).

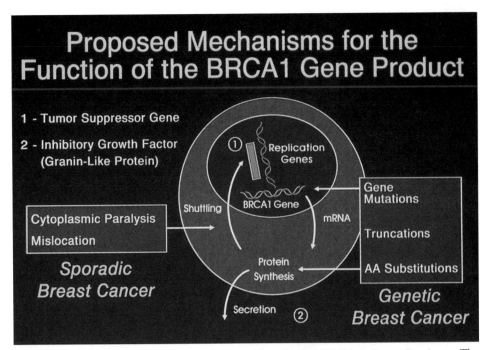

FIGURE 4 Proposed Mechanisms for the Function of BRCA-1 Gene Product The BRCA-1 gene could be either (1) a tumor-suppressor gene blocking cell replication, or (2) an inhibitory-growth factor that is secreted. In genetic breast cancer, the gene is randomly mutated, leading to truncation or shortening of the protein. This will stop the protein from functioning. Alternatively, there may be single-point mutations that cause the miscoding of the protein. In sporadic breast cancer, there may be a mislocation of the BRCA-1 gene product so that it is in the wrong place in the cell. Currently, there is a growing body of evidence to suggest that BRCA-1 assists in the repair of the damaged genome. For recent reviews on BRCA-1, see Suggested Reading in Appendix 6.

effectiveness of tamoxifen to reduce the incidence of early onset breast cancer was one of the primary goals of the National Surgical Adjuvant Breast and Bowel Project (NSABP) prevention trial. Samples are to be evaluated to determine the effectiveness of tamoxifen in BRCA-1 carriers. Currently, tamoxifen has no role in protecting women from ovarian cancer; but again, this can only be evaluated in the long-term follow-up of the prevention trial.

For the future, it is possible that basic knowledge of the BRCA-1 and the much larger BRCA-2 proteins can herald a new era of therapeutics. If the proteins are only active in the breast and also selectively inhibit ovarian cancer, then new targeted therapies—which might maintain patients at risk in an inhibited state—will be possible. This maintenance treatment would be analogous to the diabetic who, for decades, is successfully maintained on insulin injections. ∎

Suggested Reading

Komb A, Skolnick MH: Identification of the BRCA-1 breast cancer gene and its clinical implication, in DeVita VT, Hellman S, Rosenberg SA (eds): *Important Advances in Oncology*, pp 23-35. Philadelphia, Lippincott-Raven Publishers, 1996.

Statement of the American Society of Clinical Oncology: Genetic Testing for Cancer Susceptibility. *J Clin Oncol* 5:1730-1736, 1996.

Lerman C, Narod S, Schulman K, et al: BRCA-1 testing in families with hereditary breast-ovarian cancer: A prospective study of patient decision making and outcomes. *JAMA* 275:1885-1892, 1996.

Weber B: Genetic testing for breast cancer. *Sci Amer Sci Med* January/February:12-21, 1996.

Burke W, Daly M, Garber J, et al: Recommendations for follow-up care of individuals with an inherited predisposition to cancer. *JAMA* 277:997-1003, 1997.

Greene M: Genetics of breast cancer. *Mayo Clin Proc* 72:54-65, 1997.

Whittemore A, Gong G, Itnyre J: Prevalence and contribution of BRCA-1 mutations in breast and ovarian cancer: Results for three US population-based case-control studies of ovarian cancer. *Am J Hum Genet* 60:496-504, 1996.

Blackwood M, Weber B: BRCA-1 and BRCA-2: From molecular genetics to clinical medicine. *J Clin Oncol* 5:1969-1977, 1998.

Cummings S: Predisposition testing for inherited breast cancer. *Oncol* 12(8):1227-1242, 1998.

Frank T, Manley S, Olopade O, et al: Sequence analysis of BRCA-1 and BRCA-2: Correlation of mutations with family history and ovarian cancer risk. *J Clin Oncol* 16:2417-2425, 1998.

Ford D, Easton D, Stratton M, et al: Genetic heterogeneity and penetrance analysis of the BRCA-1 and BRCA-2 genes in breast cancer families. *Am J Hum Genet* 62:676-689, 1998.

Appendix 4

How Are Drugs Developed?

Ruth O'Regan, MD
Fellow
Hematology/Oncology Division
Robert H. Lurie Comprehensive Cancer Center
Northwestern University Medical School
Chicago, Illinois

V. Craig Jordan, PhD, DSc

The Western world is committed to, and profits from, a system of continuous change. A tenet of our society is: "There must be a better way to achieve success." So it is with the development of medicines to treat disease. Citizens invest in the process by buying stock in the pharmaceutical industry, whose business goal is to discover new medicines to treat disease. Without the investment, there would be very few drugs.

A Long, Costly Road

During this century, this process has been remarkably successful with the Western pharmaceutical companies, whose discoveries are initially protected by patent laws, providing society with virtually every new medicine used today. Regrettably, the process of discovery has no guarantee of success and depends on the professionals whose careers are dedicated to the search. It is, as a result, a long and very costly process, with hundreds of failures for every success. But the beneficiaries of success are the citizens who make discovery possible by investing in the process, and as a result, will live healthier and longer lives.

Nevertheless, there are legitimate concerns and criticisms about healthcare costs. Often, however, the criticism results from a lack of understanding of how drugs are discovered and how much time and dedication are involved. Drugs do not come from the government or some company that accidentally finds an obscure plant or compound. They are discovered by trained individuals who must subject their discovery to the most rigorous of tests before it can be used to treat human disease.

The issue of drug costs was raised in a letter to the *Chicago Tribune* on August 6, 1996:

Vial Thoughts

Chicago—Lately, nearly every conversation that I have had with senior citizens has started with, or soon turned to, the high cost of senior healthcare. Singled out for the most heated comments have been the high prices of medication.

Almost always overlooked in these complaints has been the point that the expense of those life-sustaining chemical morsels is largely determined by the research effort that went into discovering and determining the utility of those magic little molecules that give these pills their efficacy—and, of course, the extensive safety checking that had to be done before they could go on the market.

The price of the chemical raw materials and the manufacture of the pills are not what makes them cost so much. If that were all that was involved, in most cases, they would be dirt cheap.

It takes a lot of money to hire and equip labs, and when one considers those pills from a risk/benefit point of view, it's the biggest bargain we seniors ever got.

—*Carl E. Moore*
Emeritus Professor of Chemistry
Loyola University, Chicago

Clearly, the synthesis, packaging, and distribution of a new medicine is not the important cost. The real expense is the cost of the hundreds, perhaps thousands, of salaries for professionals whose technical skills have made a discovery possible and who have taken it from the lab to the bedside. Teams of synthetic, organic chemists, who have spent most of their lives in training programs, initially have the task of making pure samples of novel compounds that will be passed on to the biologists who will test for the activity required. Thousands of compounds will be synthesized and tested, and the task of focusing on the correct new compound will take years. But the search does not end here. Several compounds are then selected—all with good activity—but the questions must be asked: "Will the new drug be safe? Although we may be able to treat the disease, will the side effects be dangerous?"

The government sets down strict requirements that must be followed precisely before the US Food and Drug Administration (FDA) will permit clinical testing. Unfortunately, there is no exact way to predict harm to humans; but animal testing is an essential safeguard to protect citizens from the potential hazards of any new drug. For this reason, toxicology testing usually takes many years and is extremely expensive. Highly skilled experts (pathologists and toxicologists), who have spent their lives training in the discipline, will evaluate all the available safety data from the animal studies before a new compound is chosen to test in a specific disease state.

Before a drug can be tested in humans, it must be formulated. This involves the decision of how to give the drug to the patient. Questions must be addressed, such as: "Do we make one-tablet-a-day dosing? Should it be twice daily? Can we use injections? Should it be stored in the refrigerator, or away from light?" Industry pharmacists play an essential role in drug development because without their skill, any new medicine may be unacceptable to a patient or may lose its effectiveness too quickly. Only clinical trials will prove how skilled the industrial pharmacists have been.

Additionally, before the drug goes into clinical trial, a method of large-scale synthesis and a chemical manufacturing plant must be designed. It is one thing for a lone chemist to make a few teaspoons of a drug in the laboratory—this may take a week or so. It is, however, an entirely different matter to make tons of the new drug. Truckloads of raw materials must be checked for purity; then, the *final* product must be free of any impurities. Quality control is an essential and ongoing part of the drug manufacturing industry, and this is strictly monitored by the government. Still, the drug is not yet ready for sale. The government has to be convinced that the drug is safe and effective. This process can take many years.

The government sets down strict requirements that must be followed precisely before the FDA will permit clinical testing.

Clinical testing of new drugs for cancer is divided into three phases (I, II, and III). The objective and rationale for each phase in the process of drug development are briefly explained in the following sections. Each of the testing phases is performed under the strictest requirements set down by the FDA, and the pharmaceutical company is usually required to organize and pay for the testing. Additionally, all experiments, all side-effects, and measures of response must be available for scrutiny by panels of experts at the FDA. Precise recordkeeping is an absolute requirement for the approval of any drug.

Phase I Trials

The objective of a phase I trial is to evaluate the toxicity of a drug in question—often an experimental agent—and to determine a dose schedule. Phase I studies are usually conducted in previously treated patients. However, they may be conducted in untreated patients, provided no other therapeutic options exist. The organ systems expected to be targets of toxicity for the study drug should be competent or the obtained data will not be relevant in less debilitated patients. Phase I studies are not targeted at specific malignancies, and response of the malignancy to the study drug is not a major end point. However, response rates seen in certain malignancies may pave the way for phase II studies of this agent in this malignancy. The end points in phase I studies are to determine the toxicity of a given agent and to ascertain the maximum tolerated dose so that a dose schedule for phase II studies can be determined.

The starting dose of the study drug is one that is not expected to produce serious toxicity in any patient. It is usually determined as a fraction of the lethal dose in animal studies. A certain number of patients—usually less than 10—are treated at this first-dose level. If this dose is tolerated, it is then escalated in subsequent patients according to a series of preplanned steps. One common method treats a second group of patients at twice the dose of that used in the first group. A third group is then treated at a dose 67% greater than the second group, a fourth group at a dose 33% greater than the dose used in the third group, and so on, until the dose-limiting toxicity is reached. Obviously, toxicity in each group must be below a certain level for dose escalation to occur in the next group.

The phase II dosage is usually the highest dose where the incidence of dose-limiting toxicity is less than 33%. It is important to point out that doses are not escalated in the same patient due to the risk of cumulative toxicity. More precise methods of dose escalation involve the use of the drug's serum level to determine further dosage. The number of patients required and the duration of a phase I trial may be huge, depending on how high the maximum dose is above the starting dose.

Phase II Trials

Once the maximum tolerated dose is determined, the drug can be entered into phase II studies for malignancies where it has shown the most activity. The objective of phase II studies is to identify tumor types where a drug seems most active. Thus, the end point of a phase II study is the response of a certain tumor to a study drug. A large number of patients are needed to accurately evaluate a response. The study drug should first be tested in patients with malignancies most likely to have a favorable response. The most accurate information is obtained in patients with a good overall performance status, minimal disease, and minimal prior treatment. In patients with a poor performance status and extensive prior treatment, it is often not possible to give the full desired dose. In addition, a lack of activity in such patients does not necessarily indicate a similar outcome in other patients. In malignancies known to be poorly sensitive to other treatments, it is reasonable to enroll untreated patients into phase II studies.

Phase II evaluation is not appropriate when treatment with curative potential is available. The results of phase II studies may unfortunately be misleading (either overly optimistic or unduly disappointing), as the studies are not randomized and the treatment outcomes are compared with historical controls. As a result, specific statistical methods are now available to determine the required size and duration of phase II trials, based on likely response of the malignancy to the study drug. Prior to study commencement, the total number of patients necessary to achieve a certain response is ascertained. Of this total number, a proportion is analyzed early in the study to ensure that the desired response rate is being achieved. If the response rate is adequate in the initial group of patients, enrollment continues until the total number of patients is reached. This second group of patients is essential to estimate the true activity of the drug. If the desired response rate is not seen in the initial small group of patients, the trial is ended prematurely. The total number of patients required depends on the precision of the estimated response rate. The larger the number of patients, the more accurate the estimate of the response rate.

Quality-of-life aspects are becoming increasingly important as better methods of measurement become available.

Phase III Trials

Once a study drug has demonstrated desired response rates in a given cancer compared with historical controls, it must be randomized against current standard therapies or practices. The objective of these phase III studies is to determine the effects of this new treatment relative to either the natural history of or standard therapies for the malignancy in question. Phase III studies may also compare a drug believed to have similar efficacy to the standard treatment to determine if the study drug is associated with less morbidity than the standard therapy. All patients eligible for a phase III study should be able to tolerate the allocated treatment. Results obtained in a phase III trial should be of such importance that they can be applied on a national and/or international basis.

The major end points of phase III trials are measures of patient welfare. Two such end points are survival and quality of life. Response rate is more of a subjective measurement, as it does not directly translate into a survival benefit and consequently improved patient welfare. Quality-of-life aspects are becoming increasingly important as better methods of measurement become available.

In phase III studies, patients are randomized to different treatments. As previously mentioned, comparison of results with historical controls is associated with considerable bias. Randomization significantly reduces bias. Patients may be randomized to a study treatment or current standard therapy, which may be a standard drug or no treatment. In a stratified, randomized trial, patients are selected prior to randomization according to specific well-identified risk factors. This ensures equal distribution of patients with regard to these risk factors and decreases the chance of gross imbalances that cannot be adjusted at the end of the study. In a crossover study, a patient receives both the study drug and the control drug at different time intervals; therefore, patients act as their own control. Such studies are limited by a number of factors, including a change in the patient's condition over time. Factorial designs initially randomize patients to two different therapies, and then subsequently, to two further therapies. The objective of such a study is to answer two questions for the "price" of one. Large numbers of patients are needed in these studies, and the initial two treatments must have no effect on the second treatments and vice versa.

Size and duration of phase III trials are based on study objectives and end points. Follow-up must be clearly specified. Studies may be terminated prematurely due to unforeseen problems or greater-than-expected differences between the arms of the study. Target sample sizes are essential to ensure that the study is feasible and to determine when to stop accrual in the absence of premature termination. If too few patients enroll, the results may be either ambiguous or erroneous.

Significance of Trial Size

It should be possible to accrue the desired sample size in a reasonable length of time. Determination of sample size is based on the assumption that, at the conclusion of the trial, a statistical significance test will be performed comparing the treatment groups with regard to the primary end point. The study will have a null hypothesis, which presumes that there will be no difference in end points between the study drug and the control treatment. The null hypothesis will either be accepted or rejected based on statistical analysis of the study results. Through statistical means, it will be determined whether the study drug is significantly better or worse than the control drug. The significance level used in most studies is only 5 chances in 100, which means if the study drug is truly better than the control drug, the probability of this being attributable to chance is only 0.05. The number of patients enrolled dictates the likelihood of a truly significant result. If few patients are enrolled, the differences between the outcome with the study drug as compared with the control drug must be extreme to be significant. When greater numbers of patients are enrolled, smaller differences in outcome become significant at the 0.05 level. Therefore, to detect small differences between two groups, huge numbers of patients need to be enrolled, which may take many years. Tables are available which dictate how many patients need to be enrolled on both arms based on the likely difference between the arms of treatment. All phase III trials should be large enough to detect a 20% difference between the groups. Interim analysis should only be done by the data-monitoring committee and should be ignored unless noted differences are significant at the 0.0025 level.

At the end of phase III studies, if the study drug does indeed show a significant benefit in a particular malignancy, it will usually be approved for general use in that malignancy. Regrettably, these clinical trials can take a great many years to accomplish. Many drugs are abandoned along the way because they are either too toxic or do not have enough activity to be better than existing drugs.

The number of patients enrolled in a clinical trial dictates the likelihood of a truly significant result.

After FDA Approval

Once a new drug is approved by the FDA committees for a particular indication, a company can advertise the approved claim. A company cannot make claims outside approved uses. For example, if a new drug is proved to be useful to treat advanced breast cancer, a company cannot advertise or imply, for example, that it should be used for adjuvant treatment of node-negative breast cancer. This is to protect the public from unforeseen problems. This is why clinical trials are necessary—to look for the good as well as the bad effects.

A pharmaceutical company is required to invest in clinical testing to provide evidence for the desired FDA approval. The process is exemplified by the development of tamoxifen (Nolvadex), which was the only approved antiestrogen on the market in the United States between 1978 and 1997. No other company was willing to make the investment to make alternatives available because it was generally believed that the research investment would not be useful. All attention focused on chemotherapy. However, through the clinical trials' process, there has been a revolution in treatment that has dramatically improved the prognosis for women with breast cancer.

The commitment of the manufacturers to provide millions of free tablets to the clinical trial community over the past 2 decades has resulted in the additional FDA approvals noted in Chapter 3. The work was completed through National Cancer Institute-approved experimental protocols, by national organizations of physicians called the National Surgical Adjuvant Breast and Bowel Project (NSABP), the Eastern Cooperative Oncology Group (ECOG), and the Southwest Oncology Group (SWOG). Over decades, thousands of physicians and healthcare professionals volunteered their time to prove whether the best ideas for cancer treatment could provide benefits for their patients. Thousands of women with breast cancer made a commitment that they would participate to help themselves and future generations.

The key is that the driving force in this remarkable story were the physicians and scientists, not the pharmaceutical companies. The clinical researchers spotted the potential for success for helping breast cancer patients, devised the clinical protocols, and committed themselves to the process of clinical investigation. Without this voluntary commitment, there would have been no further FDA approvals for Nolvadex.

Generics

If a drug becomes generic, it will be cheaper. This is true, but the reason it is true is important. The major pharmaceutical companies discover drugs and are required to shoulder the responsibility for their safety and to prove they work in patients. The investment costs hundreds of millions of dollars and takes about a decade to complete the process. A patent protects the company so it can make the investment and effort. It also allows the company time to reclaim the overall costs in sales. Without patents and the power of

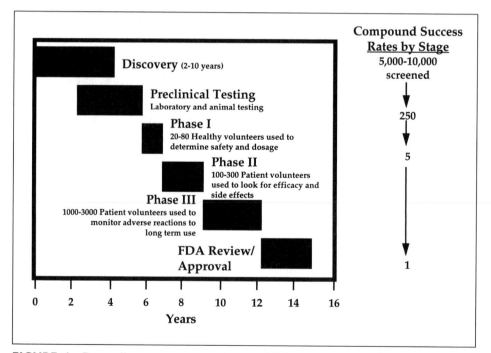

FIGURE 1 Drug discovery process to establish one new product that is FDA approved   For every new drug available, it is estimated that 5,000 to 10,000 new compounds need to be screened in the laboratory. Adapted from Pharmaceutical Research and Manufacturers of America: *PhRMA industry profile 1996: Opportunities and challenges for pharmaceutical innovation.* Washington, 1996.

the courts, no one would invest in drug discovery because someone else would steal the idea. If this were the situation, no drugs would be developed.

In contrast, a company that makes generic drugs has no commitment to new drug discovery and testing, so the price only reflects the much smaller cost of synthesis and distribution.

Without our commitment to the process of change, there would be no medicines available to treat breast cancer. The patent laws secure progress, but it is important to appreciate that the process does not stop with tamoxifen. "It is only the end of the beginning," as Winston Churchill said in 1942.

The success of tamoxifen has encouraged new ideas and initiatives that would never have been considered 30 years ago. At that time, no one was interested—but success breeds success. The profits from the success of Nolvadex have been reinvested to develop new drugs to treat breast and also prostate cancer (a disease that kills as many men as breast cancer does women). Additionally, free Nolvadex and placebo were provided for the NCI/NSABP tamoxifen prevention trial. The results of that commitment will revolutionize a high-risk woman's options and reduce her risk of breast cancer by 50%. This commitment provides a choice of novel treatment strategies for both the physician and the patient.

The development of tamoxifen as the leading cancer medicine has taken 30 years from concept to reality, so it is perhaps valuable to illustrate the time and cost of new drug development and the changes that are taking place in treatment practice. A time scale and cost estimate for the next generation of new drug development is shown in Figure 1.

Conclusion

In summary, it is clear that the inventiveness of Western society has provided enormous advantages for its citizens. However, the process of drug discovery and development takes years to safely accomplish and requires the investment of billions of dollars. Success depends upon the skill of individual scientists and physicians who have already dedicated much of their working lives training for the opportunity to contribute to the process of drug discovery and development. There are no shortcuts or quick ways to guarantee success. Nevertheless, as Carl E. Moore stated, "When one considers those pills from a risk/benefit point of view, it's the biggest bargain we seniors ever got." ■

Appendix 5

IARC Evaluates Carcinogenic Risk Associated With Tamoxifen

A working group of 17 scientists from 8 countries met at the International Agency for Research on Cancer (IARC) in Lyon during February 13-20, 1996, to review the evidence on the potential carcinogenicity of a number of pharmaceutical agents. The Working Group was chaired by Dr. George Lucier of the US National Institute of Environmental Health Sciences and Dr. Anthony B. Miller from the University of Toronto, Canada. The results will be published as volume 66 of the IARC Monographs on the Evaluation of Carcinogenic Risks to Humans. This series is recognized internationally as providing unbiased evaluations of chemicals, pharmaceutical agents, complex mixtures, industrial processes and biological and physical agents that could increase the risk of cancer in humans. This process is essentially an identification of carcinogenic hazards and is not intended as a basis for risk-benefit determination, nor for regulatory actions.

Among the agents considered at this meeting was tamoxifen, included for evaluation because of reports indicating a potential hazard in increasing the risk of endometrial cancer. Tamoxifen is recognized as an effective drug for the treatment of breast cancer. It is one of a small group of pharmaceuticals recognized by the World Health Organization as an essential drug for the treatment of this disease. It is currently being evaluated in a number of chemoprevention trials to determine whether it reduces the incidence of breast cancer in otherwise healthy women judged to be at increased risk of developing breast cancer.

The Working Group reviewed all the published scientific data on second primary tumors reported in patients who had been treated with tamoxifen for breast cancer. The group further assessed the evidence for carcinogenic effects of tamoxifen in experimental animals, and evaluated possible biological mechanisms of carcinogenesis. As none of these reports was regarded as conclusive on its own, it is the totality of the evidence that had to be considered by the Working Group in reaching their final evaluation.

Two major conclusions resulted from the evaluation process. First, there was consensus that 'there is conclusive evidence that tamoxifen reduces the risk of contralateral breast cancers,' ie, the occurrence of a second cancer in the other breast. The second conclusion was 'that there is sufficient evidence in humans of the carcinogenicity of tamoxifen in increasing the risk of endometrial cancer,' ie, a tumor originating from the inner lining of the uterus. In addition, the Working Group concluded that 'there is inadequate evidence in humans that tamoxifen affects the risk of other cancers.'

In commenting on these conclusions of the Working Group, Dr. Paul Kleihues, Director of the International Agency for Research on Cancer, said: 'Breast cancer constitutes a major threat to women's health worldwide. I am very pleased that in spite of the intense interest that this evaluation of tamoxifen has engendered in the medical and scientific community, the members of the Working Group have conducted their evaluation in accordance with the highest standards of unbiased scientific integrity.'

It is important to recognize that the findings of the Working Group do not invalidate the conclusions by clinical oncologists and surgeons that tamoxifen is a very important drug which substantially increases the survival of patients with breast cancer. No woman being treated for breast cancer should have her treatment stopped because of the conclusions of the Working Group. The risk of endometrial cancer is far lower than the benefits women with breast cancer receive from tamoxifen. However, it is important that women have access to scientific opinion on the low risk of endometrial cancer, so that they can make an informed decision on the treatment they will accept.

—http://www.iarc.fr/preleases/111e.htm

Appendix 6
Recommended Further Reading and References for Physicians and Scientists

Books

Harris J, Lippman ME, Morrow M, (eds): *Diseases of the Breast.* Philadelphia, Lippincott-Raven, 1996.

Jordan VC: *Long-Term Tamoxifen Treatment for Breast Cancer.* Madison, Wisconsin, University of Wisconsin Press, 1994.

Lindsay R, Dempster DW, Jordan VC: *Estrogens and Antiestrogens.* Philadelphia, Lippincott-Raven, 1997.

Wisemen H: *Tamoxifen: Molecular Basis of Use in Cancer Treatment and Prevention.* Chichester, John Wiley & Sons, 1994.

Reviews in Refereed Journals

Gradishar WJ, Jordan VC: The clinical potential of new antiestrogens. *J Clin Oncol* 15:480-489, 1997.

Jordan VC: Designer estrogens. *Scientific Am* 279:60-67, 1998.

Jordan VC, Gradishar WJ: Molecular mechanisms and clinical potential of new antiestrogens. *Molecular Aspects Med* 18:167-247, 1997.

Acknowledgments in Five Photo Collages

*On the following pages,
you will find photographs of
the many investigators and
clinicians, friends and colleagues,
who were important in the
discovery and development
of tamoxifen...*

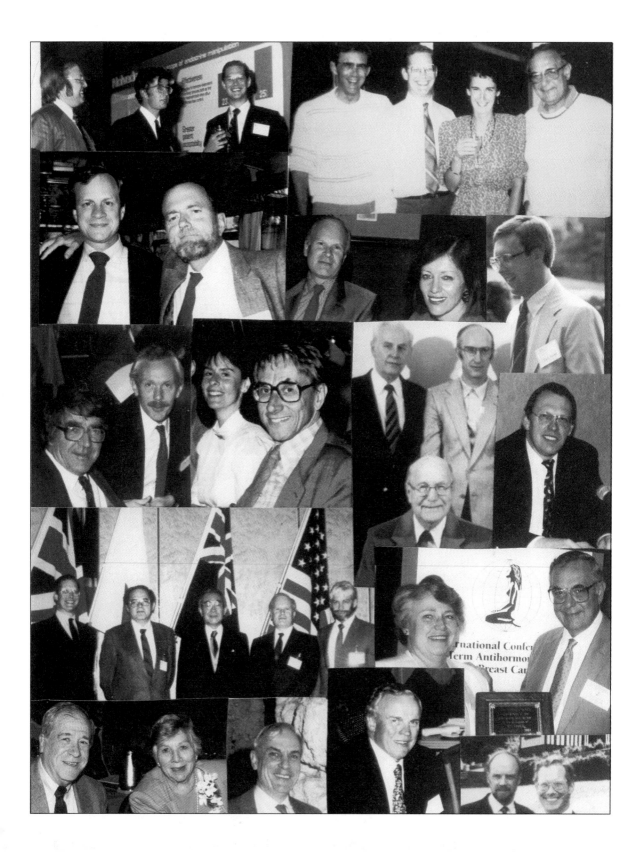

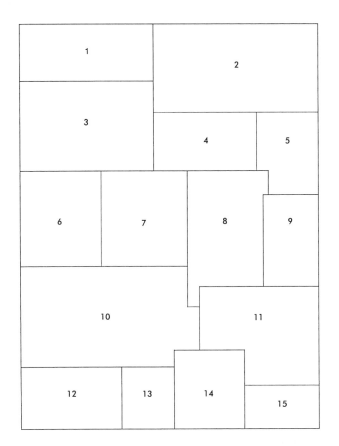

1. L to R: **Alex Pleuvry, Dr. John Patterson** (who had recently joined ICI [now Zeneca]) and the **author** at the International Congress of Chemotherapy, London 1975. Dr. Patterson became responsible at ICI for coordinating clinical trials with Nolvadex, notably the Nolvadex Adjuvant Trial Organization (NATO).

2. L to R: **Drs. Douglas Tormey**, then head of the Breast Cancer Committee of ECOG; the **author, Anna Reigel** (nee Tate); and **Paul Carbone**, Chairman of ECOG, Wisconsin, 1983.

3. **Drs. Geof Greene** (l) and the **late Bill McGuire** (r), International Congress of Chemotherapy, Budapest, 1986. Dr. Greene developed monoclonal antibodies to the estrogen receptor, and Dr. McGuire developed the concept of the progesterone receptor as a prognostic indicator.

4. **Michael Baum**, former Professor of Surgery at the Royal Marsden Hospital, London, and his wife **Judy**, attending an International Breast Cancer meeting in Florida, 1991.

5. **Dr. C. Kent Osborne**, Chief of Medical Oncology, The University of Texas Health Science Center, San Antonio, at a breast cancer meeting in Colorado, 1987. He is internationally recognized for his research on tamoxifen resistance and the treatment of hormone-dependent breast cancer.

6. **Professor Keith Griffith** (Director of the Tenovus Institute for Cancer Research, Cardiff, Wales) and **Dr. Rob Nicholson**, at an estrogen-receptor meeting in Monte Carlo, 1984. Dr. Nicholson completed some of the first laboratory studies of tamoxifen as an antitumor agent in the United Kingdom.

7. **Drs. Benita Katzenellenbogen** and **Henri Rochefort**, Steroid Biochemistry meeting, Canary Isles, 1989. Both scientists provided invaluable knowledge to our understanding of the basic aspects of estrogen and antiestrogen action.

8. **Drs. Gerald Mueller**, Lasker Professor of Oncology; **Jack Gorski,** Professor of Biochemistry; and **Harold Rusch**, Founding Director of the McArdle Laboratory and the Wisconsin Clinical Cancer Center, Wisconsin, 1985.

9. **Professor Manfred Kaufman**, Chairman, Department of Gynecology, University of Frankfurt, at a breast cancer meeting in Japan, 1994. Professor Kaufman completed pivotal studies of Zoladex for the treatment of breast cancer in premenopausal women.

10. L to R: the **author, Dr. Norman Wolmark,** now Chairman of the NSABP; **Professor O. Abe**, our host; **Professor Michael Baum**, Chairman of NATO; and **Professor John Forbes**, Chairman, Breast Committee, Australia and New Zealand Oncology Group. Pictured at a breast cancer meeting in Japan, 1986.

11. **Lois Trench-Hines**, receiving an award from **Dr. Paul Carbone**, at a breast cancer meeting in Florida, 1991, for her commitment to the early development of Nolvadex.

12. **Dr. Bernard Fisher**, then Chairman of the NSABP, with **Mrs. Louise Rusch** on the occasion of the inaugural Rusch Memorial Breast Cancer Lecture, 1991. As chairman of the NSABP, Dr. Fisher laid the foundation for current standards of breast cancer treatment in the United States. Currently, Dr. Fisher is Scientific Director at Allegheny University of Health Sciences in Pittsburgh, Pennsylvania.

13. **Professor Roger Blamey**, Chairman of Surgery at Nottingham City Hospital, England, 1990. He completed pivotal studies with Zoladex and the new pure antiestrogen in women with breast cancer.

14. **Dr. Trevor Powles**, Director of the Breast Cancer Program at the Royal Marsden Hospital, London, attending the Miami International Breast Cancer Conference, 1995. He initiated the first pilot prevention study with tamoxifen in 1986.

15. The **author** and **Dr. Richard Love**, organizer of the Wisconsin Tamoxifen study that showed tamoxifen maintains bone density in postmenopausal women. A visit to England, 1988.

Collage Number 2, composed of photos 16 through 30,
appears on the following page.

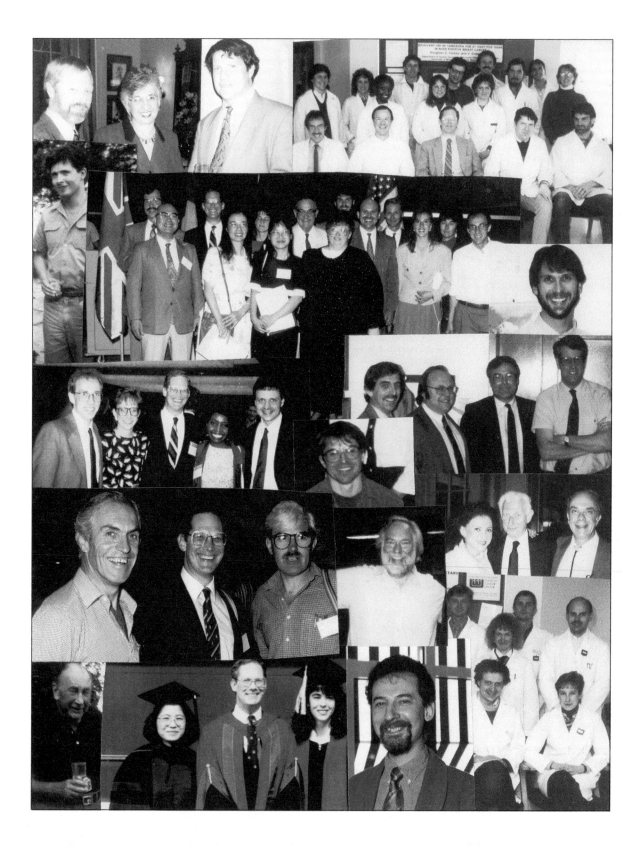

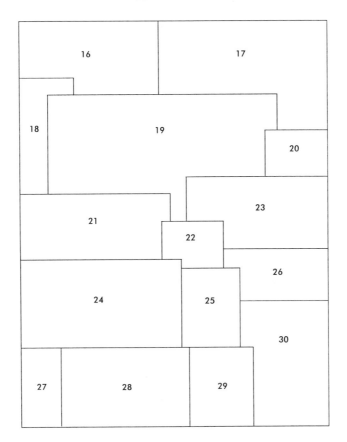

16. Some of the attendees at the Bill McGuire Memorial Dinner at the Langston House, New Braunfels, Texas, 1994. L to R: Biostatistician **Dr. Gary Clark**, who developed the concept of prognosticators for breast cancer; **Mini DeLaGarza**, administrative assistant to the **late Bill McGuire**; and **Dr. Peter Ravdin**, Associate Professor of Medicine/Oncology, The University of Texas Health Science Center, San Antonio (former Tamoxifen Team member).

17. Tamoxifen Team, 1986, University of Wisconsin. Back row, L to R: **Dawn Mirecki, Cathy Murphy, Ethel Cormier, Dave Whitford, Nancy Fritz, Marco Gottardis, Mary Janes, Mike Wolf, Richard Bain, Eric Phelps**, and **Pat Morton**. Front row, L to R: **Simon Robinson, Wade Welshons**, the **author**, Peter Ravdin, and **Rick Koch.**

18. **Professor R. Charles Coombes, MD**, Chairman of Medical Oncology, Charing Cross Hospital, London, visiting Madison, Wisconsin, 1984. Dr. Coombes did the first clinical studies with the aromatase inhibitor discovered by the Brodies at the Worcester Foundation (#46, #73).

19. Tamoxifen Team, 1991, at the International Antihormones in Breast Cancer meeting Orlando, Florida.

20. **Dr. Doug Wolf**, former PhD student, 1992. He discovered a natural point mutation of the estrogen receptor in a tamoxifen-stimulated tumor, and described a new model to explain how adjuvant tamoxifen therapy might work.

21. American Association for Cancer Research Meeting, BF Cain Memorial Award Reception, 1989. L to R: **Drs. Simon Robinson, Cathy Murphy**, the **author, Ethel Cormier**, and **Marco Gottardis**.

22. **Mike Fritsch, MD, PhD**, currently working at the National Institute of Health, Washington. He obtained his Doctor of Philosophy with **Jack Gorski** and was a postdoctoral fellow in the author's laboratory, 1991. He originally worked with **Dr. Mara Lieberman** and conducted numerous studies on the estrogen receptor and antiestrogen action.

23. ICI Pharmaceuticals, Alderley Park, 1986. **Alan Wakeling**, discoverer of the pure antiestrogens; **Alex Pleuvry**, responsible for global marketing of Nolvadex; **Barry Furr**, Director of Bioscience II and responsible for the development of Zoladex and Casodex; and **Sandy Todd**, Product Development Manager.

24. Madrid, 1986. Steroid Biochemistry Meeting. L to R: **Dr. Roger King** (who has provided fundamental insights into hormone-dependent and independent tumor growth), the **author**, and **Rob Sutherland**, who is recognized for the basic understanding of estrogen and antiestrogen action in the cell cycle.

25. **Dr. Michael Gould**, Professor of Human Oncology, University of Wisconsin, 1993. Responsible for discovering new natural products as breast cancer preventives currently being tested by **Professor Coombes** (#18).

26. BF Cain Memorial Award Dinner, 1989. **Dr. Syd Salmon**, Director of the Arizona Cancer Center and his wife, **Joannie**. In the center is **Dr. Len Lerner**, the discoverer of the first nonsteroidal antiestrogen, MER 25, and the fertility drug, clomiphene citrate.

27. The **late Dr. Olaf Pearson**, Case Western Reserve, at a breast cancer meeting in Madison, Wisconsin, 1984. Dr. Pearson did some of the first work on adrenal estrogen and was among the first to test tamoxifen in the United States.

28. Graduation, University of Wisconsin, 1991. **Dr. Shun-Yuan Jiang** (who created new breast cancer cell lines with the reintroduction of the estrogen-receptor gene), the **author**, and **Amy Stella**, former Research Assistant who has now qualified as an MD.

29. **Professor Adrian Harris**, Oxford University, at the St. Gallen Breast Cancer Meeting, Switzerland, 1992. Professor Harris used antiestrogens to reverse chemotherapeutic drug resistance and is recognized for his work on angiogenesis.

30. Partial Tamoxifen Team, 1989: Back row, L to R: **Chris Parker, Mary Lababidi, Mark Thompson**, and **John Pink.** Front row, L to R: **Marco Gottardis** and **Cathy Murphy.**

*Collage Number 3, composed of photos 31 through 43,
appears on the following page.*

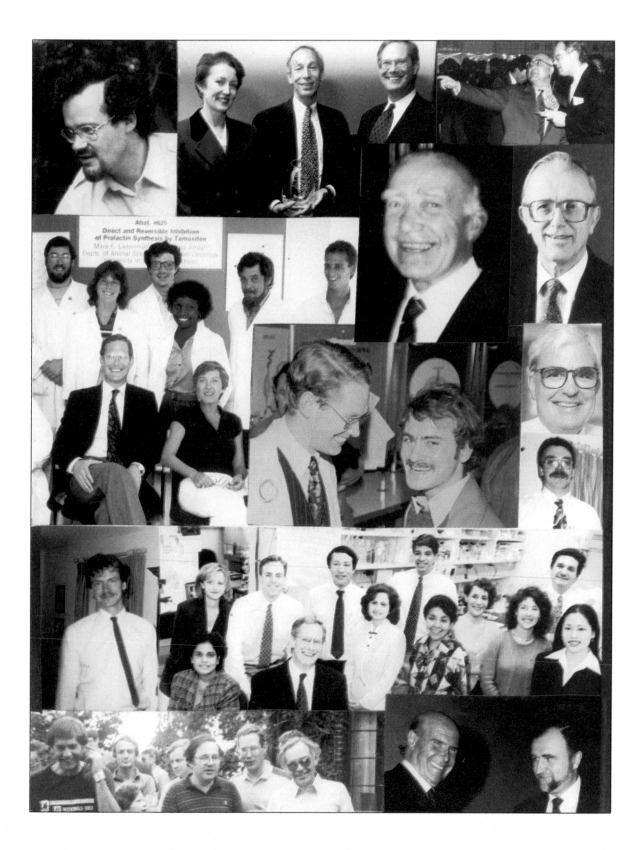

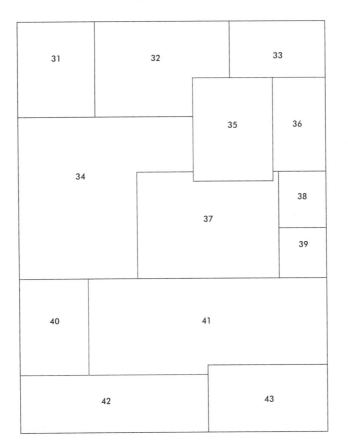

31. **Dr. John Katzenellenbogen**, Professor of Chemistry, University of Illinois, at the Meeting on Antiestrogens and Estrogens, 1984. His skill as an organic chemist has proved to be invaluable for the synthesis and identification of estrogens and antiestrogens. The biological studies were completed with his wife, **Benita** (#7), Professor of Physiology, Cell and Structural Biology at the University of Illinois.

32. Center: **Dr. Marc E. Lippman**, Director of the Vincent T. Lombardi Cancer Center, Washington, DC; the Inaugural Lynn Sage Visiting Professor, 1995. For the past 25 years, his research program has provided fundamental links between hormones and growth factors. He mapped out future biological strategies for breast cancer therapy.

33. **Professor Yuchi Iino**, Gunma University, Japan, 1993. A former member of the Tamoxifen Team (1988-89).

34. The Tamoxifen Team, 1983. Back row, L to R: **Stewart Lyman**, **Dawn Mirecki**, **Marco Gottardis**, **Ethel Cormier**, **Richard Bain**, **Eric Phelps**, the **author**, and the **late Dr. Mara Lieberman**.

35. **Dr. Edward R. Clark** (my PhD Supervisor, 1969-72), formerly of the Department of Pharmacology, University of Leeds. Pictured at the Gaddum Memorial Award Ceremony, Cambridge University, 1993.

36. **Dr. Henry Pitot**, former Director of the McArdle Laboratory, University of Wisconsin. He is one of the leading authorities on rat liver carcinogenesis and has contributed important new data on the effects of antiestrogens.

37. The **author** and **Dr. Timothy Jaspan** (then a medical student). Open Day, University of Leeds Medical School, 1976. He is now a consultant physician in Nottingham, United Kingdom. He did some of the early studies of tamoxifen and breast tumor growth in the author's laboratory in 1975.

38. **Professor Rob Sutherland**, Garvan Institute, Sydney, Australia. His distinguished career has resulted in the description of cellular antiestrogen binding sites, the reason for "tumor flare" with antiestrogen treatment, and the interaction of progestins and antiestrogens in the cell cycle.

39. **Dr. David Gibson**, postdoctoral fellow (1988-1990). He is a former member of the Tamoxifen Team, who performed the first studies to show that tamoxifen plus interferon can completely control breast cancer growth under laboratory conditions.

40. **Dr. Andreas Friedl**, a visiting fellow from Germany in 1988, and now Assistant Professor in the Department of Pathology, University of Wisconsin. A former member of the Tamoxifen Team who completed unique studies about hormone-responsive tumor growth of hormone-independent cancer cells in animals.

41. Tamoxifen Team, Northwestern University, 1996. Back row, L to R: **Dr. Claudia Tellez**, **Henry Muenzner**, **Dr. Zehan Chen**, **Dr. Malcolm Bilimoria**, **Dr. Anna Levenson**, and **Dr. Vasileios Assikis**. Front row, L to R: **Kala Tanjiori**, the **author**, **Dr. Debra Tonetti**, **Angela Cisneros**, **Jennifer MacGregor**, and **Julie Yang**.

42. L to R: **Douglas Tormey**, **Franco Cavali**, (**Helen Jordan**, age 11), **Henri Rochefort** (rear), **Geof Greene**, **Norman Wolmark**, the **author**, and **Gene DeSombre**. Madison, Wisconsin, 1984.

43. **Professor Umberto Veronesi**, Scientific Director of the European Institute of Oncology, Milan; **Dr. Gabriel Hortobagyi**, Chairman, Breast Medical Oncology, M. D. Anderson Cancer Center, Houston, Texas, 1995. Professor Veronesi has championed the use of conservative surgery as a treatment for breast cancer. He published the first studies showing the value of the approach.

Collage Number 4, composed of photos 44 through 54,
appears on the following page.

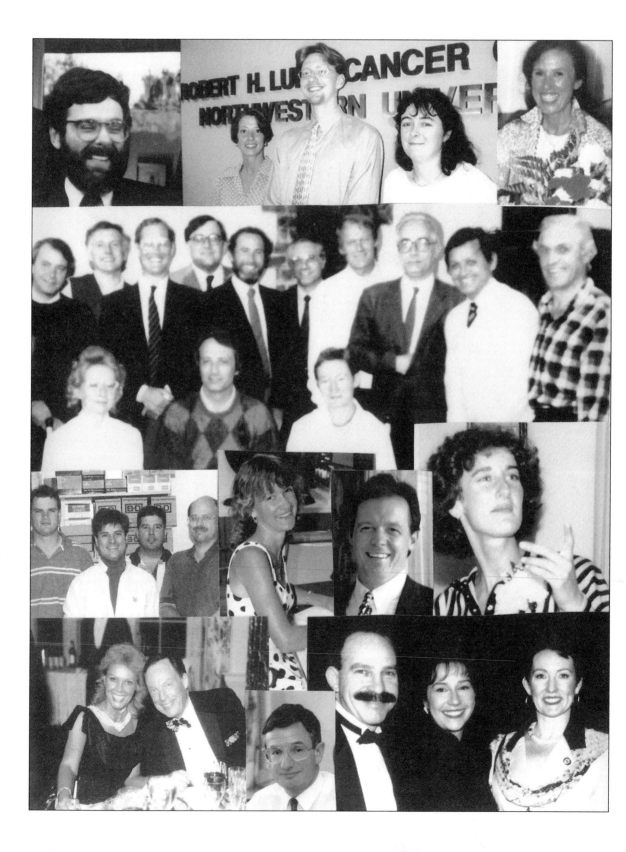

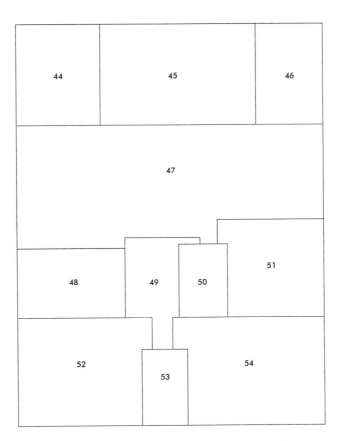

44. **Dr. Donald ("Skip") Trump**, 1986. He organized clinical studies to evaluate high-dose tamoxifen as a strategy to combat drug resistance to chemotherapy. He is currently Chief of Hematology/Oncology and Professor of Medicine at the University of Pittsburgh Cancer Institute at Montefiore University Hospital, Pennsylvania.

45. The remainder of the 1996 Tamoxifen Team at Northwestern University Medical School, Robert H. Lurie Comprehensive Cancer Center (#41). **Dr. Gale England, Michael Piette**, and **Dr. Ruth O'Regan.**

46. **Dr. Angela Brodie**, Hamburg, 1987. She is currently Professor of Pharmacology and Experimental Therapeutics at the University of Maryland. With her husband, **Harry**, she completed the first laboratory studies on the antitumor use of 4-hydroxyandrostenedione at the Worcester Foundation, 1974-76 (#73).

47. The European School of Oncology, Breast Cancer Task Force, Italy, 1986. **Dr. Franco Cavalli**, the Chairman, is seated at the front. On the left of the **author** is **Dr. Peter Walton** (Zeneca), and at right is **Dr. Aron Goldhirsch**, Chairman of the International Breast Cancer Study Group. Behind **Dr. Simone Saez** (lady seated right) is **Dr. Henig Mouridsen** from Denmark, who completed numerous clinical studies with tamoxifen.

48. The Tamoxifen Team remaining at the University of Wisconsin, 1993-95. **Matt Bong**, and **Dr. Bill Catherino**, who provided valuable insight into the molecular biology of tamoxifen resistance; **Jim Holson** and **Dr. John Pink**, who identified the first high molecular weight estrogen receptor and described the loss of estrogen receptors in breast cancer cells.

49. **Dr. Mary Lababidi**, 1990. She ran the steroid receptor laboratory at the University of Wisconsin Comprehensive Cancer Center that serves Southern Wisconsin. She also completed animal studies to demonstrate that tamoxifen prevents mammary cancer in mice.

50. **Dr. Bill Gradishar**, currently Director of Lynn Sage Breast Medical Oncology and Associate Professor of Medicine at the Robert H. Lurie Comprehensive Cancer Center at Northwestern University. Completed several recent clinical reviews of new antiestrogens with the author.

51. **Dr. Anna Riegel**, a graduate of the Department of Pharmacology and Steroid Endocrinology at the University of Leeds in the 1970s. She came to America as a Fulbright Hays Scholar to complete her PhD at the McArdle Laboratory in Wisconsin. She was the first member of the US Tamoxifen Team in 1980. She described differences between estrogen receptors bound to estradiol or 4-hydroxytamoxifen. She is currently Associate Professor of Pharmacology at Georgetown University in Washington, DC.

52. **Professor Elwood Jensen** and his wife, **Peggy**, at a General Motors Prize dinner in Washington. Professor Jensen led pioneering studies to identify the estrogen receptor, and in the late 1960s, devised the estrogen-receptor assay to predict the hormone responsiveness of breast cancer. In parallel studies with **Jack Gorski**'s group (#8), he developed models of estrogen action and subsequently isolated the receptor to make monoclonal antibodies used in clinical assays today. **Dr. Gene DeSombre** was Professor Jensen's co-investigator throughout the late 1960s and 1970s (#42). **Dr. Geof Greene** (#3) is the immunologist who trained with Professor Jensen and conducted the laboratory investigation to prepare antibodies. Professor Jensen is the former Director of the Ben May Laboratory for Cancer Research at the University of Chicago, the Medical Director of the Ludwig Institute for Cancer Research in Switzerland, and a Professor at the Institute for Hormone and Fertility Research in Hamburg, Germany. He is currently at the Karolinska Institute, Stockholm, Sweden.

53. **Dr. John Patterson**, currently Territorial Business Director for Zeneca Pharmaceuticals, Alderley Park, United Kingdom.

54. **Dr. Steven Rosen**, Director of the Robert H. Lurie Comprehensive Cancer Center, and his wife, **Candy**. **Dr. Monica Morrow** (r) is Director of the Lynn Sage Breast Center Program at Northwestern University Medical School and Northwestern Memorial Hospital.

*Collage Number 5, composed of photos 55 through 74,
appears on the following page.*

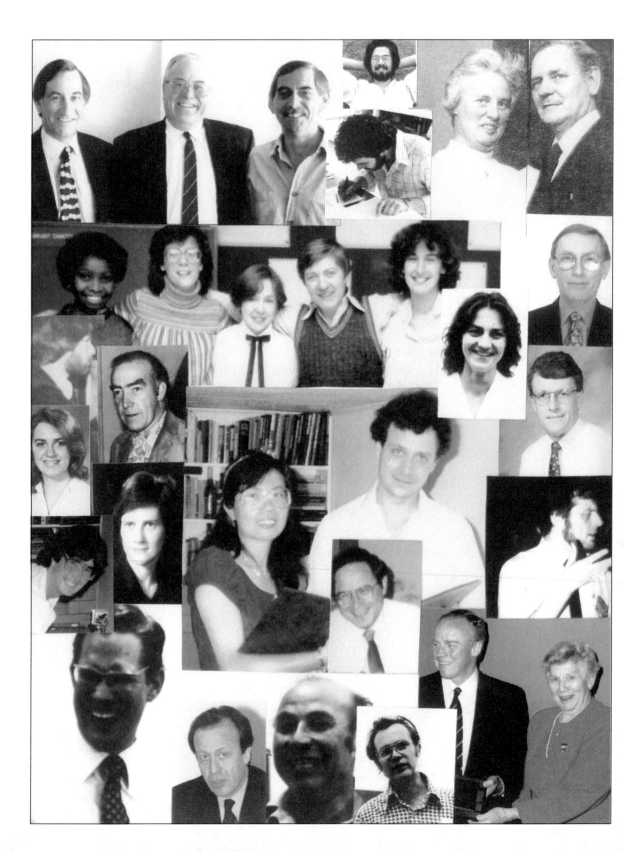

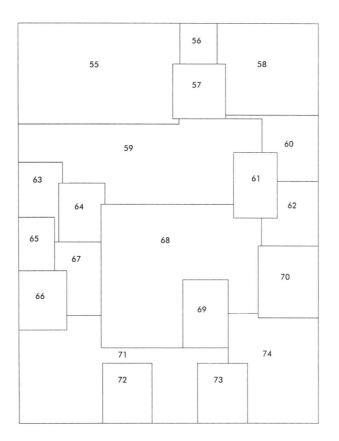

55. L to R: **Drs. Mike Dukes, Barry Furr,** and **Alan Wakeling**, Zeneca, Macclesfield England, 1996. Alan discovered the pure antiestrogen ICI 182,780. Mike Dukes has been intimately involved in the drug development. Barry Furr published reviews with the author on tamoxifen and was specifically involved with the development of Zoladex and Casodex.

56. **Graham Prestwich,** 1977, then research assistant at Leeds University. He is now National Health Trust Accounts Manager for Astra Pharmaceuticals in the north of England.

57. **Dr. Clive Dix** in 1978. He was an ICI Scholar completing his PhD with the author. He described the actions of tamoxifen as an antitumor agent in rats and defined the pharmacology of 4-hydroxytamoxifen. He is now Director of Research and Development (UK) with Glaxo Wellcome in England.

58. The **late Dr. Jean Bowler**, who synthesized the pure antiestrogens; and **Dr. Brian Newbould**, who was Research Director at ICI (Zeneca) during the late 1970s.

59. Tamoxifen (Women's) Team 1983, University of Wisconsin. In the center is **Barbara Gosden**, who completed some of the first laboratory studies to define antiestrogens with a high affinity for the estrogen receptor. Successor compounds, like raloxifene, are now being used as preventives for osteoporosis.

60. **Dr. Tony Howell**, a leading medical oncologist at the Christie Hospital, Manchester, England. He completed the first clinical studies with a pure antiestrogen to define its value as a second-line therapy after tamoxifen failure.

61. **Dr. Yvonne Dragan**, McArdle Laboratory, University of Wisconsin. She has completed essential work to define the safety of different antiestrogens. She worked in collaboration with the author and **Dr. Henry Pitot** (#36). Currently, she is an assistant professor at the Ohio State University.

62. **Dr. Timothy Kinsella**, former Chairman of the Department of Human Oncology, University of Wisconsin. Currently, he is Professor and Chairman of Radiology and Oncology at Case Western Reserve, Cleveland, Ohio.

63. **Graham Prestwich**, the author's research assistant at Leeds University (1974-1977), where we described the first studies with radioactive tamoxifen and estrogen-receptor binding. He was also part of the team that discovered the potent activity of the tamoxifen metabolite, 4-hydroxytamoxifen.

64. **Dr. Edward Clark** (1971), the author's PhD supervisor at Leeds University (1969-1972). The topic was the structure activity relationships of antiestrogens.

65. **Susan Koerner Ravatoy**, the author's research assistant at the Worcester Foundation (1972-74). We completed the first laboratory studies with tamoxifen as an antitumor agent. She is now involved in genetic testing in New York State.

66. **Susan Lagan-Fahey**, tamoxifen team during the late 1980s at Wisconsin. She was responsible for tamoxifen determinations in long-term adjuvant patients and other laboratory studies.

67. **Dr. Kathy Pritchard**, a leading medical oncologist at Sunnybrook, Toronto, Canada. Her clinical work defined the value of tamoxifen both as an adjuvant therapy and as a treatment for premenopausal women.

68. **Dr. Meei-Huey-Jeng** (with the author in 1992), who completed studies linking progestins with breast cancer stimulation. She is now Research Assistant Professor at the University of Virginia. **Dr. Marco Gottardis** (with the author in 1989) was responsible for describing laboratory models of tamoxifen-stimulated tumor growth and for the first studies to show the application of pure antiestrogens as a second-line therapy. He is currently at Bristol-Myers Squibb in Princeton, New Jersey.

69. **Dr. Norman Wolmark**, Chairman of the NSABP.

70. **Dr. Guy LeClerq**, Institute Jules Bordet, Brussels, who has completed extensive studies on the antitumor and receptor-binding properties of antiestrogens.

71. The **author** with **David Kupfer**, who completed pivotal research on the metabolism of tamoxifen, at the Worcester Foundation, 1976.

72. **Dr. Alberto Costa**, Director of the European School of Oncology, and one of the organizers of the Italian study to test the worth of tamoxifen as a preventive.

73. **Dr. Harry Brodie**, who started studies (with his wife, **Angela**, #46) on aromatase inhibitors at the Worcester Foundation, 1974.

74. **Dr. Trevor Powles**, the 1992 recipient of the Harold Rusch Memorial Breast Cancer Award, with **Mrs. Louise Rusch**, Madison, Wisconsin.

Index

A

Adam, Hugh, 41
Adjuvant Tamoxifen—
    Longer Against Shorter
    (ATLAS) trial, 45-49, 79,
    127-138, 141-144
Adjuvant Tamoxifen-
    Treatment Offer More?
    (aTTom) trial, 141-144,
    182
Adjuvant tamoxifen, 45-49,
    57-79, 87-94, 127-138,
    163-185
Age distribution, of breast
    cancer, 187-202
American Cancer Society,
    156
Aminoglutethimide, 148-150
Anastrozole (Arimidex),
    149
Antiestrogens, 34-36, 145-147
    and breast cancer, 36
    first compounds, 18,
        225-226
    ideal agents, 227
    structural formula of,
        149-150
Apolipoproteins, 211-212
Assikis, Vasileios J., 117,
    161-185, 296
Atypical hyperplasia, 118,
    212-213
Axillary lymph node status,
    effects of tamoxifen ana-
    lyzed by, 65-67, 249

B

Bain, Richard, 291, 295
Barakat, Richard R., 13, 109,
    111, 163
Baum, Michael, 287
Benign breast disease,
    196-197
Bilimoria, Malcolm M., 15,
    97, 296
Blamey, Roger, 288

Blink, Sarah, 21
Bone effects with tamoxifen
    (see Osteoporosis), 94,
    101, 211-212, 225-234
Bong, Matt, 300
Bowler, Jean, 303
BRCA-1, 159, 189-193, 237,
    240, 251, 265-270
BRCA-2, 159, 189-193, 237,
    240, 251, 265-270
Breast Cancer Prevention
    Trial (BCPT), 54, 225,
    229-232
Brodie, Angela, 149, 299
Brodie, Harry, 304

C

Cancer Care, Inc., 156
Carbone, Paul, 287
Cardiovascular effects, 73,
    98-99, 104-105, 154, 172-
    174, 229-230
Cataracts (see Ophthalmo-
    logic effects), 36-38, 103,
    158, 170-172, 218-219
Catherino, Bill, 300
Cavalli, Franco, 296, 299
Chemotherapy
    combined with tamox-
        ifen, 49, 53, 62-63, 71-
        73, 89, 94, 129, 136,
        174, 180-181
    vs tamoxifen, 58-59, 62-
        63, 73-74, 180-181, 245
Chen, Zehan, 296
Chisamore, Mike, 21
Christie Hospital, 38
Cisneros, Angela, 296
Clark, Edward R., 24, 296, 304
Clark, Gary, 291
Cole, Mary, 38
Collins, Rory, 58
Contralateral breast cancer,
    74-76, 82-84, 105-106, 207-
    222, 231
Coombes, R. Charles, 291,
    292

Cormier, Ethel, 291-292, 295
Coronary heart disease (see
    Cardiovascular effects),
    98-101, 104-105
Costa, Alberto, 228, 304
Cotton, Roy, 42
Cunliff, Barry, 42

D

Deep vein thrombosis, 211,
    214, 241-242
DeLaGarza, Mini, 291
De los Reyes, Alex, 21
DeSombre, Gene, 27, 296,
    300
Dietary factors, 195
Dix, Clive, 303
Dodds, Charles, 26, 36
Dose of tamoxifen, 48, 67-69,
    83, 119, 230, 304
Dragan, Yvonne, 304
Drug development, 225-226
    after FDA approval,
        53-56, 225, 238, 245
Drug resistance,
    mechanisms of, 141-145
    in premenopausal
        women, 175-176
Ductal carcinoma in situ
    (DCIS), and tamoxifen,
    182, 210-211, 215, 221,
    236
Dukes, Mike, 17, 303
Duncan, Gloria, 21
Duration of tamoxifen treat-
    ment, 67-71, 79-85, 90-91,
    121-123, 127-138, 141-144,
    236-238, 241

E

Early breast cancer, 58-59,
    79-85
Eastern Cooperative Oncolo-
    gy Group (ECOG), 50,
    141
Eckert, Steve, 229

Endometrial cancer and
  tamoxifen, 109-115, 117-
  124, 133-135, 155, 164-
  167, 238-239, 281-282
  aggressiveness of cancer,
    112-113, 120-121,
    167-168, 243-244
  effect of treatment
    duration, 83, 111-112,
    121-123,
  endometriosis, 118-119
  epidemiology, 117-118
  general screening issues,
    113-115
  preventive measures,
    168-170
  recommendations for
    patients, 114-115,
    166-170
  role of screening, 111
  transvaginal sonography,
    112-113
  worldwide clinical
    database, 109-115
England, Gale, 299
Environmental factors, 197
Estrogen-receptor status,
  effects of tamoxifen
  analyzed by, 79-86, 141-
  144, 229
Estrogens,
  estrogen-receptor
    hypothesis, 32-34
  estrogen target tissues,
    32-34
  physiologic role of, 31-34,
    51, 193, 198, 208,
    226-227
  role in breast cancer
    development, 43-45, 51
  role in drug resistance,
    145-147
  structural formula of, 259

F

Family history, 187-205, 216,
  230, 237
Family questions about
  tamoxifen, 159-160
Fat intake and breast cancer
  risk, 158-159

Fisher, Bernard, 288
Friedl, Andreas, 296
Fritsch, Mike, 292
Fritz, Nancy, 291
Furr, Barry, 228, 292, 303

G

Gibson, David, 14, 296
Gorski, Jack, 23-24, 32, 288,
  292, 300
Gosden, Barbara, 303
Goserelin (Zoladex), 95, 146
Gottardis, Marco, 291-292,
  295, 304
Gould, Michael, 292
Gradishar, Bill, 300
Gray, Richard, 58
Greene, Geof, 287, 296, 300
Griffith, Keith, 288

H

Haddow, Alexander, 36
Harris, Adrian, 292
Hayes, Alan, 42
Henderson, I. Craig, 15, 57,
  79, 141, 163, 165
Herbert, Greg, 21
High-density lipoprotein
  cholesterol, 102-104, 211
High-risk women, 187-202
Holson, John, 300
Horiguchi, Jun, 21
Hormonal Factors, 193-194
Hot flashes, 235-236, 285-286
Hormone-replacement
  therapy, 194, 225, 239
Howell, Tony, 304
Hozumi, Yasuo, 21
Huey-Jeng, Meei, 304
Hyperplasia (atypical), 118,
  212-213
Hysterectomy, 113-115

I

ICI 46,474, 9, 23, 25-26, 28
ICI Pharmaceuticals (see
  Zeneca), 17, 23-28, 36-38,
  41-42, 287, 292, 303
Iino, Yuchi, 295
Incidence, of breast cancer,
  187-188

Invasive cancer, 110, 114,
  118, 182, 190, 197, 211-
  214, 228-229, 252
Italian study, 209, 212, 220-
  222, 228, 304

J

Jacobson, Herb, 32
Janes, Mary, 291
Japanese women and risk, 82
Jaspan, Timothy, 296
Jensen, Elwood V., 26, 32-33,
  300
Jiang, Shun-Yuan, 292
Jordan, V. Craig, 21, 23, 31,
  41-42, 47, 53, 79, 97, 117,
  141, 145, 162, 185, 207,
  225, 228, 235, 247, 257,
  271, 283, 287-288, 292,
  295-296, 300-304

K

Katzenellenbogen, Benita,
  288
Katzenellenbogen, John, 295
Kaufman, Manfred, 288
King, Roger, 292
Kinsella, Timothy, 304
Koch, Rick, 291
Koerer Ravatoy, Susan, 304
Kupfer, David, 304

L

Lababidi, Mary, 292, 300
Lagan-Fahey, Susan, 304
Langer, Amy, 153, 161-185
LeClerq, Guy, 304
Lee, Eun-Sook, 21
Lerner, Leonard, 34, 292
Levenson, Anait, 21, 296
Leverhulm, Viscount, 41-42
Lieberman, Mara, 292, 294
Lippman, Marc E., 45-46,
  228, 257, 288, 295
Liver, 33, 231
  cancer and tamoxifen,
    85, 155, 164, 170-171,
    296
  and "fatty liver," 181-182

Lobular carcinoma in situ (LCIS), 174, 196, 212-213, 229, 231, 237, 239-240
Low-risk patients, 92, 98
Love, Richard, 102, 288
Lui, Hong, 21
Lumbar spine (see Bone effects) 102, 211, 225
Lyman, Stewart, 295

M

MacGregor, Jennifer, 21, 296
Male breast cancer, tamoxifen use in, 53, 182
Mammography, 158, 197, 201, 231
Mastectomy, 46, 63, 130, 132, 135, 193, 201, 202, 222, 240
McGuire, Bill, 287, 291
Menopausal symptoms with tamoxifen, management of (see Hot flashes) 179-180, 183-184
MER 25, 34, 292
Meta-analyses of tamoxifen (see Overviews of tamoxifen)
Metastatic disease, tamoxifen in, 64, 92-94, 99, 128, 148, 172, 175-176, 181, 247-249, 253-255, 260-261
Mirecki, Dawn, 291
Morrow, Monica, 9, 207, 228, 247, 283, 300
Morton, Pat, 291
Mueller, Gerald, 288
Muenzner, Henry, 296
Murphy, Cathy, 291-292

N

National Alliance of Breast Cancer Organizations (NABCO), 153, 156, 163, 165
National Breast Cancer Coalition, 156

National Cancer Institute (NCI), 33, 45, 54, 56, 127, 157, 159, 177, 189-191, 241, 277
National Coalition for Cancer Survivorship, 157
National Surgical Adjuvant Breast and Bowel Project (NSABP), 27, 50, 109, 127-139, 163-168, 171-179, 225, 269, 277
additional benefits of tamoxifen, 174
adverse effects of tamoxifen, 133, 242
duration of treatment, 127-139, 177-178, 184-185
patients' major concerns about tamoxifen, 164-166
Protocol B-14 study rationale and conduct, 127-139,164-168, 171-179
responsiveness of pre- vs postmenopausal women, 174-177
tamoxifen and concomitant chemotherapy, 50, 180-181
tamoxifen and endometrial cancer, 109-110, 122, 133, 166-167
tamoxifen and "fatty liver," 181-182
tamoxifen and liver cancer, 85, 155, 164, 170-171, 296
tamoxifen in noninvasive breast cancer, 182
tamoxifen vs placebo, 132
Newbould, Brian, 303
Nolvadex (see Tamoxifen)
Nolvadex Adjuvant Trial Organization (NATO), 287-288
NSABP (see National Surgical Adjuvant Breast and Bowel Project)

O

O'Regan, Ruth, 21, 27, 299
Oncogenes, role in breast cancer, 249-250, 252-253
Oophorectomy, 31, 54, 64, 89-93, 146-147, 176, 193, 207-209
Ophthalmologic effects of tamoxifen (see Cataracts), 36-38, 103, 158, 170-172, 218-219
Organizations for breast cancer patients and professionals, 156-157
Osborne, C. Kent, 147
Osteoporosis (see Bone effects and Lumbar Spine), 20, 28, 45, 49, 98-99, 102, 154, 163-185, 194, 219, 225-233, 239-240, 255, 258, 303
Overview analyses of tamoxifen, 46, 57-77, 79, 80-85, 89, 91, 97, 141, 164, 173-176, 181, 195, 198, 221, 236, 238, 244
1984 overview, 57-59
1990 overview, 57, 61-77
1995 overview, 57, 61, 65
additional benefits, 73-77
age and menopause, 63-65, 71-72
axillary lymph node status, 65-67
combined with chemotherapy, 71-73
duration of treatment, 69-71
estrogen-receptor status, 64,65
impact of, in premenopausal patients, 87-89
optimal dose, 67-69
Oxford Overview Analysis, 46, 57-77, 79-86, 164, 181, 238

P

Pap test, 114, 230
Parker, Chris, 292
Patterson, John, 287, 300

Pearson, Olaf, 292
Peto, Richard, 58
Phelps, Eric, 291, 295
Photon absorptiometry, 101, 226
Phytoestrogen products, 183-184, 254
Piette, Michael, 299
Pink, John, 292, 300
Pitot, Henry, 296, 304
Pleuvry, Alex, 287, 292
Postmenopausal women
    breast cancer risk in, 193-194
    cancer prevention in, 207-234
Powles, Trevor, 209, 228, 288, 304
Pregnancy and tamoxifen, 176, 239-240
Premenopausal women,
    breast cancer risk in, 193-194
    cancer prevention in, 207-234
    drug resistance in, 174-177
Prestwich, Graham, 303-304
Prevention of breast cancer, 45, 173, 207-234, 240-241
Primary cancer, 20, 79, 83, 85, 122, 130, 138, 143, 232, 236, 238, 241, 247, 281
Pritchard, Kathy, 304
Progesterone (PgR), 33, 64, 80-81, 112, 236, 250, 287
Protein C, S, 211
Pulmonary embolism, 211, 242
Pulsing, 232, 236-237

Q

Queen's Award for Techno-
logical Achievement, 17, 41-42, 233

R

Ragaz, Joseph, 163-185
Raloxifene, 28, 45, 159, 225, 234, 238-239, 255, 303

Rat mammary carcinoma
    model, 45-49
Ravdin, Peter M., 87-96, 291
Recurrence, 46, 50, 57-77, 79-85, 89-92, 109-110, 115, 124, 131-136, 143-145, 154, 166, 173-174, 184, 236-237, 241, 244, 247, 258
Reigel, Anna, 287
Richardson, Dora, 17, 36-37, 42
Risk factors of developing
    breast cancer, 105, 153-161, 187-205, 230-232, 237
Risks of tamoxifen treatment
    (see Tamoxifen)
Robinson, Simon, 291-292
Rochefort, Henri, 288, 296
Rosen, Candy, 300
Rosen, Steven, 300
Royal Marsden study, 93, 207-223
Rutqvist, Lars, 47, 105

S

Salmon, Joannie, 292
Salmon, Syd, 292
San Antonio Roundtable, 161-185
Selective estrogen receptor
    modulators (SERMS), 9, 28, 45, 227, 232-233, 261
Side effects of tamoxifen
    (see Tamoxifen)
St. Gallen Consensus Panel
    Recommendations, 55, 87
STAR trial, 159, 225-234, 255
Stella, Amy, 292
Stewart, Helen, 46
Stockholm study, 105, 122, 173
Study of tamoxifen and ral-
    oxifene trial (see STAR
    trial)
Susan G. Komen Founda-
    tion, 19-20, 157
Sutherland, Rob, 44, 292, 296

T

Tamoxifen (Nolvadex)
    adjuvant use of, 45-49, 57-79, 87-94, 127-138, 163-185
    age and menopause, effects analyzed by, 63-64, 193-194, 243-244
    antitumor actions of, 257-261
    approved uses and recommendations in United States, 53-56, 207
    axillary lymph node status, effects analyzed by, 65-67, 249
    bone, effects on, 94, 101, 211-212, 225-234
    cardiovascular effects, 73, 98-99, 104-105, 154, 172-174, 229-231
    chemotherapy combined with, 49, 53, 62-63, 71-73, 89, 94, 129, 136, 174, 180-181
    chemotherapy vs, 58-59, 62-63, 73-74, 180-181, 245
    clinical development of, 23-28, 41-52
    communicating with patients about, 153-162
    contralateral breast cancer, 74-76, 82-84, 105-106, 207-222, 231
    controversies on treat-
    ment duration, 127-140
    coronary heart disease
    (see Cardiovascular effects),
    effects on, 98-101, 104-105
    dose, 48, 67-69, 83, 119, 230, 304
    drug resistance, mecha-
    nisms of, 141-142, 145
    and ductal carcinoma in situ (DCIS), 182, 210-211, 215, 236

duration of treatment,
67-71, 79-85, 90-91,
121-123, 127-138,
141-144, 176-178,
236-238, 241
early breast cancer,
79-86
effectiveness of, 45, 141
and endometrial cancer,
109, 115, 117-124,
133-135, 155, 164-167,
238-239, 281-282
estrogen-receptor status,
effects analyzed by,
79-86, 31-34
family questions about,
159-160
and "fatty liver," 181-182
and hot flashes, 235-236,
285-286
and liver cancer, 85, 155,
164, 170-171
and lobular carcinoma in
situ (LCIS), 174, 196,
212-213, 237, 229, 231,
237, 239-240
in low-risk patients, 9, 92,
98
in lymph-node-negative
breast cancer, 98-99,
129, 137-138
in lymph-node-positive
breast cancer, 137, 142,
172, 177-178, 245, 50
menopausal symptoms
with, management of,
63-64, 179-180, 183-
184, 235-236, 285-286
metabolism of, 41-43
in metastatic disease,
64-65, 92-94, 99, 128,
148, 172, 175-176, 181,
247-249, 253-255,
260-261
monitoring women on,
238, 243-244
node negative, 141, 144
node positive, 144
nonbreast cancer mor-
tality with, 73-74,
172-173

ophthalmologic effects of
(see Cataracts), 36-38,
103, 158, 170-172,
218-219
optimal use of, 67-69
overviews of adjuvant
tamoxifen use (see
Overview analyses),
46, 57-77, 79, 80-85,
89,91, 97, 141, 164,
173-176, 181, 195, 198,
221, 236, 238, 244
patients' major concerns
about, 153-162, 164-
166, 235-246
pregnancy and, 176,
239-240
in premenopausal
women, 87-96, 174-177
preventive use, 45, 173,
207-234, 240-241
price of, 244, 271-280
pulsing, 232, 236-237
rationale for therapy
with, 97, 153-154
recurrence, 57, 61, 64-67
risk assessment, 239-240,
229-232, 187-206
risks associated with,
67, 79-86, 109-125, 135,
142, 153-177, 281-282
risk reduction, 80-81,
219, 239-240
serum lipids, effects on,
94, 102-104
side effects, 154-158,
164-166
site-specific effects of,
243, 258, 263
survival differences with,
133-134
Tanjiori, Kala, 296
Tellez, Claudia, 296
Thompson, Mark, 292
Todd, Sandy, 42, 292
Tonetti, Debra, 21, 296
Tormey, Douglas C., 49,
287, 296
Transvaginal untrasonogra-
phy, 112-113, 212, 230-
231

Trench-Hines, Lois, 288
Trump, Donald ("Skip"),
299
Tumoricidal actions, 85
Tumor-suppressor genes,
role of, 251-253

U

Upjohn Pharmaceuticals, 36

V

Vaginal discharge, 94, 133,
211, 242
Vangard study, 209-212
Venous thrombosis, 211, 220
Veronesi, Umberto, 296

W

Wakeling, Alan, 149-150,
292, 303
Walpole, Arthur, 23-24, 37-38
Ward, Harold, 38
Welshons, Wade, 23, 291
Whitford, Dave, 291
Wolf, Doug, 292
Wolf, Mike, 291
Wolmark, Norman, 15, 127,
163, 165, 288, 296, 304
Worcester Foundation for
Experimental Biology,
26, 149, 291, 299, 304
World Health Organization
(WHO), 26, 117, 225, 281

Y

Yang, Julie, 296
Yao, Kathy, 21
Y-ME National Breast
Cancer Organization, 157

Z

Zeneca, 17, 19, 23, 38, 41,
149, 244